Surgical Management of Urolithiasis

Stephen Y. Nakada • Margaret S. Pearle
Editors

Surgical Management of Urolithiasis

Percutaneous, Shockwave and Ureteroscopy

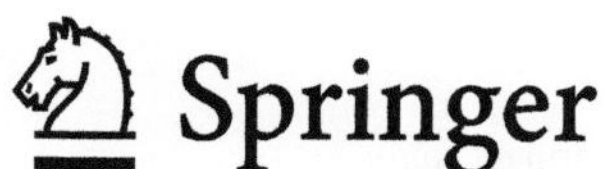

Editors
Stephen Y. Nakada, MD, FACS
Department of Urology
University of Wisconsin School of Medicine and Public Health
Madison, WI, USA

Margaret S. Pearle
Department of Urology
University of Texas Southwestern Medical Center
Dallas, TX, USA

ISBN 978-1-4614-6936-0 ISBN 978-1-4614-6937-7 (eBook)
DOI 10.1007/978-1-4614-6937-7
Springer New York Heidelberg Dordrecht London

Library of Congress Control Number: 2013937183

Printed on acid-free paper

Springer is part of Springer Science+Business Media (www.springer.com)

Preface

Surgical Management of Urolithiasis, Percutaneous, Shockwave, and Ureteroscopy provides a comprehensive and state-of-the-art overview of the major issues specific to the field of surgical urolithiasis. As a major part of general urologic practice, urolithiasis remains a significant domain in urology today. Written entirely by surgical urologists, *Surgical Management of Urolithiasis, Percutaneous, Shockwave, and Ureteroscopy* presents a comprehensive overview of all current surgical techniques, with a focus on educating urologists on the full spectrum of stone procedures. In addition to the technical issues, detailed complications are described. Basic as well as advanced techniques are presented in both a didactic and visual mode with representative endoscopic images and radiographs. Recent advancements that are not routinely a core component of surgical training programs are covered in detail. This useful text is extensively illustrated with radiographs, figures, and algorithms to highlight the clinical application of available surgical techniques.

Care of these patients and clinical conditions can be quite complex, and materials will be collected from the most current, evidence-based resources. The proposed sections of the book have been structured to review the overall scope of issues of all major categories of surgical stone therapy. This book will fill a critical need for resource materials on these topics. The book will also include practical presentations of typical patients seen in the clinical practice. This will be in the form of case presentations with expert analysis. This book is a unique and valuable resource in the field of surgical urolithiasis both for those currently in training and for those already in clinical or research practice. The book does not seek to duplicate or replace other current resources. Rather, it will create a comprehensive yet concise resource on these topics. No practicing urologist should be without it.

Madison, WI, USA — Stephen Y. Nakada, MD, FACS
Dallas, TX, USA — Margaret S. Pearle, MD, PhD

Contents

Contributors

Shadi Al Ekish Department of Urology, Rhode Island & The Miriam Hospitals, Providence, RI, USA

Jodi Antonelli Department of Urology, University of Texas Southwestern Medical Center, Dallas, TX, USA

Paurush Babbar Department of Urology, Wake Forest School of Medicine, Winston Salem, NC, USA

Sara L. Best Department of Urology, University of Wisconsin School of Medicine and Public Health, Madison, WI, USA

Naeem Bhojani Department of Urology, Indiana University School of Medicine, Indianapolis, IA, USA

Cecilia Maria Cracco Department of Urology, Cottolengo Hospital of Torino, Torino, Italy

Mitra R. de Cógáin Department of Urology, Mayo Clinic Rochester, Rochester, MN, USA

John D. Denstedt Department of Surgery, Western University, London, ON, Canada

Sammy Elsamra Division of Urology, The Warren Alpert Medical School of Brown University, Providence, RI, USA

Andrew Fuller Division of Urology, Department of Surgery, Western University, London, ON, Canada

Muhammad Waqas Iqbal Division of Urology, Department of Surgery, Duke University Medical Center, Durham, NC, USA

Adam Kaplan Department of Urology, University of California, Irvine Medical Center, Orange, CA, USA

Amy E. Krambeck Department of Urology, Mayo Clinic Rochester, Rochester, MN, USA

Jaime Landman Department of Urology, University of California, Irvine Medical Center, Orange, CA, USA

James Lingeman Department of Urology, Indiana University School of Medicine, Indianapolis, IA, USA

Michael E. Lipkin Division of Urology, Department of Surgery, Duke University Medical Center, Durham, NC, USA

Patrick Lowry Section of Laparoscopy and Endourology, Texas A&M College of Medicine, Scott & White Memorial Hospital, Temple, TX, USA

Brian R. Matlaga Johns Hopkins Medicine, The James Buchanan Brady Urological Institute, Baltimore, MD, USA

Nicole L. Miller Department of Urologic Surgery, Vanderbilt University School of Medicine, Nashville, TN, USA

Manoj Monga Department of Urology, Glickman Urologic and Kidney Institute, The Cleveland Clinic, Cleveland, OH, USA

Stephen Y. Nakada Department of Urology, University of Wisconsin School of Medicine and Public Health, Madison, WI, USA

Gyan Pareek Department of Urology, Rhode Island & The Miriam Hospitals, Providence, RI, USA

Margaret S. Pearle Department of Urology, University of Texas Southwestern Medical Center, Dallas, TX, USA

Ryan B. Pickens Department of Urologic Surgery, Vanderbilt University Medical Center, Nashville, TN, USA

Glenn M. Preminger Division of Urology, Department of Surgery, Duke University Medical Center, Durham, NC, USA

Cesare Marco Scoffone Department of Urology, Cottolengo Hospital of Torino, Torino, Italy

Michelle Jo Semins Department of Urology, University of Pittsburg Medical Center, Pittsburgh, PA, USA

Sri Sivalingam Department of Urology, University of Wisconsin Hospitals & Clinics, Madison, WI, USA

Devon Snow-Lisy Department of Urology, Glickman Urologic and Kidney Institute, The Cleveland Clinic, Cleveland, OH, USA

Prone Percutaneous Access: *Case Discussion—Caliceal Diverticular Calculi*

1

John D. Denstedt and Andrew Fuller

Abbreviations

CD	Caliceal diverticulum
CT	Computed tomography
PCNL	Percutaneous nephrolithotomy
SFR	Stone-free rate
SWL	Shock wave lithotripsy
TDPN	Transdiverticular puncture and neoinfundibulotomy
UPJ	Ureteropelvic junction
URS	Ureteroscopy
US	Ultrasound
UTI	Urinary tract infection

Since its initial description by Fernstrom and Johansson in 1976, percutaneous nephrolithotomy (PCNL) has evolved with improvements in technique and equipment to become the gold standard form of management for large stones in the upper urinary tract. It has now largely replaced open surgery in this context. Although alternatives such as supine patient positioning have emerged in the last decade, the vast majority of PCNL cases worldwide continue to be performed prone, with high stone-free rates (SFR) and a low incidence of major complications [1, 2].

The ability to safely and efficiently achieve percutaneous renal access depends on a number of factors including appropriate training, careful preoperative planning, recognition of anatomical variation, interpretation of radiological investigations, reproducible technique, and the availability of specialized instrumentation to effectively delineate and negotiate the urinary tract. Tract placement by the treating urologist without the involvement of an interventional radiologist in routine cases has been shown to be associated with excellent outcomes [3–5]. Additionally, such an approach allows PCNL to be performed as a one-stage procedure with the opportunity to place additional tracts as dictated by intraoperative findings.

This chapter summarizes what we believe to be a series of safe and effective strategies when performing percutaneous renal access. In presenting the chapter, we acknowledge that there are many effective alternate approaches to PCNL, some of which may not have been incorporated into this work. Many cases require the endourologist to safely apply a range of techniques in combination to achieve the desired outcome.

J.D. Denstedt, M.D., F.R.C.S.C., F.A.C.S. (✉)
Department of Surgery, Western University, London, ON, Canada
e-mail: john.denstedt@sjhc.london.on.ca

A. Fuller, M.B.B.S., F.R.A.C.S.
Division of Urology, Department of Surgery, Western University, London, ON, Canada
e-mail: afuller@sturology.com.au

S.Y. Nakada and M.S. Pearle (eds.), *Surgical Management of Urolithiasis: Percutaneous, Shockwave and Ureteroscopy*, DOI 10.1007/978-1-4614-6937-7_1, © Springer Science+Business Media New York 2013

Preoperative Planning

Indications

The advent of extracorporeal shock wave lithotripsy and flexible ureteroscopy has expanded the treatment options available for stones within the upper urinary tract. Despite the emergence of these technologies, PCNL remains the most appropriate and effective form of management for most large renal calculi [6]. As with any form of surgical intervention, appropriate patient selection is crucial. Table 1.1 summarizes the contemporary indications for PCNL.

While there are few absolute contraindications to PCNL, each patient scheduled for PCNL should undergo a thorough evaluation incorporating history, physical examination, and review of preoperative laboratory and radiological investigations.

History and examination should be focused to identify factors that may have implications from a surgical or anesthetic perspective. In particular, one should identify the presence of bleeding diathesis, anticoagulant therapy, recurrent urinary tract infection (UTI), chronic obstructive pulmonary disease, and morbid obesity, all of which may significantly increase the risk of perioperative complications. The presence of spinal deformity and limb contractures may complicate patient positioning and percutaneous access. In the case of morbid obesity, special equipment may be required. In high-risk patients, preoperative anesthetic assessment is mandatory prior to any contemplated intervention.

Laboratory investigations should include complete blood count, group/reserve, electrolytes, creatinine, and urinalysis/culture. Even in the context of a negative preoperative urine culture, there is evidence to support the routine administration of prophylactic oral fluoroquinolone antibiotics in reducing the risk of septic complications in the perioperative period [7].

Cross-sectional imaging with computed tomography (CT) affords the opportunity to assess the renal collecting system and plan appropriate sites of access prior to PCNL. Additionally, one may evaluate the relationship of the planned site of access to surrounding structures including colon, liver, spleen, and pleura. This is particularly important in the context of previous abdominal surgery, where the risk of retrorenal colon (Fig. 1.1) is higher [8]. Patel and colleagues [9] demonstrated the value of multiplanar CT reconstructions in defining the morphology of the intrarenal collecting system, calyceal orientation, stone location, and anatomical variants such as caliceal diverticulum.

Table 1.1 Indications for PCNL

Indications for PCNL
Staghorn calculi
Stones >2 cm in size
Lower pole stones >1 cm
Cystine stones
Failure of other treatments
Associated anatomical anomalies (UPJ obstruction, Caliceal diverticulum, horseshoe kidney)

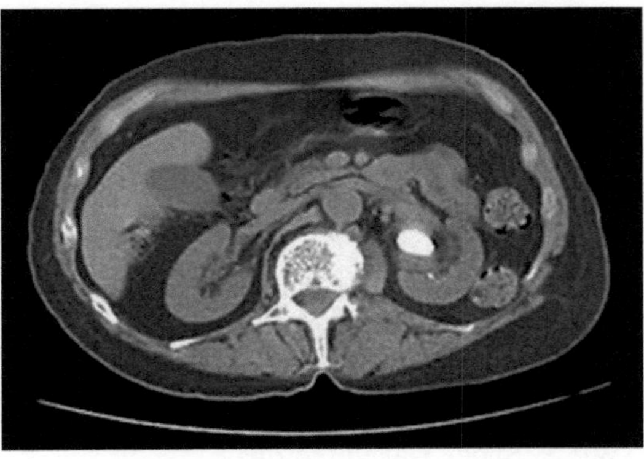

Fig. 1.1 CT demonstrating retrorenal colon. *Reproduced from Ko R, et al. Percutaneous nephrolithotomy made easier: a practical guide, tips and tricks. BJU Int 2007;101:535–539* (*Figure 1*)

Technique of PCNL

Anatomical Considerations

A detailed understanding of the intrarenal vascular anatomy, calyceal orientation, and perirenal visceral relationships is essential in minimizing the likelihood of morbidity related to PCNL.

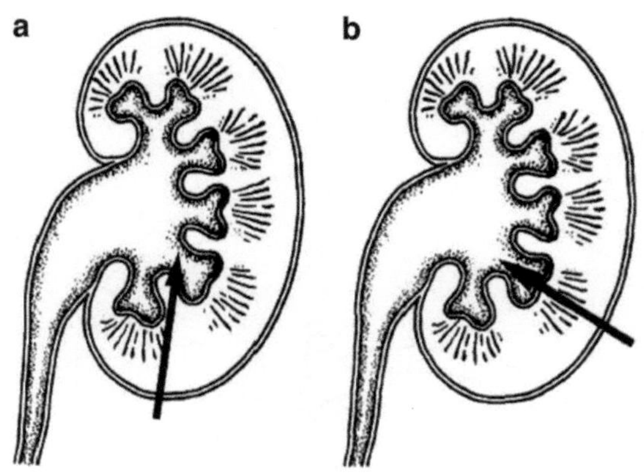

Fig. 1.2 (**a**, **b**) Puncture into the infundibulum (*left*) risks injury to the interlobar and arcuate branches of the renal artery. *Reproduced from Sampaio FJB. Renal Anatomy. Urol Clin North Am 2000;27(4):585–607 with permission (Figures 17a, 18a)*

After arising from the lateral aspect of the aorta at a level between the first and second lumbar vertebrae, the main renal artery divides into anterior and posterior divisions. The renal parenchyma supplied by each of these branches is separated on the lateral aspect of the kidney by Brodel's line. This location represents the optimal location to traverse the kidney during percutaneous access. The anterior division branches into 4 segmental arteries which supply the anterior and polar aspects of the kidney. The posterior division supplies the reminder of the kidney. Segmental arteries divide further into interlobar (infundibular), arcuate, and interlobular vessels. Entering the caliceal fornix in the correct orientation (end on rather than side on) as demonstrated in Fig. 1.2 serves to minimize the risk of inadvertent vascular injury by avoiding the interlobar and arcuate vessels which run in proximity to the caliceal infundibulum and medullary pyramids respectively [10].

Access via a posterior calix is desirable as it facilitates direct access to the collecting system to allow initial passage of guidewires with subsequent nephroscopy and stone removal. The posterior calices are at a 30° oblique angle to the vertical plane with the patient positioned prone. Additionally, the upper and lower pole calices adopt a 10° offset in the cranial and caudal plane respectively. This has particular implications when positioning the fluoroscopic unit during access which will be discussed in more detail later.

Particularly in the context of large stones at the ureteropelvic junction (UPJ), staghorn calculi and stones located in the upper pole calix, supracostal access and upper pole puncture may be the optimal approach for efficient stone removal [11–13]. When performing such access it is essential to appreciate the proximity of the pleural reflection and lung base to the trajectory of the planned access. The pleura is attached to the medial half of the 12th rib and medial three quarters of the 11th rib [14]. The lower border of the lung lies at the 10th intercostal space. Irrespective of the phase of respiration, the likelihood of intrathoracic complications is much higher with a supra-11th rib approach [15, 16]. Where possible, supra-12th puncture should be used as the approach to the upper pole due to the lower risk of pleural and pulmonary complications [17]. To avoid damage to the intercostal neurovascular structures in a supracostal approach, one should remain as close as possible to the upper border of the rib.

Patient Positioning

Many of the challenges associated with prone positioning can be managed with appropriate attention to detail and planning. One should be aware of the risk of peripheral nerve compression injuries and brachial plexus traction injuries in this position [18]. The patient's upper limbs should be positioned on arm boards with the shoulders abducted to 90° and the elbows flexed to 90°. The cervical spine should be in a neutral position. Padding should be placed to support the chest to assist with ventilatory function. In consultation with the anesthetic staff, the surgeon should confirm that the face and eyes are padded appropriately.

Fluoroscopic access techniques require the placement of a ureteral catheter through which contrast may be injected to outline the collecting

Table 1.2 Instrument list for prone PCNL

• Flexible cystoscope
• 0.035″ Guidewire
• 5 Fr ureteric catheter
• Contrast media
• Access needle
• Fascial incising needle
• 0.035″ Hydrophilic tip guidewire
• Kumpe catheter
• 0.038″ Extra stiff guidewire
• Balloon dilator
• 30 Fr Amplatz working sheath
• Rigid nephroscope
• Rigid graspers
• Lithoclast/Ultrasonic device
• Flexible nephroscope
• 2.4 Fr Nitinol basket
• 18 Fr Councill catheter

system. In most cases, flexible cystoscopy and cannulation of the ureteric orifice can easily be achieved with the patient prone. This approach offers several advantages over cystoscopy in the supine or dorsal lithotomy position. In particular, one avoids the need for a second patient transfer and the associated risk of ureteral catheter displacement.

Equipment

Preoperative planning, particularly with regard to ensuring the availability of specialized equipment is essential to the successful performance of PCNL. Before gaining access, one should confirm the availability of all necessary equipment (Table 1.2). A number of patient factors may necessitate specialized equipment. In particular, when treating obese patients, it may be necessary to use a longer access needle, working sheath, and/or rigid nephroscope. A larger skin incision is also occasionally required to facilitate access to the working sheath. Commercially available balloon dilation devices range in length from 12 to 15 cm. When this is insufficient, the use of serial Amplatz dilators is a useful means of gaining additional length.

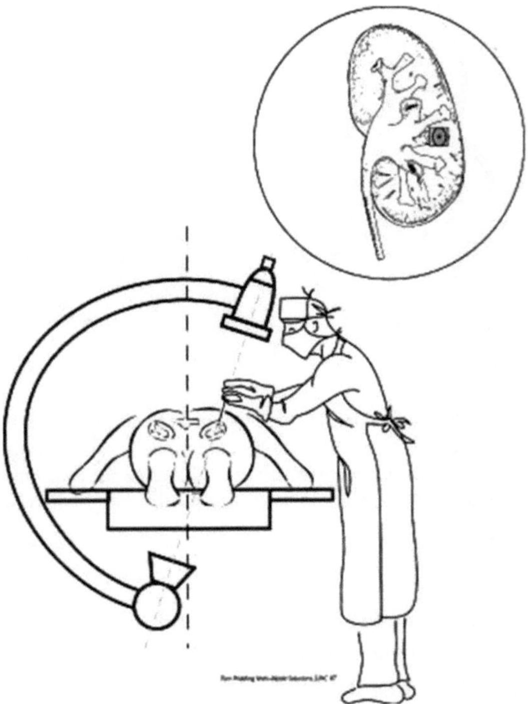

Fig. 1.3 The C-arm rotation toward the surgeon to align the needle tip with the desired entry calix. The *inset* shows the "bull's eye" appearance of the needle on the fluoroscopy monitor. *Reproduced from Ko R, et al. BJU Int 2007;101:535–539 with permission (Figure 3)*

Access Techniques

Several image-guided techniques have been described to facilitate antegrade renal access including biplanar fluoroscopy, ultrasound, and CT. In experienced hands, each technique provides safe and efficient access to the renal collecting system [19–24].

Fluoroscopy

Both the "bulls eye" and triangulation techniques represent effective means of achieving renal access.

When utilizing the "bulls-eye" technique, correct orientation of the C-arm is essential in order to visualize the targeted posterior calix end on. The C-arm is rotated approximately 20–30° from the vertical, towards the surgeon in the axial plane (Fig. 1.3). For upper and lower pole stones, it is then angled cranially or caudally respectively by approximately 10°. Although posterior calices generally appear less radio-opaque relative to anterior calices after contrast injection, if there is uncertainty, one can inject air with a 10 cc syringe through the ureteric catheter to identify preferential filling of the posterior calices.

A hemostat should then be used to localize the tip of the desired calix at the skin level. A 15 cm, 18 G needle is inserted at this point and advanced carefully under fluoroscopic guidance in expiration. The hemostat should be used to grasp the needle to maintain the surgeon's hands outside the field. An appropriate trajectory is confirmed by the appearance of the needle end-on (Fig. 1.3). Entry of the needle tip into the renal parenchyma may be confirmed by movement of the needle consistent with the phase of respiration. At this point, the C-arm should be rotated away from the surgeon at approximately 10° from the horizontal plane to provide depth perspective and to facilitate precise placement of the needle into the tip of the targeted calix (Fig. 1.4). Once the renal parenchyma has been entered, one should not alter the trajectory of the needle so as to avoid inadvertent cortical laceration.

Likewise, the triangulation technique relies on biplanar fluoroscopy to direct needle trajectory [20, 21]. As described by Miller and associates [21], the renal collecting system is opacified with contrast and the C-arm is moved between two positions parallel and oblique relative to the line of puncture. When the C-arm is aligned parallel, the needle trajectory may be adjusted in a medial or lateral direction. In the oblique plane, alterations in the craniocaudal axis should be made. Correct needle placement using this technique can only be achieved when the surgeon is able to maintain orientation in one plane whilst altering the other. When the needle appears to be in satisfactory alignment in both planes, the puncture is completed using the oblique view with the patient maintained by the anesthetist in the expiratory phase of respiration. The oblique view is advantageous in this scenario as it provides depth perspective to the operator.

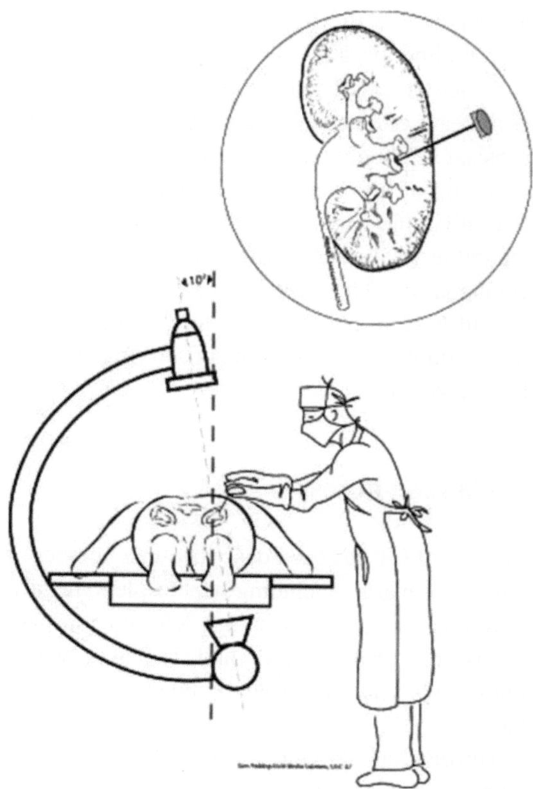

Fig. 1.4 C-arm rotation away from the surgeon to gauge the correct depth perception and to guide the needle tip into the entry calix. The *inset* shows the profile appearance of the needle on the fluoroscopy monitor. *Reproduced from Ko R, et al. BJU Int 2007;101:535–539 with permission (Figure 4)*

Ultrasound-Guided Puncture

Several investigators have demonstrated the feasibility of ultrasound (US)-guided access to the renal collecting system [22, 23]. Relative to fluoroscopy, this approach offers the advantage of no ionizing radiation and the ability to identify surrounding structures such as colon, liver, and spleen. In addition to standard B-mode ultrasonography, power Doppler US has been advocated as a means of defining and avoiding the renal vasculature, with resultant reductions in blood loss [25]. As with any form of percutaneous renal access, the use of ultrasound requires structured training, particularly in developing the skills to recognize the normal sonographic appearance of the renal collecting system and surrounding viscera.

Where access has been placed by ultrasound as a means of emergent drainage in a patient with sepsis, one should confirm placement of the tube at the tip of a posteriorly oriented calix prior to tract dilation to minimize the likelihood of segmental arterial injury. When the location of percutaneous renal access is deemed inadequate, one should have a low threshold to re-puncture in a more suitable location after opacifying the collecting system.

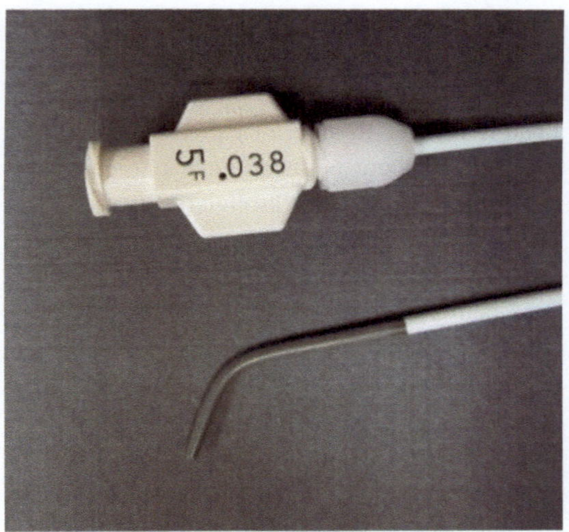

Fig. 1.5 Angled-tip angiographic catheter

CT-Guided Access

The use of CT has been described in a number of clinical scenarios including hepatosplenomegaly, retrorenal colon, severe spinal deformity, urinary diversion, renal ectopia, and in cases where fluoroscopic and ultrasound-guided renal access has failed [26]. In these cases, the precise definition of surrounding structures provided by CT facilitates accurate and safe needle placement.

The patient is usually positioned prone and noncontrast images are taken to define the position of the targeted calculus as well as the position of the kidney relative to surrounding organs. Although contrast administration may be unnecessary in cases of moderate to severe hydronephrosis, it may assist in cases where the collecting system is not dilated. This procedure relies on the involvement of an interventional radiologist, however close collaboration with the referring urologist is useful, particularly when deciding upon the most suitable calix to expedite stone removal.

Dilation and Tract Placement

Once the tip of the needle has been placed into the renal collecting system, the stylet should be removed. An angled-tip 0.035 in. Sensor guidewire (Boston Scientific, Natick, MA) is passed through the needle and coiled within the renal pelvis. A 1cm incision is made at the level of the skin to allow for subsequent passage of a balloon dilation device. If possible, the wire should be directed down the ureter and coiled in the bladder. This process may be facilitated by an angled-tip angiographic catheter (Fig. 1.5—Kumpe catheter, Cook Urological, Bloomington, IN) which can be used to steer the guidewire down the ureter. The catheter may be advanced over the wire allowing exchange for a 0.038 in. extra stiff wire over which a balloon or serial Amplatz dilation may occur.

Dilation can be safely achieved with either Amplatz serial dilators or a balloon device. One-stage balloon dilation is quicker than the use of Amplatz dilators, although it has been suggested by Lopes and colleagues [27] that this technique may pose a higher risk of hemorrhagic complications. In a follow up study conducted on behalf of the Clinical Research Office of the Endourological Society, no such association was found on multivariate analysis taking into consideration factors such as previous surgery, stone location, stone size, patient comorbidities, and the use of anticoagulant medications [28].

Particularly in patients who have undergone previous renal surgery or who have had recurrent pyelonephritis, there may be significant perinephric fibrosis. A fascial incising needle [Cook Medical, Bloomington, IN] is often useful in this situation to facilitate balloon dilation (Fig. 1.6) [19, 21]. An alternative approach is to use serial Amplatz dilators [19].

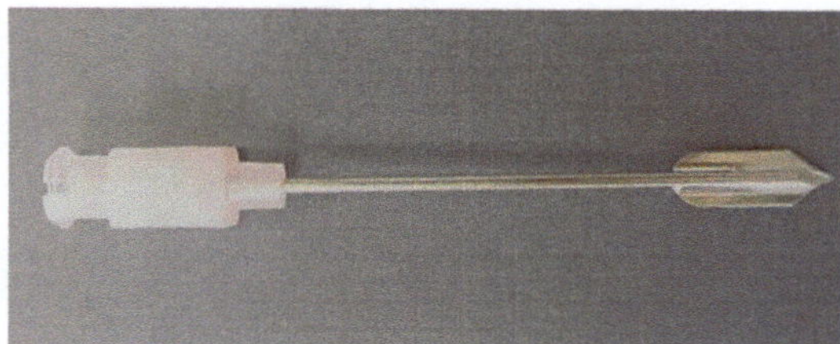

Fig. 1.6 Fascial incising needle

Once the tract has been dilated to 30 Fr, an Amplatz working sheath can be placed over the balloon. To avoid laceration of the collecting system, particular care should be taken when advancing the sheath to ensure the tip does not extend beyond the radiopaque marker on the distal aspect of the balloon. In the case of a supracostal puncture, it is essential that the working sheath remains within the renal collecting system for the duration of the procedure. Migration of the sheath out of the kidney risks considerable extravasation of irrigating fluid and hydrothorax. In such cases, a chest radiograph in recovery is useful to identify and preemptively manage intrathoracic complications.

Rigid Nephroscopy using 0.9 % saline as irrigation should be performed at this point to confirm the adequacy of sheath placement within the collecting system. If necessary, blood clot may be removed with rigid graspers. During stone fragmentation, one should avoid excessive torque on the working sheath as this is associated with a higher risk of intraoperative and postoperative hemorrhagic complications.

Case Discussion

Stones in a Caliceal Diverticulum

A 24-year-old female immigrant from Myanmar presented with a 3 year history of intermittent right sided flank pain. She was otherwise in good health and was prescribed no regular medications. There was no family history of urolithiasis.

After initially being diagnosed and treated with SWL for a presumed right lower pole renal calculus, she was referred with ongoing symptoms and residual stone for consideration of percutaneous stone removal. Noncontrast CT (Fig. 1.7) was arranged to provide further anatomical detail. This demonstrated a 12mm calculus at the lower aspect of the left kidney with minimal overlying parenchyma. An intravenous pyelogram (Fig. 1.8a, b) was performed and confirmed the presence of stone within a caliceal diverticulum (CD). The patient was counseled regarding the options for surgical management including retrograde ureteroscopic and antegrade percutaneous approaches. Although laparoscopic management has been described in this context [29, 30], this option was not felt appropriate in this scenario due to the location of the calculus in the posterior aspect of the renal parenchyma. The patient consented to PCNL.

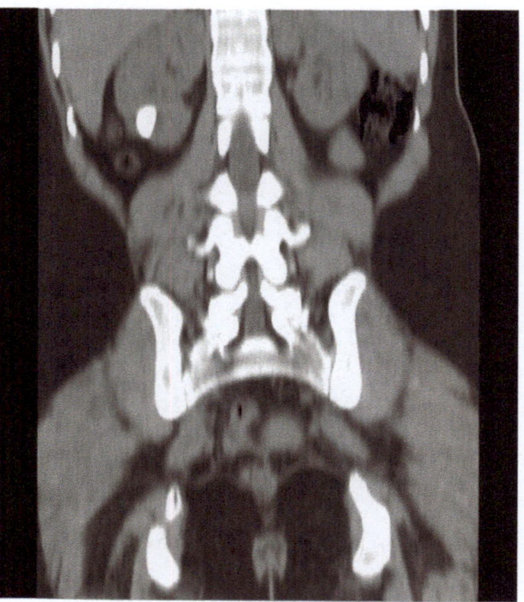

Fig. 1.7 Low-dose noncontrast CT in coronal section demonstrating a peripherally located calculus with minimal overlying renal parenchyma

Procedure

Under general anesthesia, the patient was positioned prone on the operating table. Flexible cystoscopy was performed in the prone position. A 0.035 in. wire was inserted through the right

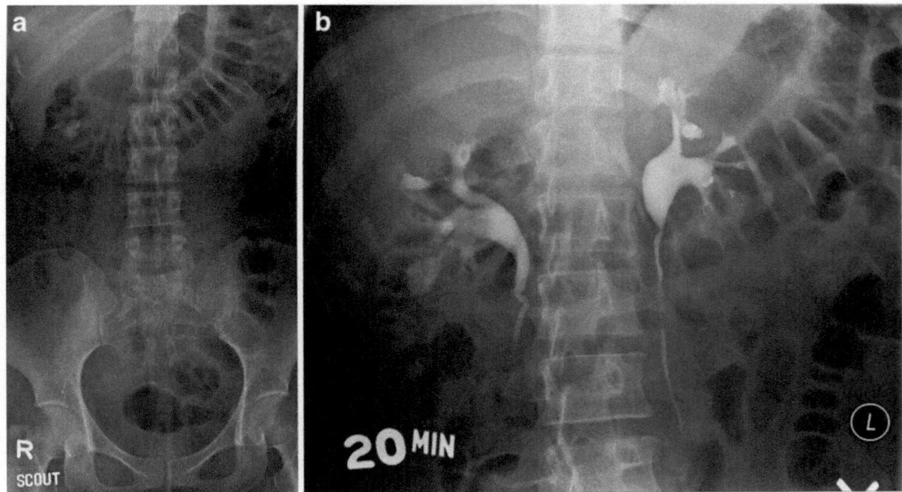

Fig. 1.8 (**a**, **b**) Intravenous pyelogram demonstrating stone within a right caliceal diverticulum arising from the mid-pole calix

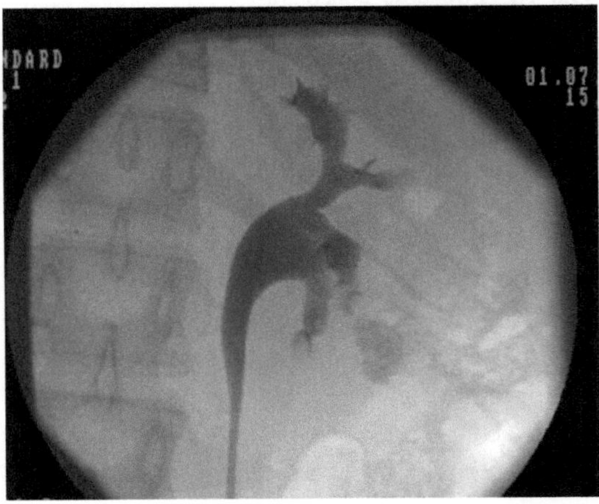

Fig. 1.9 Intraoperative retrograde pyelogram demonstrates stone within a caliceal diverticulum arising from the mid pole calix

ureteric orifice and advanced to the level of the right renal pelvis. A 5 Fr ureteral catheter was advanced over the wire under fluoroscopic guidance. Retrograde injection of contrast revealed stone within a caliceal diverticulum (Fig. 1.9).

Utilizing the "bulls-eye" technique, the diverticulum was punctured with an 18 G needle. An angled-tip 0.035 in. hydrophilic guidewire was then advanced through the puncture needle. The diverticular neck was identified with retrograde contrast injection and was able to be cannulated with the wire. The wire was coiled in the renal pelvis and a 5 Fr Kumpe catheter was inserted to direct the wire down the right ureter and to facilitate exchange for an extra stiff guidewire over which dilation could be performed. The tract was dilated with a balloon device to 30 Fr, allowing placement of a working sheath. Rigid nephroscopy confirmed the adequacy of access. Multiple stones were evacuated from the diverticulum. Once complete stone removal was confirmed, the infundibular neck was readily seen and dilated with a 6–10 ureteral balloon dilation device. This facilitated advancement of the rigid nephroscope into the main portion of the renal collecting system. No further stones were identified.

An 18 Fr Councill tip catheter was advanced over the wire and placed across the diverticular neck (Fig. 1.10). The patient tolerated the procedure well and made an uneventful recovery. After radiological confirmation complete stone removal, the nephrostomy tube was clamped and removed on the second postoperative day. Subsequent stone analysis demonstrated the stone to be calcium oxalate in composition.

Discussion

Caliceal diverticula are peripherally located cavities lined with nonsecretory transitional stratified epithelium [31]. Communication with the main

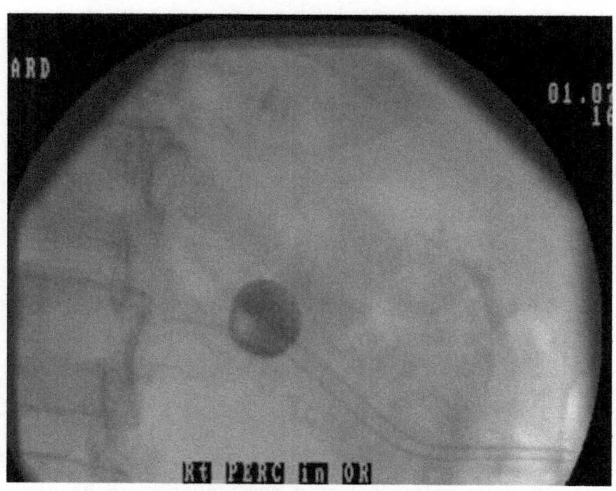

Fig. 1.10 At the completion of stone removal, a Councill catheter was placed across the diverticular neck with its tip in the main portion of the collecting system

portion of the renal collecting system is via a neck of variable width. Urine usually enters the cavity by retrograde passive filling. Although a proportion of patients with CD are asymptomatic, calculi may form with resultant pain, hematuria, or urosepsis.

Prior to the emergence of endoscopic stone surgery, treatment options for CD included partial nephrectomy, diverticulectomy, or deroofing [32]. Ureteroscopy (URS), extracorporeal shock wave lithotripsy (SWL), laparoscopy, and PCNL have now virtually replaced open surgical approaches. SWL presents as an attractive minimally invasive option however results are generally regarded as inferior with SFR [33]. Thirty-one percent of patients treated with SWL for CD stones required salvage with either URS or PCNL [34]. Laparoscopic techniques have been described with excellent SFR although the role of laparoscopy appears to be mainly in the management of stones within anteriorly located or thin walled CD. The gold standard for the management of CD is PCNL [35]. Most series report achieving SFR of approximately 80–90 % percent [36, 37]. As a result, PCNL is now widely considered the treatment of first choice for most patients.

Before contemplating percutaneous management, cross-sectional imaging with CT should be performed in all cases to ensure the diverticulum is posterior and amenable to direct percutaneous access. With the aid of a flexible cystoscope, a guidewire may be passed into the renal pelvis under fluoroscopic guidance and 5 Fr open-ended ureteral catheter positioned to allow for contrast injection to delineate the anatomy of the intrarenal collecting system. One should carefully examine the retrograde pyelogram images. In some cases, it may be possible to identify the diverticular neck and filling of the diverticulum.

Access to the diverticulum in the prone position may be achieved using the bulls-eye or triangulation techniques described previously. Ideally, once the tip of the access needle is placed into the diverticulum, one should attempt to negotiate a guidewire through the lumen of the diverticular neck. This maneuver may be facilitated by the use of a steerable, angled catheter (Fig. 1.5). If the neck cannot be identified preventing guidewire advancement into the renal pelvis, or the diverticulum is not large enough to allow curling of the guidewire, a transdiverticular puncture and neoinfundibulotomy (TDPN) is a useful means of salvage and is associated with excellent stone- and patient-related outcomes [37].

Using fluoroscopic guidance, a combination of anterior-posterior and oblique projections may be utilized to direct a Neff set (Cook Urological, Bloomington, IN) puncture needle through the wall of the diverticulum, out its back wall and into the renal collecting system (Fig. 1.11). At the completion of stone fragmentation and extraction, the neck of the diverticulum may be dilated with a ureteral balloon device. The nephroscope can then be advanced to the renal pelvis to ensure complete stone removal. At the completion of the case, a 16 or 18 Fr Councill catheter may be placed over the guidewire and through the neoinfundibulum to act as a nephrostomy tube. The nephrostomy tube should remain in place for 2–3 days postoperatively, followed by a trial of clamping and removal in the absence of pain or fever.

Other investigators have described alternative techniques such as a single-stage approach, where a puncture is made directly in to the CD, using the calculi as target without the use of retrograde contrast. The guidewire is coiled in the cavity without any attempt to communicate the CD with the urinary system [38]. The main drawback of this technique is that slippage or loss of the guidewire can occur with a resultant loss of access.

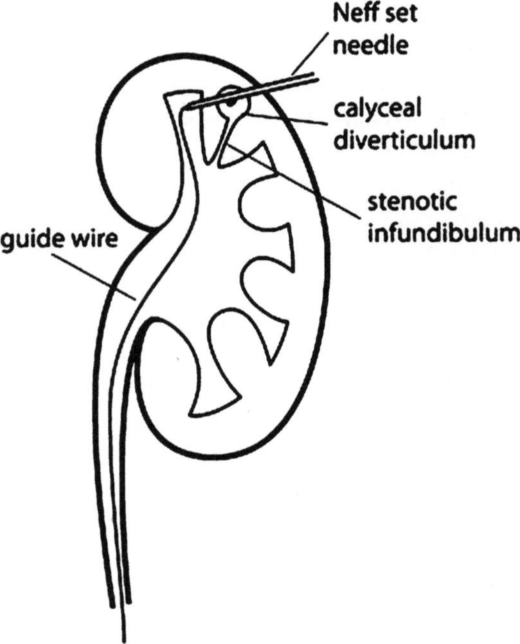

Fig. 1.11 Transdiverticular puncture and creation of a neoinfundibulotomy. *Reproduced from Méndez-Probst CE, et al. J Endourol 2011;25(11):1741–1745 with permission (Figure 1)*

Table 1.3 Key take-home messages: prone percutaneous access

• Appropriate preoperative evaluation incorporating history, physical examination, and review of radiological investigations is essential to the successful performance of PCNL
• Percutaneous renal access must be achieved through the tip of the desired calix to minimize the risk of significant renal vascular injury
• One should aim to puncture a posteriorly oriented calix where possible to facilitate access to the collecting system
• Upper pole access should be approached via a tract at the upper border of the 12th rib. Supra 11th rib punctures are associated with a significantly higher rate of pulmonary complications
• When supracostal access is necessary, one should ensure the sheath remains within the collecting system at all times to prevent extravasation of irrigation fluid into the thoracic cavity

The single-stage approach has the added disadvantage of precluding second look nephroscopy as access to the collecting system is not achieved. We propose that the safety and success of PCNL in this context can be maximized by adhering to the principles outlined in Table 1.3.

References

1. Duvdevani M, Razvi H, Sofer M, Beiko DT, Nott L, Chew BH, Denstedt JD. Contemporary percutaneous nephrolithotripsy: 1585 procedures in 1338 consecutive patients. J Endourol. 2007;21(8):824–9.
2. de la Rosette J, Assimos D, Desai M, Gutierrez J, Lingeman J, Scarpa R, Tefekli A. The clinical research office of the endourological society percutaneous nephrolithotomy global study: indications, complications, and outcomes in 5803 patients. J Endourol. 2011;25(1):11–7.
3. Tomaszewski JJ, Ortiz TD, Gayed BA, Smaldone MC, Jackman SV, Averch TD. Renal access by urologist or radiologist during percutaneous nephrolithotomy. J Endourol. 2010;24(11):1733–7.
4. El-Assmy AM, Shokeir AA, Mohsen T, El-Tabey N, El-Nahas AR, Shoma AM, et al. Renal access by urologist or radiologist for percutaneous nephrolithotomy—is it still an issue? J Urol. 2007;178(3 Pt 1): 916–20. discussion 920.
5. Watterson JD, Soon S, Jana K. Access related complications during percutaneous nephrolithotomy: urology versus radiology at a single academic institution. J Urol. 2006;176(1):142–5.
6. Management of ureteral calculi: EAU/AUA nephrolithiasis panel. 2007 [cited 2012 Feb 10]. Available from: http://www.auanet.org/content/clinical-practice-guidelines/clinical-guidelines/main-reports/uretcal07/chapter1.pdf.
7. Mariappan P, Smith G, Moussa SA, Tolley DA. One week of ciprofloxacin before percutaneous nephrolithotomy significantly reduces upper tract infection and urosepsis: a prospective controlled study. BJU Int. 2006;98(5):1075–9.
8. Hopper KD, Sherman JL, Luethke JM, Ghaed N. The retrorenal colon in the supine and prone patient. Radiology. 1987;162(2):443–6.
9. Patel U, Walkden RM, Ghani KR, Anson K. Three-dimensional CT pyelography for planning of percutaneous nephrostolithotomy: accuracy of stone measurement, stone depiction and pelvicalyceal reconstruction. Eur Radiol. 2009;19(5):1280–8.
10. Sampaio FJ. Renal anatomy: endourologic considerations. Urol Clin North Am. 2000;27(4):585–607.
11. Sukumar S, Nair B, Ginil KP, Sanjeevan KV, Sanjay BH. Supracostal access for percutaneous nephrolithotomy: less morbid, more effective. Int Urol Nephrol. 2008;40(2):263–7.
12. Lang E, Thomas R, Davis R, Colon I, Allaf M, Hanano A, et al. Risks, advantages and complications of intercostal vs subcostal approach for percutaneous nephrolithotripsy. Urology. 2009;74(4): 751–6.
13. Raza A, Moussa S, Smith G, Tolley DA. Upper-pole puncture in percutaneous nephrolithotomy: a retrospective review of treatment safety and efficacy. BJU Int. 2008;101(5):599–602.
14. Sinnatamby CS. Last's anatomy. Regional and applied. 10th ed. Edinburgh: Churchill Livingstone; 1999.

15. Munver R, Delvecchio FC, Newman GE, Preminger GM. Critical analysis of supracostal access for percutaneous renal surgery. J Urol. 2001;166(4):1242–6.
16. Hopper KD, Yakes WF. The posterior intercostal approach for percutaneous renal procedures: risk of puncturing the lung, spleen and liver as determined by CT. AJR Am J Roentgenol. 1990;154(1):115–7.
17. Yadav R, Gupta NP, Gamanagatti S, Yadav P, Kumar R, Seith A. Supra-twelfth supracostal access: when and where to puncture? J Endourol. 2008;22(6):1209–12.
18. Papatsoris A, Masood J, El-Husseiny T, Maan Z, Saunders P, Buchholz NP. Improving patient positioning to reduce complications in prone percutaneous nephrolithotomy. J Endourol. 2009;23(5):831–2.
19. Ko R, Soucy F, Denstedt JD, Razvi H. Percutaneous nephrolithotomy made easier: a practical guide, tips and tricks. BJU Int. 2008;101(5):535–9.
20. Steinberg PL, Semins MJ, Wason SE, Matlaga BR, Pais VM. Fluoroscopy-guided percutaneous renal access. J Endourol. 2009;23(10):1627–31.
21. Miller NL, Matlaga BR, Lingeman JE. Techniques for fluoroscopic percutaneous renal access. J Urol. 2007;178(1):15–23.
22. Desai M. Ultrasonography-guided punctures-with and without puncture guide. J Endourol. 2009;23(10): 1641–3.
23. Basiri A, Ziaee AM, Kianian HR, Mehrabi S, Karami H, Moghaddam SM. Ultrasonographic versus fluoroscopic access for percutaneous nephrolithotomy: a randomized clinical trial. J Endourol. 2008; 22(2):281–4.
24. Ghani KR, Patel U, Anson K. Computed tomography for percutaneous renal access. J Endourol. 2009; 23(10):1633–9.
25. Tzeng BC, Wang CJ, Huang SW, Chang CH. Doppler ultrasound-guided percutaneous nephrolithotomy: a prospective randomized study. Urology. 2011;78(3): 535–9.
26. Matlaga BR, Shah OD, Zagoria RJ, Dyer RB, Streem SB, Assimos DG. Computerized tomography guided access for percutaneous nephrostolithotomy. J Urol. 2003;170(1):45–7.
27. Lopes T, Sangam K, Alken P, Barroilhet BS, Saussine C, Shi L, et al. The clinical research office of the endourological society percutaneous nephrolithotomy global study: tract dilation comparisons in 5537 patients. J Endourol. 2011;25(5):755–62.
28. Yamaguchi A, Skolarikos A, Buchholz NP, Chomón GB, Grasso M, Saba P, et al. Operating times and bleeding complications in percutaneous nephrolithotomy: a comparison of tract dilation methods in 5,537 patients in the clinical research office of the endourological society percutaneous nephrolithotomy global study. J Endourol. 2011;25(6):933–9.
29. Miller SD, Ng CS, Streem SB, Gill IS. Laparoscopic management of caliceal diverticular calculi. J Urol. 2002;167(3):1248–52.
30. Wyler SF, Bachmann A, Jayet C, Casella R, Gasser TC, Sulser T. Retroperitoneoscopic management of caliceal diverticular calculi. Urology. 2005;65(2):380–3.
31. Kottász S, Hamvas A. Review of the literature on calyceal diverticula, a hypothesis concerning its etiology and report of 17 cases. Int Urol Nephrol. 1976;8(3):203–12.
32. Marshall VR, Singh M, Tresidder GC, Blandy JP. The place of partial nephrectomy in the management of renal calyceal calculi. Br J Urol. 1975;47(7):759–64.
33. Turna B, Raza A, Moussa S, Smith G, Tolley DA. Management of calyceal diverticular stones with extracorporeal shock wave lithotripsy and percutaneous nephrolithotomy: long-term outcome. BJU Int. 2007;100(1):151–6.
34. Streem SB, Yost A. Treatment of caliceal diverticular calculi with extracorporeal shock wave lithotripsy: patient selection and extended followup. J Urol. 1992;148(3 Pt 2):1043–6.
35. Canales B, Monga M. Surgical management of the calyceal diverticulum. Curr Opin Urol. 2003;13(3): 255–60.
36. Krambeck AE, Lingeman JE. Percutaneous management of caliceal diverticuli. J Endourol. 2009;23(10): 1723–9.
37. Mendez-Probst CE, Fuller A, Nott L, Denstedt JD, Razvi H. Percutaneous nephrolithotomy of calyceal diverticular calculi: a single centre experience. J Endourol. 2011;25(11):1741–5.
38. Kim SC, Kuo RL, Tinmouth WW, Watkins S, Lingeman JE. Percutaneous nephrolithotomy for caliceal diverticular calculi: a novel single stage approach. J Urol. 2005;173(4):1194–8.

2 PCNL: Supine Technique

Cesare Marco Scoffone and Cecilia Maria Cracco

Introduction

After more than 30 years, percutaneous stone removal still stands the test of time as treatment of choice for large and/or complex urolithiasis. In fact, instead of becoming obsolete over the decades, percutaneous nephrolithotomy (PCNL) underwent considerable evolution since its introduction in 1976, progressively acquiring a new configuration and accordingly improving its efficacy and safety in expert hands. The old static procedure has become a technically updated and really mini-invasive approach thanks to a great deal of consistent advances regarding imaging techniques, anesthetic skills, patient positioning, renal access creation, antegrade and retrograde use of semirigid and flexible endoscopes with better technology and vision, choice among a variety of accessories and intracorporeal lithotripsy devices, and postoperative renal drainage [1, 2].

The rather recent debate on patient positioning certainly contributed to the new life of PCNL [3, 4]. The prone position was the one used by Goodwin and collaborators when they gained the first percutaneous renal access in 1955, and by Fernström and Johansson when they described the percutaneous pyelolithotomy technique in 1976; therefore, it became the traditional one. Of course the prone position provides a wide surgical field for renal puncture and adequate nephroscopic manipulation, easier upper pole puncture with a lower risk of lung, pleura, and liver/spleen injury, a good distension of the collecting system and feasibility of bilateral procedures.

On the other hand, the anesthetic concerns of the prone position (especially in morbidly obese patients, those with compromised cardiopulmonary status or skeletal deformities) and the difficulty of obtaining a combined antegrade and retrograde access to the renal cavities when needed are issues that have been overlooked for a long time. A lot of modified positions have been proposed over the years, including the reverse lithotomy position of Lehman and Scarpa, the lateral decubitus of Grasso and Kerbl and the supine position of Valdivia Urìa, but none of them ever threatened the supremacy of the usual prone position until recently. In particular, Valdivia Urìa described already in the late 1980s his experience with the supine approach for PCNL, publishing consistent clinical data on the efficacy and safety of this technique, but his results did not obtain the deserved consensus within the endourological community [3, 5].

The idea of combining percutaneous and retrograde approach during the same surgical procedure is not new at all. Initial blind attempts were described in the early 1980s with the transcutaneous retrograde nephrostomies of Hawkins-Hunter and of Lawson [6, 7]; few years later a simultaneous nephroscopic and ureteroscopic access with the patient in the "reverse lithotomy

C.M. Scoffone (✉) • C.M. Cracco
Department of Urology, Cottolengo Hospital of Torino, Torino, Italy
e-mail: scoof@libero.it

S.Y. Nakada and M.S. Pearle (eds.), *Surgical Management of Urolithiasis: Percutaneous, Shockwave and Ureteroscopy*, DOI 10.1007/978-1-4614-6937-7_2, © Springer Science+Business Media New York 2013

position" was occasionally needed to solve particular clinical situations [8]. In the late 1980s Ibarluzea and coworkers progressively changed the supine Valdivia position associating a modified lithotomic arrangement of the lower limbs, giving birth to the handy and ergonomic Galdakao-modified supine Valdivia (GMSV) position, which appeared in the Spanish literature in 2001 but only in 2007 in an international publication [5]. The GMSV position optimally supports ECIRS (Endoscopic Combined IntraRenal Surgery), a novel combined antegrade and retrograde approach to the upper urinary tract for the treatment of large and/or complex urolithiasis, involving the synergic use of rigid and flexible endoscopes, various accessories and lithotripsy energies, and a synergic cooperation among all the operators (two surgeons, anesthesiologist, scrub nurse, nurses, radiology technician) with the relative armamentaries [2–5, 9–15]. This was really the first time that retrograde ureteroscopy was employed not only as an occasional complement to PCNL bur rather as an essential part of it, with an indefeasible active role for an optimal outcome. Scoffone and Scarpa made a big effort for popularizing ECIRS in the GMSV position [9] via congresses, publications, and live surgeries. The same did Daels [10] and Hoznek [11], who largely contributed to the technical standardization and improvement of ECIRS, whereas Frattini gained a wide experience with this combined approach in children with optimal results [12].

The supine positions for PCNL are not the unique alternatives to the prone position, as demonstrated by the bulk of recent literature [3, 13], proposing lateral, flank, split-leg modified lateral, flank prone, prone flexed, supine oblique, semisupine positions, and many others. The relevant aspect is that all these authors made their proposals in a common effort to improve their surgical percutaneous practice. Of course, feasibility, efficacy, and safety of PCNL performed in any alternative position have been compared to those of the prone PCNL, by now with substantially equivalent urological outcomes (in terms of stone-free rates, operative time, hospital stay, complication rates).

Among the advantages of PCNL performed in the GMSV position we number anesthesiological, management and urological advantages, which have been widely reported [2–5, 9–15]. The cardiovascular, ventilatory, neuroendocrine, and pharmacokinetic problems of the prone position [9, 14] are overcome in the supine positions, with better access to the airways and the cardiovascular system. This is particularly true for special patients, including children, elderly, obese, kyphotic/scoliotic, and debilitated patients. Management advantages include easy and comfortable patient positioning, no need for intraoperative repositioning of the anesthetized patient (with less need of nurses in the operating room, less occupational risk due to shifting of heavy loads, less risk of pressure injuries due to inaccurate repositioning responsible for ligament lesions, visual problems, and neurological deficits, a single definitive sterile draping of the patient), the possibility for the surgeon to work sitting down and with his hands out of the fluoroscopic field. Urological advantages include an easier puncture of the kidney lying nearer to the skin, the possibility of an Endovision-assisted renal puncture and tract dilation, a demonstrated decreased risk of colon injury, a great versatility in the combined stone manipulation, a better descending drainage and retrieval of stone fragments from lithotripsy because of the downward position of the Amplatz sheath, low intrarenal pressures implying less pyelovenous backflow and of postoperative infectious risk.

Description of the Supine Technique

We will focus our attention on two issues which characterize ECIRS, combining supine PCNL and retrograde access to the upper urinary tract: patient positioning and organization of the operating room and the role of retrograde ureteroscopy during PCNL.

Patient Positioning and Organization of the Operating Room

The posterior axillary line is drawn on the skin with the patient standing; subsequently the patient undergoes general anesthesia in the supine position.

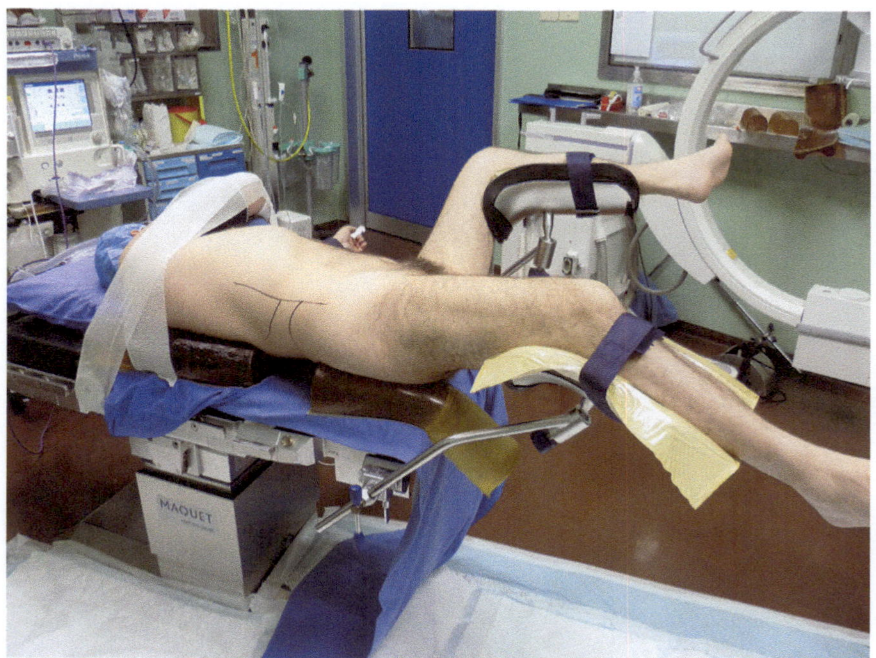

Fig. 2.1 Patient in the GMSV position, with the two jelly pillows under the thorax and the ankle

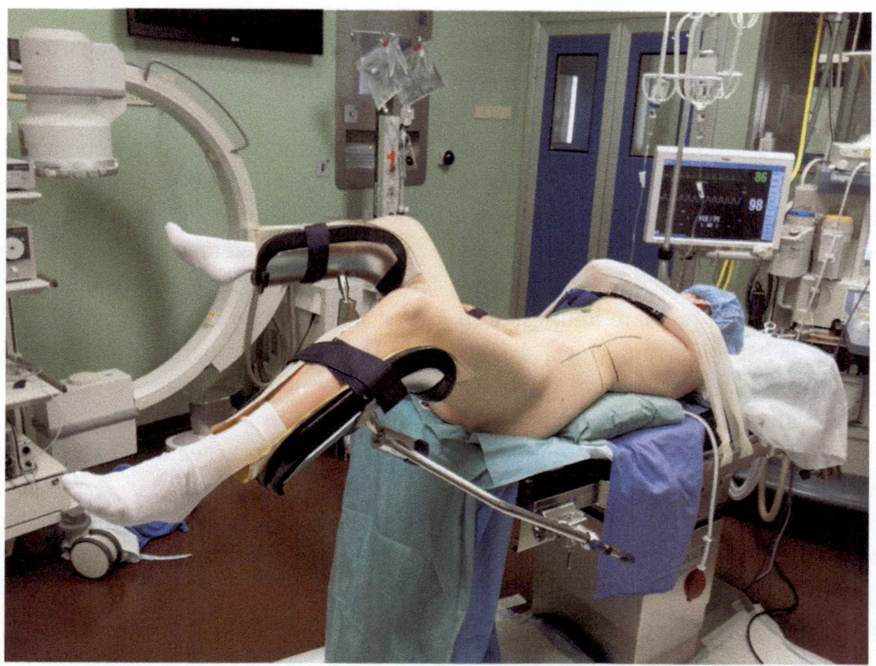

Fig. 2.2 Patient in the GMSV position, with the inflatable balloon under the flank

The flank to be operated leans out of the border of the operating table and has to be raised and slightly rotated by a single underlying 3-l saline bag, or by two separated jelly pillows put under the thorax and the ankle (Fig. 2.1), or by a particular balloon that can be inflated and deflated according to the requirements after inserting its flat part under the back of the patient (Fig. 2.2).

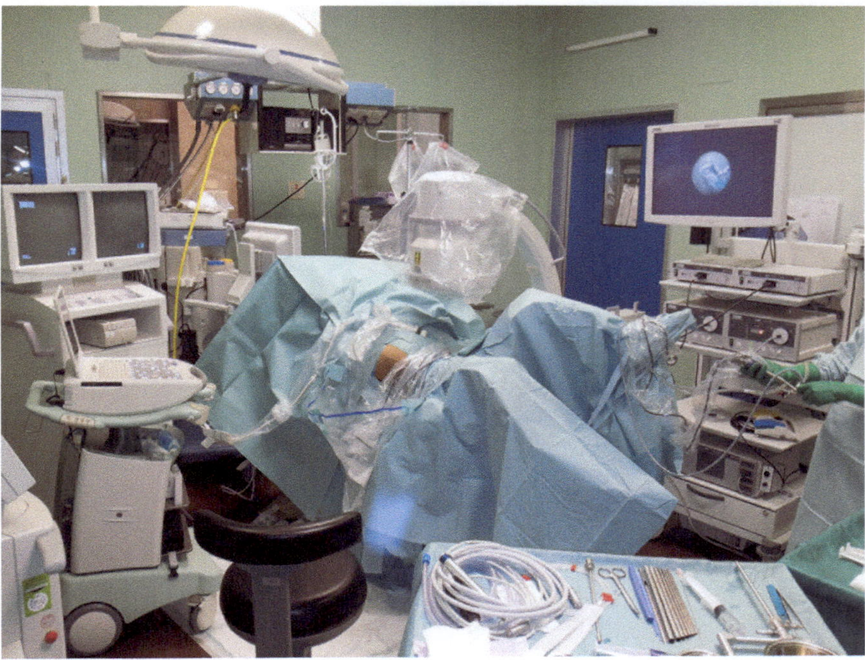

Fig. 2.3 Sterile draping of the patient and organization of the operating room

The ipsilateral arm is laid on the thorax, while venous access is assured on the contralateral arm; the remaining landmarks, i.e., 12th rib and iliac crest, are then drawn of the skin (Figs. 2.1 and 2.2). Subsequently the lower limbs are arranged in a modified lithotomic position, typical of the GMSV position, with the leg of the operated side extended and the contralateral one well abducted. Care is taken to prevent pressure injuries, accurately padding the legs stirrups (Figs. 2.1 and 2.2). Once the positioning of the patient is completed a single sterile draping is applied, standardized according to the individual requirements (Fig. 2.3). Both percutaneous and retrograde accesses should be simultaneously accessible, the movements of the endoscopic instruments not hindered (Fig. 2.4), all the monitors (endoscopic, ultrasound, fluoroscopic) visible by both surgeons, and the rest of the armamentarium (like lithotripsy energy sources) handy for the operators. This means that also the organization of the operating room should be standardized according to the space available, and common schemes should be followed (Fig. 2.3).

Preliminary Retrograde Ureteroscopic Evaluation

The possibility of obtaining a combined approach to the upper urinary tract allows to do something more than the cystoscopic application of a guidewire and of a ureteral catheter for pyelography or renal cavities distension with saline, which is the first step of prone PCNL.

The initial retrograde ureteroscopic control follows a mandatory preoperative CT scan, and allows to assess:

- The anatomical features of the lower urinary tract.
- The anatomical features of the ureteral meatus and of the ureter (a thin or a spastic ureter would need smaller caliber ureteroscopes and/or ureteral sheaths).
- The presence of ureteral stones or strictures to be contextually treated.
- Pyelic and calyceal morphology, in normal conditions as well as in known congenital renal malformations or outcomes of previous renal surgeries.

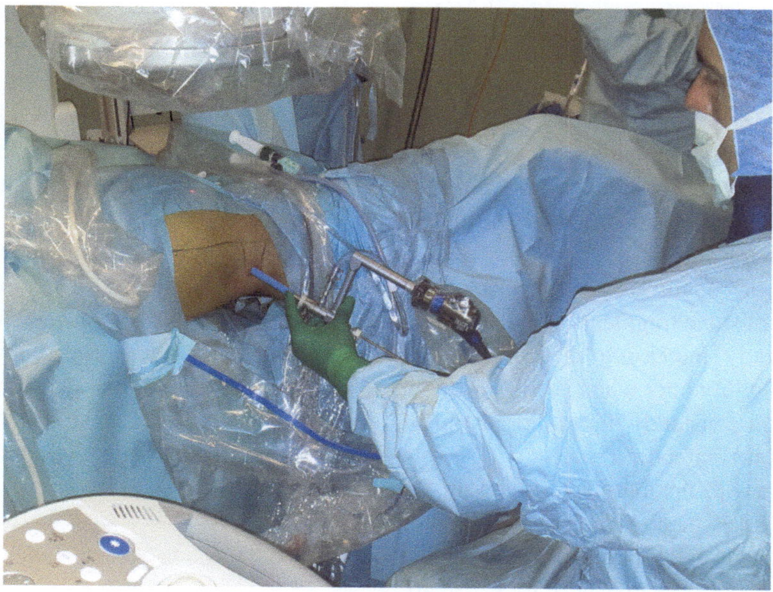

Fig. 2.4 The resulting freedom of movements of the rigid nephroscope in the GMSV position

- Stone accessibility, position, mobility, hardness, and peculiarities (intraparenchymal calcifications rather than Randall's plaques), with a possible change in indication from percutaneous to ureteroscopic treatment.
- The course of the Endovision-assisted fluoroscopic and ultrasound-guided renal puncture, with the possibility of controlling/correcting the exiting of the needle through the tip of the renal papilla after passing through the Brodel's avascular line, thus minimizing the risk of bleeding (Fig. 2.5).
- The course of the Endovision-assisted percutaneous tract dilation and of the Amplatz sheath application, minimizing radiation exposure.
- The preparation of the "kebab" (skewered) patient for absolute procedural safety: the guidewire entering the kidney through the percutaneous tract is retrogradely extracted with forceps and exits through the external urethral meatus; vice versa, the main guidewire (or an auxiliary one) may be inserted via the ureteroscope and externalized through the Amplatz sheath.

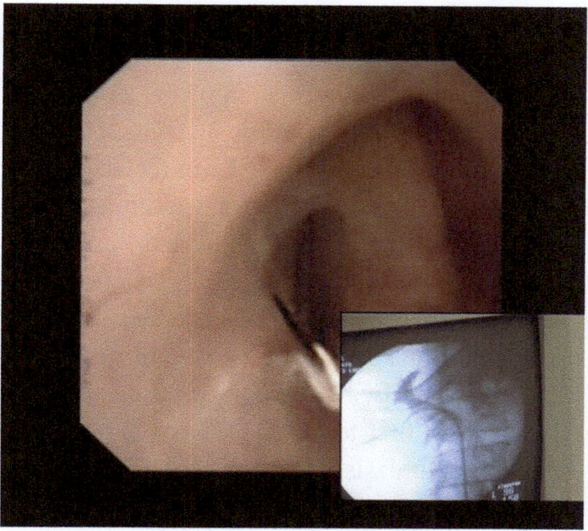

Fig. 2.5 Endovision-assisted renal puncture, with the entry of the needle within the renal cavities through the tip of the renal papilla

Intraoperative Retrograde Ureteroscopy

Nowadays we can exactly acknowledge all the critical PCNL steps that may greatly benefit from a retrograde ureteroscopic assistance:

- Retrieval of stone fragments from calices parallel to the access tract or within narrow infundibula by means of flexible ureteroscopy, retrograde in situ laser lithotripsy, or dislodgement in sites more suitable for antegrade lithotripsy (this avoids the need for multiple percutaneous tracts and related hemorrhagic risk, optimizing stone-free rates).
- Control of the ongoing lithotripsy, avoiding the descent of stone fragments along the ureter and transiently increasing the irrigation to improve visibility only when needed, without the risks of a constantly high intrarenal pressure and related infectious risks.
- Cooperation with flexible nephroscopy in the final visual assessment of the stone-free status (with reduced intraoperative fluoroscopic exposure and postoperative need for CT scan), with the possibility of completing the procedure or of planning kind and timing of a second look treatment of the residual stone burden, and in the decision for a tubeless procedure (in absence of bleeding or upper urinary tract perforation/lesion).
- Final endoscopic evaluation of the meatus, the ureter, and the ureteropelvic junction in order to decide for a stentless PCNL (in the absence of edema, bleeding, clots, stone fragments, wall lesions, or strictures) or about the timing of a double J stent (short- or long-term application).

According to our personal experience (unpublished data), in a series of 55 consecutive patients who underwent ECIRS in our Department during 2011 and the first term of 2012 for large and/or complex urolithiasis ureteroscopy was carried out in 84 % of cases (76 % semirigid 6–7.5 Ch ureteroscopy, 37 % associated flexible ureteroscopy, 7 % only flexible ureteroscopy, 44 % of total flexible ureteroscopies, 10 % application of a ureteral sheath). The stone-free rate after a first treatment was 90, 94 % after a second early treatment (second PCNL or retrograde ureteroscopy). The mean operative time was 88 min including patient positioning. The Endovision aid to the renal puncture was feasible in 29 % of the procedures, the combined treatment of ureteral stones, calculi in calices parallel to the percutaneous tract or impacted in infundibula, calyceal diverticula and double districts in 48 % of cases. Evaluation for final application of a double J stent lead to a 35 % of stentless (but not tubeless) ECIRS; of the 65 % ECIRS concluded with the application of a double J stent 50 % had a string for facilitated removal after few days [1–3]. There were no ureteral lesions at all, and an overall complication rate of 5.5 % (two fevers responsive to antibiotic treatment and one self-limiting bleeding). Therefore, the complication rate of ECIRS is not the sum of those of PCNL and retrograde ureteroscopy; on the contrary, retrograde ureteroscopy contributes to minimize the more relevant PCNL complications (mainly bleeding and infection).

Conclusions

For sure ECIRS is not the unique new gold standard for percutaneous renal stones treatment, but may be is a candidate, representing a new comprehensive attitude of the urologist toward the various PCNL steps, exploiting the surgeon's versatility for an optimal outcome in terms of safety and effectiveness. Among the merits of ECIRS we recognize the large amount of thorough critical analysis of the PCNL procedure triggered by its proposal, as demonstrated by the bulk of literature published on this argument, which has led to the standardization of each surgical step for a shorter learning curve and a better replicability, and extended its positive influence on the standardization of the prone procedure as well. The GMSV position allowing ECIRS is very handy and ergonomic, but first of all very safe from an anesthesiological point of view. In conclusion, ECIRS passwords are "synergy, versatility, and standardization," for an optimal outcome of the percutaneous treatment of large and/or complex renal stones.

References

1. Preminger GM. Percutaneous nephrolithotomy: an extreme technical makeover for an old technique. Arch Ital Urol Androl. 2010;82(1):23–5.
2. Cracco CM, Scoffone CM, Scarpa RM. New developments in percutaneous techniques for simple and

complex branched renal stones. Curr Opin Urol. 2011;21(2):154–60.
3. Miano R, Scoffone CM, De Nunzio C, Germani S, Cracco C, Usai P, et al. Position: prone or supine is the issue of percutaneous nephrolithotomy. J Endourol. 2010;24(6):931–8.
4. Cracco CM, Scoffone CM, Poggio M, Scarpa RM. The patient position for PNL: does it matter? Arch Ital Urol Androl. 2010;82(1):30–1.
5. Ibarluzea G, Scoffone CM, Cracco CM, Poggio M, Porpiglia F, Terrone C, et al. Supine Valdivia and modified lithotomy position for simultaneous anterograde and retrograde endourological access. BJU Int. 2007;100(1):233–6.
6. Hunter PT, Hawkins IF, Finlayson B, Nanni G, Senior D. Hawkins-Hunter retrograde transcutaneous nephrostomy: a new technique. Urology. 1983;22(6):583–7.
7. Lawson RK, Murphy JB, Taylor AJ, Jacobs SC. Retrograde method for percutaneous access to the kidney. Urology. 1983;22(6):580–2.
8. Lehman T, Bagley DH. Reverse lithotomy: modified prone position for simultaneous nephroscopic and ureteroscopic procedures in women. Urology. 1988;32(6):529–31.
9. Scoffone CM, Cracco CM, Cossu M, Grande S, Poggio M, Scarpa RM. Endoscopic combined intrarenal surgery in Galdakao-modified supine Valdivia position: a new standard for percutaneous nephrolithotomy? Eur Urol. 2008;54(6):1393–403.
10. Daels F, González MS, Freire FG, Jurado A, Damia O. Percutaneous lithotripsy in Valdivia-Galdakao decubitus position: our experience. J Endourol. 2009;23(10):1615–20.
11. Hoznek A, Rode J, Ouzaid I, Faraj B, Kimuli M, de la Taille, et al. Modifeid supine percutaneous nephrolithotomy for large kidney and ureteral stones: technique and results. Eur Urol. 2012;61(1):164–70.
12. Frattini A, Ferretti S, Dinale F, Salsi P, Granelli P, Campobasso D, Cortellini P. Supine percutaneous nephrolithotripsy in children: technical aspects. J Endourol Part B, Videourology. 2012;26(2): doi:10.1089/vid.2012.0001.
13. Cracco CM, Scoffone CM. ECIRS (Endoscopic combined intrarenal surgery) in the Galdakao-modified Valdivia position: a new life for percutaneous surgery? World J Urol. 2011;29(6):821–7.
14. Scoffone CM, Cracco CM. Percutaneous nephrolithotomy: opinion—supine position. In: Knoll T, Pearle MS, editors. Clinical management of urolithiasis. Springer: Heidelberg; 2013. p. 117–21.
15. Scoffone CM, Cracco CM, Poggio M, Scarpa RM. Endoscopic combined intrarenal surgery for high burden renal stones. Arch Ital Urol Androl. 2010; 82(1):41–2.

Percutaneous Access to the Kidney: Endoscopic

3

Adam Kaplan and Jaime Landman

Introduction

The "make or break" component of a successful percutaneous nephrolithotomy (PCNL) is proper access to the renal collecting system. Thoughtful and accurate access during PCNL will minimize complications, and will optimize the outcomes of the procedure. It is easily argued that safe and direct access to the kidney presents the greatest challenge of PCNL.

Since the inception of percutaneous access to the kidney over 50 years ago, fluoroscopy and more recently, ultrasound, have remained the standard imaging modalities for obtaining renal access [1]. While effective in most cases, many urologists find the traditional methods of obtaining access technically daunting. These challenges result in the requirement of collaboration with an interventional radiologist to gain access, or in some cases, the use of alternative and sub-optimal strategies for stone treatment. In recent years, we have combined traditional two dimensional access modalities such as fluoroscopy and ultrasound imaging with direct endoscopic visualization for access. The application of direct ureteroscopic vision to visualize the needle penetrating into the renal collecting system during access allows the majority of urologists (who are very familiar with renal endoscopy) to greatly facilitate proper needle deployment.

In this chapter, we will detail the "Endoscopic PCNL," a technique that combines flexible ureteroscopy with fluoroscopy to obtain precise and safe renal access in the desired calyx under direct vision. The flexible ureteroscope has become increasingly more advanced and ubiquitous in clinical practice over the past decade. As such, it provides a new adjunct modality to assist in the otherwise very challenging, technically demanding, and potentially dangerous endeavor of direct puncture of the renal collecting system.

PCNL was initially described by FernstrÖm and Johansson in 1976 and has remained the gold standard for treatment of large renal stones [2–4]. As most practitioners know, direct puncture into the kidney is not without its difficulties and risks. The procedure often requires multiple needle punctures, which can lead to bleeding, perforation of bowel, and damage to the collecting system. Occasionally, urologists fail to gain access despite multiple attempts. Gaining access to the kidney can be particularly challenging in the case of a non-dilated collecting system, in patients with a large stone burden, in cases of aberrant renal anatomy, in patients with an allergy to angiographic contrast material, or with obesity or previous renal surgery.

Several modifications of the original technique of PCNL have occurred over the years in an attempt to decrease complications. Retrograde access, an idea introduced in the 1980s by Hunter and Lawson's groups, sought to use the principle

A. Kaplan • J. Landman (✉)
Department of Urology, University of California, Irvine Medical Center, Orange, CA, USA
e-mail: landmanj@uci.edu

S.Y. Nakada and M.S. Pearle (eds.), *Surgical Management of Urolithiasis: Percutaneous, Shockwave and Ureteroscopy*, DOI 10.1007/978-1-4614-6937-7_3, © Springer Science+Business Media New York 2013

of going from known to unknown [5, 6]. Using fluoroscopy, the desired calyx can be accessed retrograde. A 5 F ureteral catheter and wire are guided to the calyx of choice, which is then punctured with a sharp 160-cm needle passed through the catheter. Then, under fluoroscopy the needle is passed under the ribs to the skin. The needle can be exchanged for a wire, and a tract is then dilated. While this technique and several modifications were successful in obtaining renal access in 89–100 % of cases, there were significant limitations [7–10]. In cases of large stones, the tracts made were often long and tortuous making the procedure more difficult [11].

With advances in imaging and materials technology, the ureteroscope has evolved into a highly functional, nimble, and relatively durable instrument. Image quality continues to rapidly improve, particularly with the introduction of distal sensor ureteroscopes. Endoscope diameter continues to diminish, albeit not with the distal sensor ureteroscopes. Contemporary ureterosopes incorporate a functional working channel with a diameter adequate to accommodate instruments such as a 200 μm laser fiber or nitinol instruments while maintaining outstanding active and passive deflection characteristics. Indeed, with contemporary ureteroscopes, it is feasible to routinely achieve access to every calyx in almost every case [12–14].

The routine incorporation of a ureteral access sheath has also become an important part of the urologist's armamentarium. These lubricious and wide caliber sheaths can be passed into the renal pelvis, allowing for excellent high-flow and low-pressure drainage of the kidney. Deployment of an access sheath during PCNL procedures also allows for stone fragments to pass down the ureter and out of the patient. Contemporary access sheaths come in a wide range of lengths and diameters and several features that enable easy deployment in most ureters. The incorporation of a hydrophilic coating, a tapered dilator and kink resistant materials and a funnel-shaped ergonomic entry port make deployment of today's access sheath very easy in most patients [15]. Using an access sheath, the ureteroscope can easily and atraumatically be passed up and down the ureter [16–19]. It is the advances in ureteroscope technology and contemporary access sheaths that have made Endoscopic PCNL possible, efficient and, in many cases, safer than the traditional approach.

The first endoscopic PCNL was reported by Grasso and Colleagues in 1995 after attempted access under fluoroscopy in seven patients failed [20]. Kidd and Conlin used endoscopy to obtain access in three cases as well [21]. Of the ten patients reported, most were obese and/or presented an anatomic challenge; endoscopy was used as a last resort. These procedures were done without the use of an access sheath. In 2003, Landman and colleagues reported the application of a ureteral access sheath during PCNL [15]. This offered the advantage of a better retrograde dilation of the collecting system, which would facilitate needle access and passage of the guidewire between large stones. Studies of renal pelvic pressures showed that placement of an access sheath provides for maximum flow of the irrigant while maintaining a low intrarenal pelvic pressure [18]. Additionally it would expedite through and through wire placement, provide drainage stone fragments, and allow for rapid and atraumatic placement of the ureteroscope throughout the case.

Clayman and colleagues later described the current Endoscopic PCNL technique after his initial experience at the University of Texas, Southwestern Medical Center in 2005, which involved placement of a ureteral access sheath and placement of a ureteroscope at the onset of the case to facilitate needle placement. The advantages of precise placement of the nephrostomy needle and direct visualization of the tract dilation and sheath placement were immediately apparent, and the technique was refined over the subsequent 100 PCNL cases [22]. Since then, access sheath placement and endoscopy have become an integral part of PCNL at the author's institution.

Details of the Procedure

Positioning

The patient is positioned prone on spreader bars with legs abducted. This allows for simultaneous access to the flank and genitalia. Both areas are prepped and draped (Figs. 3.1 and 3.2).

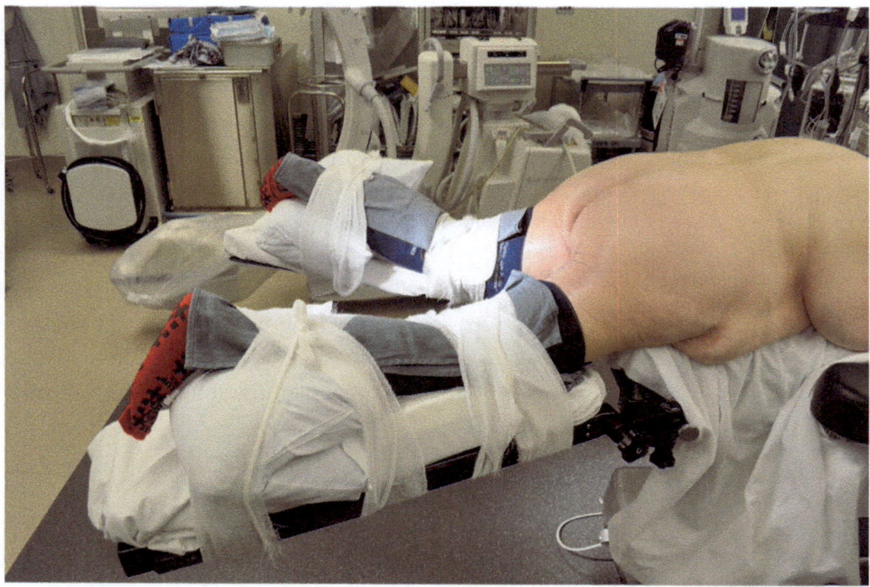

Fig. 3.1 Patient positioning. Patient is positioned prone with spreader bars to allow for endoscopic access from below

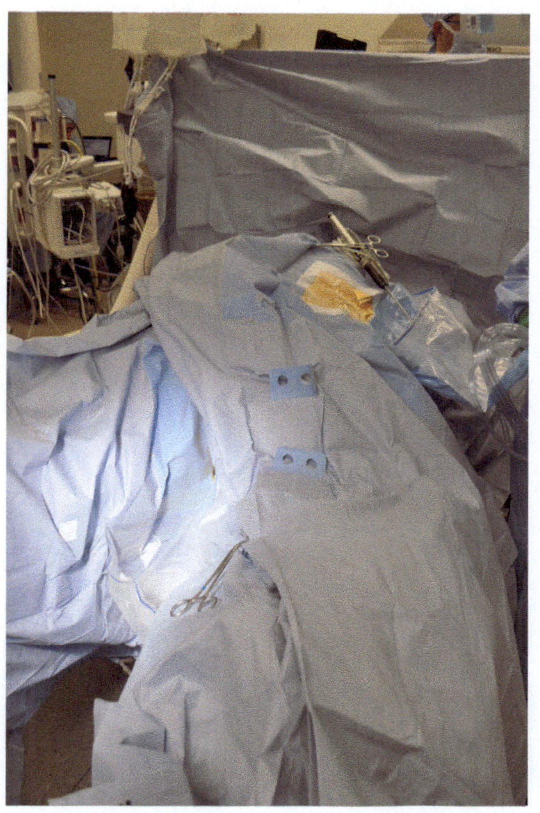

Fig. 3.2 Patient positioned in prone position with spreader bars with drapes in place

Ureteral Access

Proper setup of the back table is of paramount importance when performing complex endoscopy (Table 3.1, Fig. 3.3). A flexible cystoscope is inserted into the bladder and a 0.035″ floppy tip hydrophilic glidewire is advanced up the ureter under fluoroscopic guidance. An 8 F/10 F coaxial dilater is advanced over the glidewire. The 8F coaxial dilator is removed and the 10 F dilator is used to perform a retrograde pyelogram. A floppy tip guidewire and a 0.035″ superstiff wire are advanced through the 10 F sheath to the collecting system. The superstiff wire will be the working wire. The 10 F sheath is removed and the guidewire is coiled and fixed to the drapes near the upper thigh with a Kelly clamp. This will function as a safety wire. A 12 F Foley catheter is placed in the bladder for drainage.

A ureteral access sheath is passed over the working wire until the distal tip rests at the level of the ureteropelvic junction. Access sheath size will depend on the size and sex of the patient, the stone burden and the size of the ureteroscope. Men will often require a 55 cm sheath where as a 35 cm sheath will reach the UPJ in most women.

Table 3.1 Instrument setup guide

Operating room
Fluoroscopy-compatible operating room table
Leg spreader bars
C-arm fluoroscopy with monitor
Video tower setup with light source, camera, and monitor
Standard surgical tray (includes #11 scalpel blade and kelly clamps)
Flexible cystoscope/nephroscope (16 F standard)
Flexible ureteroscope
Rigid nephroscope (26 F offset lens)
Lithotripsy equipment and supplies including grasping forceps, stone baskets, and laser fiber
Pressurized warming irrigation system
Disposable
0.035-in. 150-cm nitinol hydrophilic guidewire—straight tip and/or angled tip
0.035-in. 150-cm floppy-tip Bentson guidewire
0.035-in. 145-cm super-stiff guidewire
0.035-in. 260-cm floppy-tip Bentson exchange guidewire
5 F open-ended ureteral catheter
8 F/10 F coaxial dilator-introducer set
Ureteral access sheath (35 or 55 cm, 9.5/11 F or 12/14 F)
18-G 15-cm conical tip, percutaneous renal trocar needle
5-mm fascial incising needle (Cook Urological, Spencer, IN, USA)
30 F nephrostomy dilating balloon catheter with 30 F renal access sheath
12 F Foley catheter
10 mL Luer lock syringe
Optional
Sureseal II® Side arm self-sealing adapter (Applied Medical Corp., Rancho Santa Margarita, CA, USA)

Diameter ranges from an inner/outer diameter of 9.5 F/11 F to 14 F/16 F. A larger sheath should be used for larger ureteroscopes and in cases of significant stone burden. That said, if the sheath does not pass easily, a smaller diameter sheath should be chosen. In cases where the patient already has a ureteral stent in place prior to the procedure, we routinely advance a 14/16 F access sheath without difficulty to the level of the UPJ. The working wire is removed once the sheath is in place and the ureteroscope is advanced into the renal pelvis through the access sheath.

Renal Access

A double contrast nephrogram is performed via the ureteroscope. Ten to twenty milliliters of dilute contrast material is followed by injection of 2–5 cc of air. The use of contrast and air helps map the calyceal system. With the patient in the prone position, the ureteroscopist can find the most posterior calyx by following the air bubble. The air bubble can also be seen on fluoroscopy. An upper pole posterior calyx is selected by the ureteroscopist. In some cases, the stone may hinder advancement of the ureteroscope or access to the desired calyx. A 200 μm Holmium laser fiber can be used to fragment the stone to allow passage of the ureteroscope.

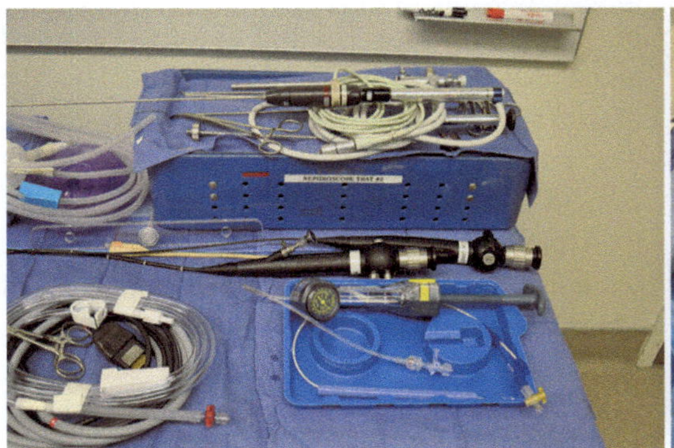

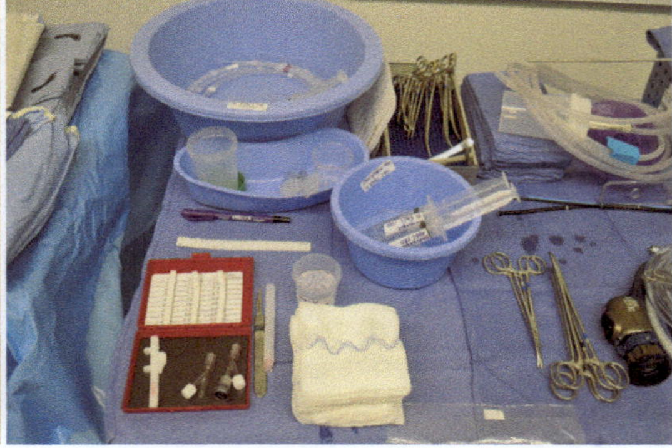

Fig. 3.3 Well-organized back table for ureteroscopy and PCNL

With the fluoroscope at a 90° anterior–posterior position, the same calyx is found by the surgeon obtaining flank access. An 18 G nephrostomy needle is advanced towards the tip of the ureteroscope, which is radiopaque on fluoroscopy. Once the needle has been advanced 4–6 cm, its trajectory is fixed. The C-arm is rotated to 25–30° posterolateral-oblique position. The needle is advanced and its position is monitored under fluoroscopy.

The needle is monitored under fluoroscopy and then visualized with the ureteroscope as it punctures the collecting system. The ureteroscopist can watch the needle traverse the fornix of a posterior calyx and ensure that it is not passed too deeply so as to perforate the anterior wall of the calyx.

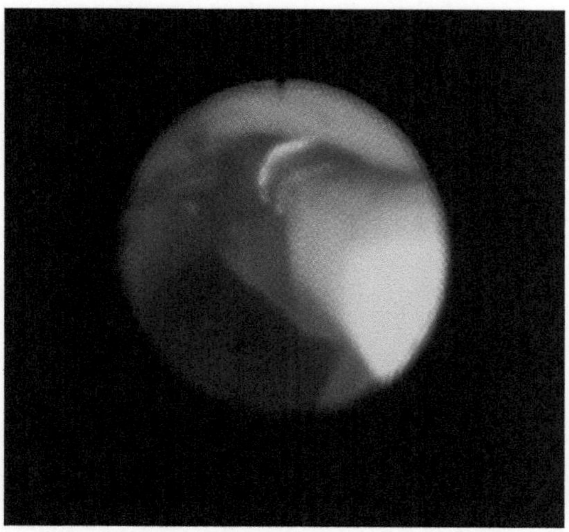

Fig. 3.4 The balloon dilator is seen dilating the renal parenchyma, under direct ureteroscopic vision

Creation of Access Tract

Once the needle is in position, the needle obturator is removed. Under direct vision and fluoroscopic guidance, a 0.035″ hydrophilic glidewire is passed through the needle and directed down the ureter alongside the access sheath or coiled in the renal pelvis. Alternatively, an angled glidewire can be maneuvered using a torquing tool such that it is advanced into the access sheath and delivered at the urethral end of the sheath. This process is very much facilitated by transiently pulling the access sheath down into the proximal ureter. In this manner, the UPJ can be used as a funnel to bring the wire into the ureter and then the access sheath. Once this through and through access has been gained, the 8 component of the 8–10 dilator can be passed down through the entire system and the angled glide wire changed to a superstiff wire. We typically advance the wire such that the floppy end is at the flank site so that it can be used for retrograde ureteral catheter deployment at the end of the procedure. The sheath can then be re-advanced up the ureter and into the renal pelvis by inserting the obturator and advancing the entire unit. The wire within the access sheath is maintained for perfect through-and-through access.

The needle puncture site is enlarged to a 1.0 cm incision with a #11 blade and the nephrostomy needle is removed. A 5 mm fascial incising needle is passed over the antegrade wire parallel to the skin incision. Tract dilation is performed under direct endoscopic visualization and fluoroscopic control. A 30 F dilating balloon with a backloaded 30 F working sheath is advanced over the superstiff wire. The tip of the balloon can be seen entering the calyx on ureteroscopy. The balloon is then inflated under direct vision. Fluoroscopy can be used to insure complete inflation of the balloon. The working sheath is passed over the balloon and rotated under ureteroscopic guidance until all the edges of the sheath are visible in the collecting system. Using direct vision, we have found it very easy to deploy the balloon and outer sheath with millimeter precision. We have therefore been able to very easily and routinely avoid dilating too deeply and traumatizing the infundibulum and deploying the outer sheath in the renal parenchyma. The balloon is deflated and withdrawn (Figs. 3.4, 3.5, 3.6).

Once access is obtained, the surgeon has many options available including rigid and flexible nephroscopy, ureteroscopy, ultrasound, suction, hydraulic devices, and graspers to evacuate the stone burden and manipulate the wires. If through-and-through access has not yet been obtained a 260 cm exchange wire can be advanced retrograde through the ureteral access

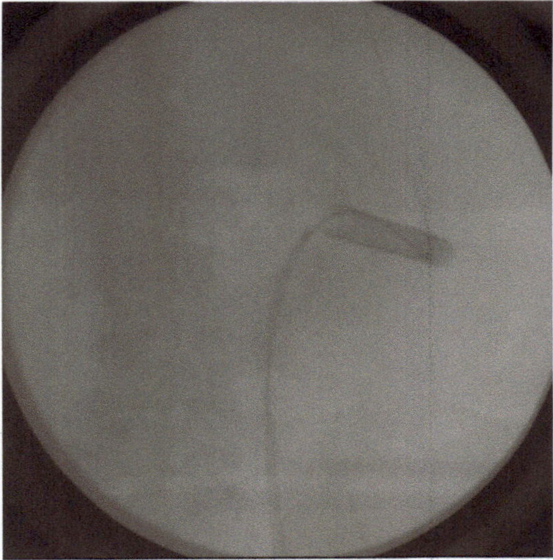

Fig. 3.5 Fluoroscopic view of ureteroscope and access sheath during tract dilation

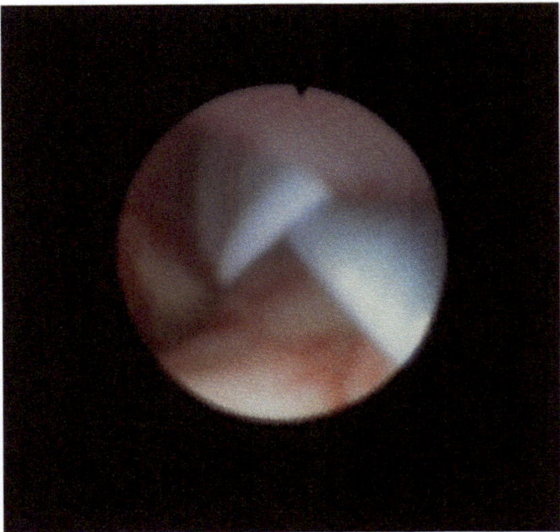

Fig. 3.6 Ureteroscopic view of access sheath in position

sheath to the renal pelvis and grasped with the nephroscope forceps and removed through the 30 F sheath.

A Safer Method of Obtaining Access

Considering the danger of direct puncture to the renal collecting system, safety is the foremost concern of the surgeon gaining access. Direct visualization of the collecting system provides several advantages in this regard.

Table 3.2 Potential advantages of endoscopic-guided PCNL

Direct visual targeting of the desired calyx
Decreased fluoroscopy needed for needle localization
Visual confirmation of needle trocar placement, dilation, and tract creation
Facilitate placement of antegrade guidewire for through-and-through access
Simultaneous antegrade and retrograde approach for complex or large stone burdens in difficult-to-access areas (middle pole calyx)
Ability to clear stone fragments proximal to the renal access in a retrograde fashion
Ability to clear ureter stones
Increased success of supracostal percutaneous access
Decreased risk of pleural injury

Targeting a posterior calyx became easier and safer with adjunct ureteroscopy. In a similar fashion to traditional PCNL, air could be injected directly into the collecting system. With the patient prone, air will rise to the most posterior position in the kidney, thereby marking a posterior target. This can be visualized under fluoroscopy as well as under direct vision, providing a target and a method for orientation for the ureteroscopist. The needle can then be passed directly toward the tip of the ureteroscope under fluoroscopy, insuring that the puncture is directly into the calyx of choice. Safe and precise placement of the nephrostomy needle in a posterior calyx with fewer needle punctures would prove beneficial in reducing blood loss, pain, incidence of post-op fever, and sepsis (Table 3.2).

Perforation of the anterior collecting system is a common complication of traditional PCNL. Often, the needle is passed to deeply or scything the desired calyx. This increases the risk of further parenchymal injury and bleeding, as well as perforation of the colon or duodenum. Many times after dilating an access tract and inserting the nephroscope with traditional access techniques, the guidewires are seen to be perforating the collecting system; often the surgeon can be fooled by the paths needles and wires take under fluoroscopy or ultrasound alone. Direct visualization with an ureteroscope allows the surgeon to see whether the needle has passed too deep or outside the collecting system. Passing wires into the collecting system or down the ureter can be done quickly and with confidence under direct vision.

A retrospective analysis at the University of California, Irvine, comparing Endoscopy Assisted PCNL versus the standard fluoroscopy-guided technique showed a decrease in estimated blood loss (158 cc vs. 211 cc, $p=0.03$) and decreased postoperative transfusion rates (7.8 % vs. 21.4 %, $p=0.05$). Stone free rates, perioperative complications, embolization rates, narcotic usage, and renal function (measured by glomerular filtration rate) were identical. There was a trend towards decreased retreatment rates with endoscopic guidance (24 % vs. 36 %, $p=0.19$), and a trend towards a longer operative time (227 min vs. 208 min, $p=0.1$) [23].

Patients who underwent endoscopic-guided PCNL with upper pole access had fewer pulmonary complications compared to reports in the literature of standard PCNL. Of 111 consecutive cases, 93 % used an upper pole access, and 75 % had a supracostal puncture. All patients received a postoperative chest x-ray, and 11 % had a pleural effusion. Three percent developed a pneumothroax and two patients required a chest tube for clinically significant effusions (none for pneumothorax). This was compared to a meta-analysis of supracostal access by Lingeman et al. of 1,580 patients who underwent PCNL, 30 % of which had upper pole access. The overall incidence of pleural complications was 14.8 % with 4.1 % of these complications requiring intervention [24].

As a whole, urologists have lower access-related complications than radiologists when obtaining renal access. However the learning curve for standard PCNL is steep, requiring 24–60 procedures to obtain proficiency [25–27]. As such, only 11 % of urologists obtain their own access. The use of endoscopy can help flatten the learning curve, allowing more urologists to feel comfortable and confident obtaining access effectively and safely.

Stone Retrieval in Endoscopic PCNL

If safe access to the kidney is the primary goal of PCNL, the secondary goal is optimal stone clearance. Large staghorn calculi are particularly suited for Endoscopic PCNL, as this technique allows the safest opportunity for upper pole posterior access. Furthermore, all renal calyces, in even the most complex collecting system, can be accessed with ureteroscopy if needed throughout the case [28].

In traditional PCNL, a second needle puncture and dilated tracts may be required to adequately access a stone that cannot be visualized with from the vantage of the first puncture. Ureteroscopy has proved helpful for accessing and inspecting these calices that were otherwise inaccessible, obviating the need for a second PCNL tract in many cases. In fact, the ureteroscope can be used to visualize these inaccessible stones and fragment them in situ, or mobilize these stones so that they can be presented to a rigid nephroscope for expeditious extraction or rapid fragmentation. Essentially, the access sheath becomes the equivalent of an additional access site without the associated risks of renal bleeding and pleural disruption.

Placement of an ureteroscope and access sheath allows for retrograde irrigation and dilation of the targeted collecting system [15]. Additionally, if necessary, ureteroscopic laser lithotripsy can reduce pre-puncture stone burden to allow for ideal caliceal placement and complete entry of the sheath into the collecting system. This has its own benefits, including reduced extravasation of irrigation into the retroperitoneum and decreased manipulating of the tract. With the sheath in proper position, stones are less likely to migrate into the retroperitoneum.

Challenges of Endoscopic PCNL

Endoscopic PCNL is not without its drawbacks. First and foremost, the procedure requires a second operator who is skilled at ureteroscopy. The ureteroscopy must be performed with the patient in the prone position, which can be initially disorienting and takes practice. Considering that most urologists are comfortable with flexible ureteroscopy, this limitation will be less of an issue moving forward. The length of the Endoscopic PCNL is on average 19 min longer than the standard PCNL performed in expert hands. It may, however, prove quicker and more efficient in the hands of a surgeon less skilled in obtaining access.

Conclusion

The safety and efficacy of PCNL can be enhanced by concurrent ureteroscopic access. Endoscopically guided percutaneous renal access provides the advantage of minimize renal punctures, optimizing the position of the access to a superior pole posterior calyx, improved stone clearance, and reduced complications. The technique involves the placement of a ureteral access sheath and a flexible ureteroscope with the patient in the prone position. Under direct vision with the ureteroscope as well as fluoroscopic guidance, direct renal access can be obtained in a similar manner to standard PCNL, but with the advantage of direct visualization of the needle puncture and tract dilation. Challenging cases of aberrant anatomy, obesity, or large stone burden may be particularly suited to endoscopic access.

References

1. Goodwin WE, Casey WC, Woolf W. Percutaneous trocar (needle) nephrostomy in hydronephrosis. J Am Med Assoc. 1955;157(11):891–4.
2. Fernström I, Johansson B. Percutaneous pyelolithotomy. A new extraction technique. Scand J Urol Nephrol. 1976;10(3):257–9.
3. Morris DS, Wei JT, Taub DA, Dunn RL, Wolf Jr JS, Hollenbeck BK. Temporal trends in the use of percutaneous nephrostolithotomy. J Urol. 2006;175(5):1731–6.
4. Skolarikos A, Alivizatos G, de la Rosette JJ. Percutaneous nephrostolithotomy and its legacy. Eur Urol. 2005;47(1):22–8.
5. Hunter PT, Hawkins IF, Finlayson B, Nanni G, Senior D. Hawkins-Hunter retrograde transcutaneous nephrostomy: a new technique. Urology. 1983;22(6):583–7.
6. Lawson RK, Murphy JB, Taylor AJ, Jacobs SC. Retrograde method for percutaneous access to kidney. Urology. 1983;22(6):580–2.
7. Hawkins Jr IF. Retrograde percutaneous nephrostomy. Crit Rev Diagn Imaging. 1987;27(2):153–65.
8. Spirnak JP, Resnick MI. Retrograde percutaneous stone removal using modified Lawson technique. Urology. 1987;30(6):551–3.
9. Morrisseau PM, Trotter SJ. Retrograde percutaneous nephrolithotomy: urological treatment of a urological problem. J Urol. 1988;139(6):1163–5.
10. Leal JJ. Percutaneous removal of renal and ureteral stones with and without concomitant transurethral manipulation by a urologist using antegrade and retrograde techniques without a radiologist's assistance. J Urol. 1988;139(6):1184–7.
11. Munch LC. Direct vision modified Lawson retrograde nephrostomy technique using flexible ureteroscope. J Endourol. 1989;3:411–7.
12. Grasso M, Bagley D. Small diameter, actively deflectable, flexible ureteropyeloscopy. J Urol. 1998; 160(5):1648–53. discussion 1653–4.
13. Traxer O. Flexible ureterorenoscopic management of lower pole stone: does the scope make the difference? J Endourol. 2008;22(9):1847–50. discussion 1855.
14. Afane JS, Olweny EO, Bercowsky E, Sundaram CP, Dunn MD, Shalhav AL, McDougall EM, Clayman RV. Flexible ureteroscopes: a single center evaluation of the durability and function of the new endoscopes smaller than 9 Fr. J Urol. 2000;164(4):1164–8.
15. Landman J, Venkatesh R, Lee DI, Rehman J, Ragab M, Darcy M, Sundaram CP. Combined percutaneous and retrograde approach to staghorn calculi with application of the ureteral access sheath to facilitate percutaneous nephrostolithotomy. J Urol. 2003; 169(1):64–7.
16. Delvecchio FC, Auge BK, Brizuela RM, Weizer AZ, Silverstein AD, Lallas CD, Pietrow PK, Albala DM, Preminger GM. Assessment of stricture formation with the ureteral access sheath. Urology. 2003;61(3): 518–22.
17. Monga M, Best S, Venkatesh R, Ames C, Lieber D, Vanlangendock R, Landman J. Prospective randomized comparison of 2 ureteral access sheaths during flexible retrograde ureteroscopy. J Urol. 2004;172(2):572–3.
18. Rehman J, Monga M, Landman J, Lee DI, Felfela T, Conradie MC, Srinivas R, Sundaram CP, Clayman RV. Characterization of intrapelvic pressure during ureteropyeloscopy with ureteral access sheaths. Urology. 2003;61(4):713–8.
19. Auge BK, Pietrow PK, Lallas CD, Raj GV, Santa-Cruz RW, Preminger GM. Ureteral access sheath provides protection against elevated renal pressures during routine flexible ureteroscopic stone manipulation. J Endourol. 2004;18(1):33–6.
20. Grasso M, Lang G, Taylor FC. Flexible ureteroscopically assisted percutaneous renal access. Tech Urol. 1995;1(1):39–3.
21. Kidd CF, Conlin MJ. Ureteroscopically assisted percutaneous renal access. Urology. 2003;61(6): 1244–5.
22. Khan F, Borin JF, Pearle MS, McDougall EM, Clayman RV. Endoscopically guided percutaneous

renal access: "Seeing is believing". J Endourol. 2006; 20(7):451–5.

23. Sountoulides PG, Kaufmann OG, Louie MK, Beck S, Jain N, Kaplan A, McDougall EM, Clayman RV. Endoscopy-guided percutaneous nephrostolithotomy: benefits of ureteroscopic access and therapy. J Endourol. 2009;23(10):1649–54.
24. Lingeman JE, Matlaga BR, Evan AP. Surgical management of upper urinary tract calculi. In: Wein AJ, Kavoussi LR, Novick AC, Partin AW, Peters CA, editors. Campbell-Walsh urology. 9th ed. Philadelphia: Saunders Elsevier; 2007. p. 1431–507.
25. Watterson JD, Soon S, Jana K. Access related complications during percutaneous nephrostolithotomy: urology versus radiology at a single academic institution. J Urol. 2006;176(1):142–5.
26. de la Rosette JJMCH, Laguna MP, Rassweiler JJ, Conort P. Training in percutaneous nephrostolithotomy—a critical review. Eur Urol. 2008;54(5): 994–1001.
27. Tanriverdi O, Boylu U, Kendirci M, Kadihasanoglu M, Horasanli K, Miroglu C. The learning curve in the training of percutaneous nephrostolithotomy. Eur Urol. 2007;52(1):206–11.
28. Ankem MK, Lowry PS, Slovick RW, del Rio Munoz A, Nakada SY. Clinical utility of dual active deflection flexible ureteroscope during upper tract ureteropyeloscopy. Urology. 2004;64(3):430–4.

4 Percutaneous Stone Removal: Case Discussion on Stones in a Horseshoe Kidney

Muhammad Waqas Iqbal, Michael E. Lipkin, and Glenn M. Preminger

Technique

Prior to surgery, all patients are extensively counseled regarding the likelihood of complete stone clearance, the need for drainage tubes, possible complications and the need for ancillary and staged procedures. The preoperative work up includes imaging, typically with a noncontrast computed tomography (NCCT). On occasion an intravenous pyelogram is obtained in complicated cases to better delineate calyceal anatomy. Routine preoperative laboratory studies include a complete blood count, basic metabolic panel, PT/INR and PTT. A type and screen is also obtained. A urinalysis and a urine culture are collected. Positive urine cultures are generally treated for 7–10 days prior to the procedure with culture-specific antibiotics. Culture-negative patients receive perioperative antibiotic prophylaxis with ampicillin and an amino glycoside with two subsequent doses.

The technique of stone removal is modified according to location, size, number, presumed composition, presence of any anatomical abnormality, previous urinary tract reconstruction and whether a percutaneous access is already in place prior to proceeding to the operating room.

M.W. Iqbal, M.D. (✉) • M.E. Lipkin, M.D.
G.M. Preminger, M.D.
Division of Urology, Department of Surgery, Duke University Medical Center, Durham, NC, USA
e-mail: muhammad.iqbal@duke.edu

Percutaneous access is described elsewhere in detail in this text. Briefly we obtain access in the prone position. We use a 30 Fr balloon dilator to establish the tract. A 30 Fr Amplatz sheath is placed over the balloon. Single or multiple tracts are placed depending upon the characteristics of the stone(s). Once access is obtained, a 25 Fr rigid nephroscope is used to visualize the stone and to assure appropriate tract placement within collecting system. Once the stones are visualized there are multiple devices for intracorporeal lithotripsy available to fragment the stones. A combination of devices can be utilized for optimal stone removal. For stones less than a centimeter in size, a rigid grasper may be placed through nephroscope and used to remove the stone intact.

We typically use an ultrasonic lithotripter during our PNL due to some of the advantages discussed below. One of the primary advantages of an ultrasonic lithotripter is the ability to suction out stone fragments during lithotripsy and to suction out blood clots in the collecting system to improve visualization during the case. The tip of the ultrasonic probe is placed in contact with the stone and activated with a foot pedal, and suction is intermittently applied to remove small fragments. The suction can be controlled by placing a clamp on the suction tubing and releasing it when suction is desired. This also prevents system from collapsing and prevents accumulation of air bubbles at the tip of the lens.

Calyceal calculi or proximal ureteric stones lying at awkward angles not accessible through rigid scopes often require flexible ureteroscopy

S.Y. Nakada and M.S. Pearle (eds.), *Surgical Management of Urolithiasis: Percutaneous, Shockwave and Ureteroscopy*, DOI 10.1007/978-1-4614-6937-7_4, © Springer Science+Business Media New York 2013

or nephroscopy for successful stone treatment. The stones may be grasped using a flexible basket and displaced into the renal pelvis, where they can be fragmented using rigid instruments. In cases where the stone cannot be easily displaced or captured in a basket, a holmium laser fiber can be passed through the flexible scope and laser lithotripsy can be performed. Once the stone fragments have been removed, all the calices and proximal ureter may be visually inspected with rigid/flexible instruments to document stone-free status. This may be guided and confirmed by fluoroscopic imaging.

We perform the majority of our procedures without leaving a nephrostomy tube in place. The 6 Fr open-ended ureteral catheter that is placed in the beginning of the procedure to aide in access is left in place overnight. In patients with a collecting system injury, significant residual stone burden requiring a second-stage percutaneous procedure or lower urinary tract diversion, a 10 Fr nephrostomy tube is left in place. For a patient who had a proximal ureteral stone or ureteropelvic junction stone treated with significant inflammation, an internal ureteral stent is placed in an antegrade fashion.

There are several methods and devices for intracorporeal lithotripsy. These include ultrasonic, pneumatic, or combined devices, electrohydraulic lithotripsy and laser.

Ultrasonic Lithotripsy

Ultrasound was first described to fragment kidney stones in 1953 [1]. The basic unit of an ultrasonic lithotripter consists of a power generator, an ultrasound transducer and a probe (Fig. 4.1). Ultrasonic probes come in various sizes ranging from 2.5 to 6 Fr. The 2.5 Fr probes are solid and contain no hollow center for suction. The ultrasonic generator utilizes piezoelectric crystals located in the hand piece to generate ultrasonic waves (23,000–27,000 Hz) from electric energy. These are transmitted along the hollow metal probe as longitudinal and transverse vibrations. When the vibrating tip is brought in contact with stone, the calculus is fragmented. The stone fragments are suctioned out

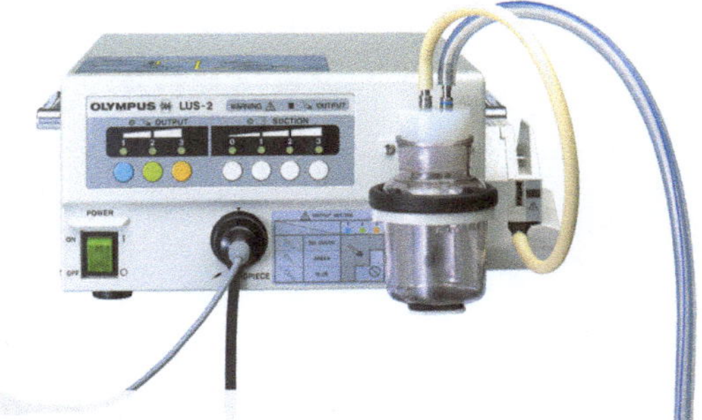

Fig. 4.1 Olympus LUS-2®. Ultrasonic lithotripter

through the hollow probe by connecting it to suction tubing [2]. The circulation of irrigant helps to keep the temperature along the probe from rising significantly. It is important to keep irrigation running during ultrasonic lithotripsy to prevent the probe from overheating and malfunctioning. Normal saline is generally used as an irrigant during the procedure.

Ultrasonic lithotripters have proven to be efficacious at treating renal stones. In one large series of 800 patients reporting on percutaneous removal of renal calculi using ultrasonic lithotripsy, the success rate was over 95 %. One limitation of this study was that stone size and location were not reported and success was not clearly defined [3]. In a more recent randomized study comparing an ultrasonic lithotripter (LUS-2 Olympus, Inc., Melville, New York) to a combined pneumatic/ultrasonic lithotripter(Lithoclast Ultra (Microvasive, Natick, Massachusetts and EMS, Bern, Switzerland),in patients undergoing percutaneous nephrolithotomy, the ultrasonic lithotripter demonstrated significantly longer stone-clearance times(43.7 min vs. 21.1 min, $p=0.036$). Similarly the average rate of stone clearance for ultrasonic device was 16.8 mm^2/min versus 39.5 mm^2/min for the combination unit ($p=0.028$). Both groups had similar stone location, burden and composition. However, the stone-free rates and complications rates were comparable for the two devices [4].

Another study involving 82 patients with renal calculi looked at long-term complications of ultrasonic lithotripsy using DMSA renal scan; nine patients had residual stones. At mean follow-up of

22 months recurrence was noted in two patients. There was no evidence of hypertension or urinary tract infection related to the procedure. A cortical scar was noted in only 1 kidney and no arteriovenous fistulas were found [5].

Ultrasonic lithotripsy is a safe energy source. It has been shown in rabbit and canine models not to cause significant changes in urothelium even when the probe tip is placed in direct contact with the urothelium [6]. However there is risk of thermal damage if probe becomes overheated. In a study looking at long-term effects on rat bladders comparing pneumatic versus ultrasonic lithotripsy, 71 % of bladders where ultrasonic energy was used were edematous and hemorrhagic versus none for pneumatic. In 57 % of the bladders that were treated with an ultrasonic probe, there was evidence of microscopic inflammation. This was only seen in 22 % of the bladders in which the pneumatic probe was used. Additionally 85 % of ultrasonic and only 22 % of pneumatic treated bladders developed microscopic stones in the bladder wall at 30 days after treatment [7]. Although ultrasonic lithotripsy has been shown to be safe, caution should still be used to avoid contact with the urothelium whenever possible to avoid these complications.

A disadvantage of ultrasound lithotripsy is that probe must be rigid to transmit sound waves, as flexible probes cannot transmit sound waves without loss of significant energy. Therefore, ultrasonic lithotripsy cannot be performed through flexible scopes. Another disadvantage of ultrasonic lithotripsy is, it does not work well on harder stone compositions such as calcium oxalate monohydrate, uric acid and cystine stones.

Ballistic Lithotripsy

Ballistic lithotripters utilize energy from a source to generate physical displacement of a projectile. They include pneumatic and electro-kinetic energy probes. When the projectile (probe) comes in contact with the stone, it transfers its energy to the stone and this leads to fragmentation. These fragments then need to be removed with another device, such as a grasper or via suction through an ultrasonic probe.

Ballistic lithotripters have many advantages over other lithotripters. Ballistic devices utilize probes that are generally reusable and very durable [8]. Ballistic devices are especially effective at the initial fragmentation of large and hard stones. Ballistic lithotripters are also relatively safe compared to other lithotripters. It has been demonstrated in the bladder and ureter that there is less risk of urinary tract perforation compared to EHL, ultrasonic lithotripters and laser lithotripsy [9]. There is also no risk of thermal injury.

The major disadvantages of ballistic lithotripsy are an additional device is required to remove stone fragments and the probes are rigid. The rigid probes prevent ballistic lithotripters from being used with flexible endoscopes. Bending of the probe can significantly reduce tip displacement and velocity [10] which may compromise stone fragmentation.

There are two main types of ballistic lithotripters, pneumatic and electrokinetic.

Pneumatic Energy

The Swiss LithoClast® (EMS, Nyon, Switzerland) was the first ballistic device introduced. It uses compressed air from a generator connected to a compressed air tank or central air supply to move a metal projectile, which in turn moves a metal probe at a frequency of 12 cycles/s and a pressure of three atmospheres, resulting in a jackhammer like effect on stones [11]. The probes are available in sizes ranging from 0.8 to 3 mm. A modification to the Lithoclast, the Lithovac device (EMS, Nyon, Switzerland), was made to allow suction to remove fragments from 2 to 3.5 mm in size [12]. This device suffered from problems with clogging from stone fragments during suction. The advantage pneumatic lithotripters is its efficiency to break calculi of all compositions [13, 14].

Pneumatic lithotripters have been safely and effectively used in both ureteric and renal calculi. Murthy et al. used Swiss Lithoclast in 114 patients with ureteral stones and reported the stone fragmentation rate was 93.4 %. There were no major complications, although 25 % patients had uncomplicated urinary tract infections or hematuria [15]. In another study, the Swiss Lithoclast was used to treat stones during PNL, ureteroscopy and cystolitholapaxy. The authors reported that it was effective for stones of varying compositions including calcium oxalate monohydrate, calcium phosphate, cystine, struvite, and uric acid stones. All renal and bladder stones were fragmented to completion and, complete stone fragmentation was achieved in 95 % ureteral stones [16] Denstedt and colleagues reported on the use of the Swiss Lithoclast during PNL in 45 patients. A variety of stone compositions were included in this report including 16 calcium oxalate/phosphate, 17 struvite, 8 uric acid, and 4 cystine calculi. The Lithoclast was able to fragment the hard stones rapidly and successfully. In three cases where ultrasound was initially used, the ultrasonic probe had to be replaced by the Lithoclast to fragment stones that were resistant to lithotripsy. The authors did note that unlike harder stones, struvite stones are better treated with ultrasonic lithotripsy. There were no intraoperative complications related to the Lithoclast and there were no collecting system perforations. None of the patients required transfusion [17]. A randomized, prospective trial compared two pneumatic lithotripters, the Swiss Lithoclast and the LMA Stonebreaker (Cook Medical, Bloomington, IN). The Stonebreaker had a significantly faster stone fragmentation rate; however, there was no difference in stone-free rate between the two lithotrites (54 % for the Stonebreaker vs. 39 % for the Lithoclast). The authors reported no device-related complications in either group [18].

In addition to being effective at stone fragmentation, pneumatic lithotripters are safe. Unlike ultrasonic lithotripters, pneumatic lithotripsy is not associated with the production of heat during use. Both animal and clinical studies have attested this fact. Denstedt and colleagues studied the tissue effects of the pneumatic LithoClast on pig bladders and ureters. They found areas of focal hemorrhage in places where the Lithoclast had been in contact with the urothelium, but there no ureteral perforations or late tissue fibrosis visualized [19].

Electrokinetic Energy

Electrokinetic lithotripters use a hand set with the capability of generating an electromagnetic field, which then vibrates a probe at 15–30 cycles/s. These vibrations are transmitted to the end of the probe to provide a jackhammer effect on the stone similar to the pneumatic devices. This requires electrical power for adequate functioning. Alternatively, some electrokinetic devices use electricity to power a motor that displaces a probe thereby creating the same jackhammer effect.

Electrokinetic devices have been shown to be as effective at stone fragmentation as pneumatic devices. One study compared a new electrokinetic device (Combilith® Walz; Rohrdorf, Germany) to a pneumatic lithotripter (Swiss Lithoclast) in both an in vitro model and clinically. In the in vitro model, there was no difference in stone fragmentation; however, stone displacement was significantly less for the electrokinetic lithotripter. In the clinical trial portion of the study, 22 ureteral stones were treated with the Lithoclast and 35 with the Combolith Walz. There was no difference between the devices for stone fragmentation, stone-free rates or complications [20].

In another study comparing the electrokinetic and pneumatic devices, Wang et al. compared two portable handheld lithotrites the electrokinetic EMS Swiss Lithobreaker (EMS, Nyon, Switzerland) and the pneumatic LMA Stonebreaker, which runs on CO_2 cartridges. One centimeter spherical BegoStone phantoms were placed on a 2 mm mesh sieve and fragmented underwater using 2 mm probes in an in vitro percutaneous model. The number of shocks required to clear the stone phantoms through the sieve were 430±97 for the Lithobreaker compared to 29±3.7 for the Stonebreaker. Similarly, the time required to clear the stones was significantly less for the Stonebreaker, 122±56 s compared 484±79 s. The electrokinetic device had significantly higher tip displacement and slower tip velocity compared to the pneumatic device [21].

Laser Lithotripsy

LASER (Light amplification by stimulated emission of radiation) allows considerable energy in the form of photons to be transmitted in a highly concentrated fashion. They require a medium for generation and are named after that medium. In general, lasers cause stone fragmentation by two effects. The pulsed lasers, when applied to the stone surface causes release of electrons and the generation of a plasma bubble. This plasma bubble expands, followed by its collapse, generating a shockwave that causes stone fragmentation, a mechanism known as Photo acoustic effect [22]. The coumarin laser is an example of a pulsed dye laser. The holmium laser actually works by a process known as the photo-thermal effect, whereby the laser causes vaporization of stone; the shock wave produced by holmium laser is weak [23].

Currently, the holmium laser is the most commonly used laser in the treatment of stones. It has been demonstrated to be very safe when compared to EHL probes [24]. The zone of thermal injury in contact with urothelium for the holmium laser extends 0.5–1 mm. In addition, it is highly absorbed by water thereby allowing the heat to dissipate and increasing the safety profile. By comparison, EHL probes can cause tissue injury even when activated several millimeters away from the urothelial wall. Laser safety has been evaluated in a pig model using a 1,000 μ holmium laser fiber at 70 W:(3.5 J_20 Hz). The laser was fired at close to but not in contact with the mucosa of the renal pelvis and calices, lasting for about 1 h. The pigs were sacrificed on the next day and the kidneys harvested to evaluate any histological changes in the glomeruli or basal membrane. No significant changes were seen in the glomeruli or tubules [25].

Holmium laser fibers are available in 200, 365, 550 and 1,000 μm diameter sizes. The 365, 550 and 1,000 μm fibers are amenable for rigid scopes. Additionally 200 and 365 μm fibers may be employed through flexible instruments to reach points not accessible via rigid instruments as well as the ureter. The main disadvantages of the holmium lasers use in percutaneous stone removal is the cost and the inability to remove fragments made while performing lithotripsy. The cost can be reduced by using reusable fibers. Much like ballistic lithotripters, a second device, whether it be a grasper or an ultrasonic probe, is needed to remove fragments created by the laser. The main advantage of the holmium laser is its ability to fragment all types of stones regardless of composition, including uric acid, calcium oxalate monohydrate and urate stones. However, it can produce a drilling action in very hard stones. In order to maximize lithotripsy efficiency, care should be taken to paint the surface of the stone and not bury the tip of the fiber or drill into the stone. An additional advantage the holmium laser has is it can be passed through both rigid and flexible instruments.

Another advantage of the holmium laser is it produces significantly smaller fragments than other lithotrites, reducing the need for extracting the fragments. Teichman et al. compared stone fragmentation results for electrohydraulic lithotripsy, pneumatic lithotripsy, 320 μm pulsed dye lasers and 365 μm holmium:YAG laser, in an in vitro model utilizing stones composed of calcium hydrogen phosphate dihydrate, calcium oxalate monohydrate, cystine, magnesium ammonium phosphate and uric acid. For holmium lithotripsy energy was started at 0.5 J. at 6 Hz. If fragmentation was not efficient, the energy or frequency was increased incrementally until a desired effect was achieved, not exceeding a maximum of 1.0 J. at 15 Hz. The mean fragment size generated by the holmium:YAG laser was significantly smaller compared to the other lithotrites for all stone compositions. There were no fragments greater than 4 mm for holmium lithotripsy [26].

Vasser et al. utilized holmium:YAG energy in contact mode using 272, 365, 550 and 940 μm laser fibers at energy settings of 0.2, 0.5, 1.0 or 1.5 J to measure stone mass loss of calcium oxalate monohydrate calculi in an in vitro model, delivering a total of 1 kJ at each setting. There was no significant difference in fragment size distribution among various fiber diameters or energies. The authors also found that for a given fiber diameter stone loss increased as energy/

pulse increased to 1.0 J. For a given energy setting stone loss increased as fiber size decreased, with exception to 272 μm fiber, for which stone loss was inefficient at 1.0 J per pulse or greater [27].

Typically, a 1,000 μm fiber is utilized during PNL. The efficiency of different energy settings using a 1,000 μm fiber has been evaluated. Sun et al. compared two energy settings for the holmium laser during PNL performed to treat staghorn calculi. The authors used a 1,000 μm holmium laser fiber and compared settings of 30 W (3.0 J/10 Hz), and 70 W (3.5 J/20 Hz). All patients had successful PNL. The average lithotripsy time for the higher power group was significantly shorter (44 ± 11.5 min vs. 69 ± 14.8 min; $p < 0.05$). There were no major complications and there were no reported renal pelvic perforation or ureteropelvic junction injury. There was no significant difference in the mean drop in hemoglobin or blood transfusion requirements between the two groups. Both groups had similar stone-free rate at discharge (83.6 % vs. 84.4 %) and at 3 months (87.3 % vs. 87.9 %). The glomerular filtration rate of the treated kidney, reexamined 6 months after the operation, had improved significantly (45.12 mL/min vs. 31.91 mL/min; $p < 0.05$) [25].

In another large series Jou et al. utilized a 30 W, 1,000 μm, holmium:YAG laser fiber to treat 334 patients with upper tract calculi [28]. The average stone size was 3.3 ± 1.8 cm. In 3.9 % of cases an additional pneumatic lithotripter was used. The overall stone-free rate was 83.7 %. The reported complications included postoperative urinary tract infections in 7.2 % of patients and transfusions in 2.0 % of patients. The holmium:YAG laser was effective against all kinds of stones.

When using the laser to perform lithotripsy during PNL, there can be concern about the requirement of additional instruments to remove stone fragments. Michel et al. reported results of an innovative device using a Ho:YAG laser in combination with simultaneous suction in an in-vitro model and compared it to standard ultrasonic lithotripsy. The authors used a 365 μm to perform laser lithotripsy at a setting of 2 J and 8 Hz. The mean time until complete disintegration and removal of all fragments via suction was 1.106 ± 0.357 min for ultrasonic group and 0.687 ± 0.33 min for holmium laser litotripsy/suction group ($p = 0.0139$) [29].

There are several key technique points in using the holmium laser to perform lithotripsy during PNL. The fiber tip should extend at least 2 mm from tip of nephroscope to prevent damage to the scope itself. Further, tip should be visible at all times during activation to prevent injury to both the scope and the surrounding urothelium. The fiber tip should be kept at least 2 mm from the urothelium. The laser should never be activated with the tip inside the scope. Finally, the laser fiber should never be passed through a deflected scope, as it may damage the inner working channel. Our preferred setting for holmium laser during PNL is 0.2 J and 50 Hz for smaller stones. However, for larger stones we prefer to use 1 J and 20 Hz. The lower energy, higher frequency settings typically create smaller fragments or dust that will flush out with the irrigant. The higher energy settings produce larger fragments which can then be removed with a rigid grasper or a basket. In addition to treating intrarenal calculi during PNL, we utilize the holmium laser through flexible scopes to treat proximal ureteral stones.

Electrohydraulic Lithotripsy

EHL was first described and developed by Russian engineers in 1950. The probe is made up of a central metal core and two layers of insulation with another metal layer in between them. EHL probes essentially works as an underwater spark plug, the electric current is transmitted to the tip, where as it moves across the gap between the metal layers. An intense amount of heat is generated which leads to the vaporization of water and development of cavitation bubbles. This generates a primary shock wave that radiates spherically in all directions. This is followed by a collapse of the cavitation bubbles resulting in generation of a secondary shockwave, or high speed micro jets, depending upon the distance from stone [30]. The probe has to be placed in close proximity to the stone for the shock waves to be effective. EHL does not convert the stone into dust and the fragments produced need to be removed by grasping forceps or can be washed away with irrigation.

EHL probes are flexible and are available in varying sizes from 1.6 to 9 Fr sizes. They can be used through flexible ueteroscopes or nephroscopes to obtain access to stones not accessible with rigid instruments. EHL probes are effective for fragmenting all kinds of urinary calculi, including uric acid, cystine and calcium-oxalate monohydrate. The significant problem leading to the decrease use of this mode of lithotripsy is the tissue damage associated with blast waves. EHL is rarely used today during the percutaneous management of renal calculi.

Combined Probes

CyberWand®

The CyberWand® (Gyrus ACMI, Southborough, MA) (Fig. 4.2) is considered a dual ultrasonic lithotripter. It employs two separate ultrasonic probes that vibrate at two frequencies with a single hand piece. The inner probe is fixed, has a 2.1 mm hollow lumen and vibrates at 21,000 Hz. The lumen is connected to a suction tube for aspiration of fragments. The outer probe is free to move in a reciprocating fashion and is pushed outward by a sliding piston driven by the vibratory energy of the inner probe. The outer probe returns to its initial position by resistance from a coil spring. The vibratory frequency of outer probe is 1000 Hz and it is also thought to have some ballistic action on stones.

The "Large Stone" pedal activates both the inner and outer probe. The inner probe drills into the stone, where as the outer probe acts as a jack hammer to break up the stone. The "Small Stone" pedal only activates the inner probe which acts similar to a standard ultrasonic lithotripter. For best results, the "Large Stone" pedal is used. Overall, the CyberWand appears to be efficacious in management of kidney stones as compared to other devices [31]. In an in vitro model CyberWand had stone penetration time almost twice as fast as the LithoClast Master (EMS, Nyon Switzerland) [32]. Krambeck and associates performed a multicenter, randomized controlled trial comparing the CyberWand to the LUS-II (Olympus America, Inc., Melville, NY), a single lumen ultrasonic lithotripter [33]. A total of 57 patients undergoing PNL were included. The presence of hard stones and stone surface area was similar between the two groups. There was no difference in time to clearance of the target stone (Cyberwand 15.8 min vs. LUS-II 14.2 min) and target stone-clearance rate (Cyberwand 61.9 mm^2/min vs. LUS-II 75.8 mm^2/min). Fifteen of the 25 (60.0 %) Cyberwand and 20 of the 32 (62.5 %) LUS-II patients were stone-free after the initial PNL. There were no intraoperative complications reported in either treatment group. Postoperative complications were similar between the groups and no patients in either group required a blood transfusion. Device malfunction occurred in 32 % of the CyberWand group and 15.6 % of the LUS-II group. Of note, after completion of enrollment for this study, a new probe was introduced for the CyberWand. The authors utilized the new probe in 23 patients and found no device malfunction. However, the stone-clearance rate for the original CyberWand was 61.9 mm^2/min but for the new probe was 39.3 mm^2/min.

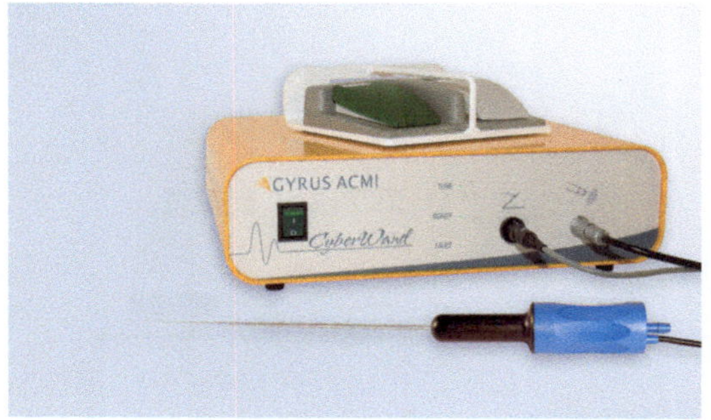

Fig. 4.2 CyberWand®, Gyrus ACMI, Southborough, MA

The major disadvantage of the CyberWand is it is a very loud device with a mean decibel level of 92 dB. This is much higher than the Olympus LUS -II ultrasonic lithotripter at 65 dB, or a Holmium LASER at 60 dB [34]. Another disadvantage is the probes are single use and can be relatively expensive.

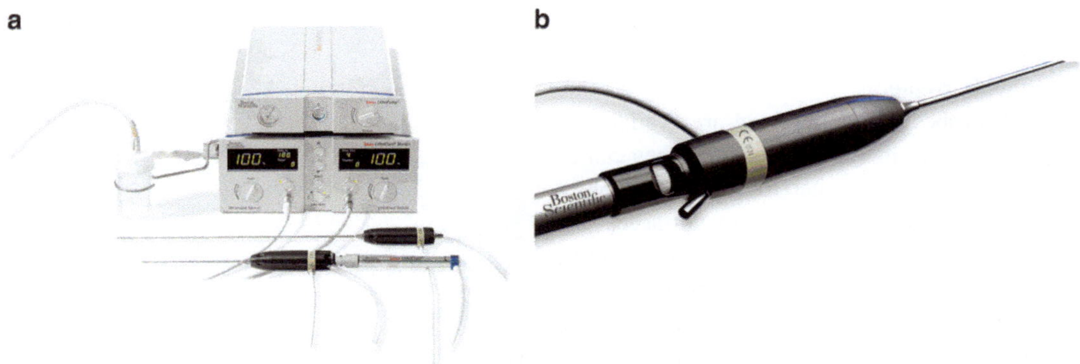

Fig. 4.3 (a, b) LithoClast Ultra® (Boston Scientific, North America)

LithoClast Ultra®/LithoClast Master® and LithoClast Select® with Vario® and Lithopump®

The LithoClast Ultra® (Boston Scientific Corp., Natick, MA) (Fig. 4.3a, b) also known as LithoClast Master® (EMS, Nyon, Switzerland) is a device that combines pneumatic and ultrasonic lithotripsy. The pneumatic probe is mounted on top of the ultrasonic probe and runs through the central lumen of the ultrasonic probe, with its tip positioned just inside the ultrasonic probe. The lumen of the ultrasonic probe continues to function as a suction device for stone retrieval. The frequency of pneumatic probe can be set between 2 and 12 Hz, while the ultrasonic frequency may be varied between 24,000 and 26,000 Hz. The foot pedal is designed so that the surgeon can operate either the pneumatic probe or ultrasonic probe in isolation, or the two of them in concert.

This combined lithotripter has been found to be more effective at stone removal than either individual device alone in in vitro studies. One study compared Swiss Lithoclast, LUS-2, and Lithoclast Ultra to fragment and retrieve begostone phantoms in an in vitro model. The combination pneumatic/ultrasound unit was more efficient than either the pneumatic or ultrasound devices alone at fragmenting and clearing the stones, with a mean time of 7.41 min compared with 12.87 min for the ultrasound and 23.76 min for pneumatic lithotrite. Additionally, the ultrasound device alone was significantly faster than the pneumatic unit. The average fragment size for the combination lithotripter was 1.67 mm versus 3.67 mm and 9.07 mm for the ultrasound and pneumatic lithotrites [35]. Hofmann and associates found stone disintegration times to be half for combination compared to individual modalities, when checked in an in vitro model [36]. Pietrow and colleagues randomized 20 consecutive patients with similar stone burden to ultrasound or LithoClast Ultra combination lithotripsy [4]. They found time to complete disintegration and stone extraction was two times higher in pure ultrasound compared to combination.

Lehman and associates prospectively randomized 30 patients undergoing PNL to either ultrasonic or combined ultrasonic and pneumatic lithotripsy. Patients in both groups had similar stone location and burden. There was no difference in stone retrieval times, mean operative times or estimated blood loss between the two groups. However, the combination lithotripter was much faster for stone fragmentation in the hard stones (calcium oxalate monohydrate, cystine or calcium phosphate), but slower in soft stone group [37].

One of the limitations of the Lithoclast Ultra was the suction would clog due to the angle the suction tubing inserted into the hand piece. The Lithoclast Select® (Boston Scientific Corporation, Natick, MA), comes with a new ultrasonic hand piece known as Vario® (EMS, Nyon, Switzerland) and a new suction attachment called the Lithopump® (EMS, Nyon, Switzerland). The Vario ultrasonic hand piece was specifically designed to overcome the problems of clogging by having a less acute angle for the suction piece when pneumatic probe is in place as well as a fenestrated outlet. The Lithopump® is an adjustable suction device that works in conjunction with LithoClast Master/Select. The pump is activated only when the ultrasound is activated which has the potential of improving vision during lithotripsy and obviates the need for an assistant to control the suction with a clamp on the suction tubing. Optimally lithotripsy can be started with pneumatic probe in place to quickly fragment the stone, followed by removal of pneumatic device and suction of fragments with ultrasonic portion.

Zhu and colleagues compared the Swiss lithoclast (44 patients, group 1), Swiss Lithoclast Master (54 patients, group 2), low power (0.5–1.0 J, 6–10 Hz) holmium:YAG laser (56 patients, group 3) and high-power (1–3 J, 10–30 Hz.) holmium:YAG laser (38 patients, group 4) (using 365 μ fiber) for the percutaneous management of proximal ureteral calculi. The stone size was similar among the groups with mean of 16.3 ± 2.4 mm. Mean operative time for different groups were 118 ± 17 min, 81 ± 10 min,85 ± 14 min, 110 ± 16 min respectively. The Lithoclast Master and low power holmium laser group had statistically shorter operative times. No statistically significant differences between groups were recorded with respect to blood loss and postoperative hospital stay. Stone-free rates were 81.8 % with the pneumatic lithotriptor, 92.9 % with the Swiss Lithoclast Master, 88.9 % with the low-power holmium:YAG laser, and 78.9 % with the higher power holmium:YAG laser. Of note, there was a 16 % incidence of ureteric stricture in patients whom the holmium laser was used at high energy settings at 1 year of follow-up [38].

The Cyberwand has been compared with LithoClast Master in in vitro studies. Kim and associates used an in vitro model where the devices were mounted upright with the probe tip up, in a modified irrigation sheath. A gypsum stone was centered on the probe tip and a mass was placed on top of stone to provide a constant force. They found the CyberWand to be significantly faster compared to LithoClast Master with a twofold more rapid stone penetration time, 4.8 ± 0.6 s versus 8.1 ± 0.6 s, for lithoclast Master [31]. Louie and associates compared the Lithoclast Ultra with the Vario hand piece with the CyberWand in a cystolithopaxy model using bego and ultracel –30 soft stones. This study found the CyberWand at large stone settings to be significantly faster than Lithoclast Ultra or small stone settings for soft stones; however, it failed to break the harder bego stones on four separate instances. In particular, CyberWand probes repeatedly fractured at the probe solder joint, a manufacturing fault that has reportedly been corrected. There was no difference in clearance time for fragments between the Cyberwand and Lithoclast Master with Vario hand piece [39].

Portable Devices

Stone Breaker®

The LMA StoneBreaker® (Cook, Bloomington, IN) is a portable pneumatic lithotripter which uses a small compressed CO_2 cartridge as its energy source. One full cartridge allows delivery of over 80 shocks while providing pressure of up to 2.9 MPa at probe tip. Probe tips come in 1, 1.6 and 2 Fr sizes.

Rane et al. evaluated the clinical efficacy of StoneBreaker for renal, ureteric and bladder stones. For the 49 patients undergoing PNL, mean stone size was 2.8 cm, with 33 staghorn or partial staghorn and 16 renal pelvic stones. Forty-three stones were successfully cleared with a single puncture and six required multiple punctures. All stones were successfully fragmented. The average number of shocks for fragmentation with subsequent successful clearance was 34 (2–76) [40].

In a randomized control trial comparing the StoneBreaker to the Swiss Lithoclast in patients undergoing PNL, 46 patients were randomized to the StoneBreaker and 31 to the Lithoclast. The mean stone size was 369.0 ± 188.1 mm² and 432.2 ± 298.5 mm² respectively. The stone fragmentation rate was significantly faster for the StoneBreaker 6.46 ± 4.16 mm²/s versus 3.59 ± 2.87 mm²/s for the Lithoclast. Total lithotripsy time, which included the time to fragment the stone, time to retrieve the fragments, and the time to remove debris with an ultrasonic lithotripter, was faster for Stone breaker 671.3±489.6 s, compared with the Lithoclast 1012.5±629.1 s. The setup time was significantly shorter and ease to use device was better for StoneBreaker. There were no significant differences in stone-free rate or stone composition between the two groups. The authors postulated that the reason for the improved times with the StoneBreaker included the ease of use as well as the higher power at the probe tip (31 bar of pressure compared with 3 bar for the Lithoclast). There were no device-related complications [18].

Lithobreaker® (EMS, Nyon, Switzerland)

The EMS Swiss Lithobreaker® (EMS, Nyon, Switzerland) is a new cordless, handheld portable electrokinetic lithotripter that is activated by a hand switch. It has 1 and 2 mm probes that can be utilized for PNL or ureteroscopy.

Wang et al. compared the EMS Swiss Lithobreaker to the StoneBreaker in an in vitro model. They compared tip velocity and displacement characteristics using the 2 mm probe for a percutaneous model with 10 mm spherical BegoStone phantoms. For both probes the electrokinetic device had significantly higher tip displacement and slower tip velocity. For the percutaneous model, the electrokinetic device required a significantly higher number of shocks to clear a stone, 484 impulses compared to 29 impulses with pneumatic device . This was attributed to the electrokinetic device having lower tip velocity and the fact that it has a continuous impulse mode which means impulses can be fired more rapidly even with the probe not in contact with the stone. Additionally clearance times were significantly less for StoneBreaker at 122 s versus 430 s [21].

Summary

A variety of intracorporeal lithotripters are available, with ultrasonic and pneumatic devices being most commonly used because of safety and effectiveness. While the pneumatic devices are effective in breaking all kinds of stone, they need separate instrumentation for stone fragment retrieval. Ultrasonic devices provide continuous suction for aspiration of fragments but may not be as effective on harder stone types. Combination lithotripters are available and seem to have better performance in vitro; however, further randomized studies will be needed to determine which device is the most efficient for percutaneous stone removal.

Digital Rigid Nephroscope

The standard rod lens nephroscope (Fig. 4.4) has been in use since the inception of PNL. Olympus Invisio® Smith (Olympus Medical, Melville, NY) digital nephroscope is similar to a digital ureteroscope, with the tip of the scope bearing a 1 mm ultra-miniature metal oxide semiconductor (CMOS) imaging sensor and dual light-emitting diodes (LED) . The fully integrated CMOS imaging sensor and LED illumination eliminates the need for bulky external gadgetry. The Invisio weighs 470 g, approximately half of a standard nephroscope (939 g). The scope has a large working channel (15 Fr) and allows insertion of a variety of instruments. In vitro studies have demonstrated the digital image to be superior in resolution compared to a standard nephroscope [41].

Stone Retrieval Devices

A number of stone retrieval devices are available in the market including 3- and 2-prong graspers. Stones up to 1 cm in diameter can be extracted

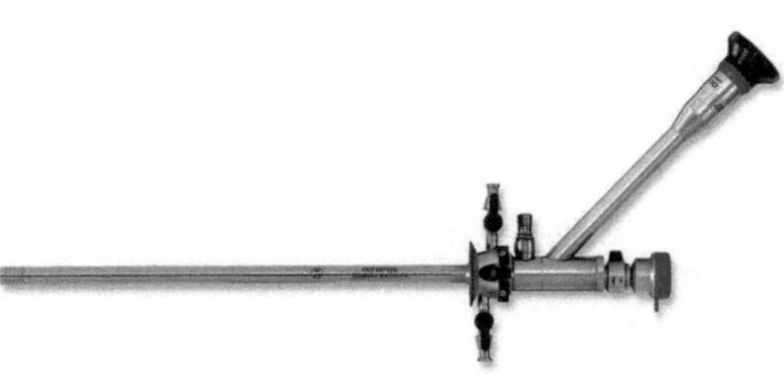

Fig. 4.4 Olympus rigid nephroscope

intact through a 30 Fr Amplatz sheath. Larger stones require fragmentation before extraction. It is important to consider that the grasper tip adds to the size of stone, making wired baskets a potentially better instrument for removal of larger stones. Risk of damage to the urothelium is another potential problem during stone retrieval with 3-prong graspers. All three prongs may not be visible through the nephroscope, making inadvertent injury more likely compared to 2-prong graspers.

Perc N-Circle® (Cook, Bloomington, IN)

It is a zero tip, 10 Fr, 39 cm-long handheld basket by Cook®. It is specifically designed for PNL and works similar to a ureteroscopic N-Circle basket. The nitinol composition provides strength and flexibility.

Hoffman et al. compared the Storz 3-prong grasper and Cook Perc N-Circle in an in vitro study using a percutaneous renal model. The mean stone extraction time was 25.3 s for Perc N-Circle and 35.1 s for 3-prong grasper [42].

The Roth-Net Retrieval Device® (US Endoscopy, Mentor, OH)

The Roth-Net retrieval device (US Endoscopy, Mentor, OH) is a 5.4 F percutaneous stone retrieval device, deployed through the working channel of a nephroscope to remove multiple small kidney stones. The device consists of a woven nylon mesh with a 1-mm open spacing. The net is 2 cm wide and 4 cm long.

In a study Khanna and associates deployed 15 calculi with sizes ranging between 2 and 3 mm ex vivo percutaneously into a porcine kidney and then compared Cook Perc-N circle to Roth-Net retrieval. The authors found that the average number of stones retrieved with the Perc-N-Circle was 1.5 per attempt, whereas the average number with the Roth-Net was 8. The calculi could be easily released by opening the Roth-Net device, and no endoscopic evidence of trauma to the urothelium was noted [43].

Antiretropulsion Devices

Stone retropulsion is a practical problem encountered during lithotripsy. Apart from doing an antegrade ureteroscopy to retrieve stone fragments or use of a ureteral balloon occlusion catheter one of new devices utilized for prevention of stone migration is Accordion®.

Accordion® (PercSys, Palo Alto, CA)

It is a 2.9 Fr, hydrophilic coated device to prevent stone retropulsion. Wosnitzer et al. retrospectively evaluated the ability of this device to prevent antegrade stone migration during PNL. The device was deployed retrograde at UPJ and attached to an open-ended catheter. A standard PNL was carried out with ultrasonic lithotripsy. The device prevented stone fragment migration in all except one patient (3 %) [44].

Take Home Points

1. A variety of devices are available for intracorporeal lithotripsy during PNL. In general, these devices are safe and effective. Combined lithotripters may be more efficient at removing harder stones.
2. The device should only be activated with the probe under direct vision. Contact with the urothelium should be avoided whenever possible and kept to a minimum.
3. The fixation of the stone against the urothelium with the probe may provide more effective lithotripsy by trapping the stone and keeping it in a single place. However, care should be taken not to exert undue pressure, especially in the renal pelvis and proximal ureter, as it may cause perforation.
4. The aim should be to generate fragments with size less than 2 mm or dust for suction devices. Single or combined energy probes may be utilized to fragment and retrieve all the fragments.

Stones in locations that are difficult to access with a rigid lithotripter may be displaced to a

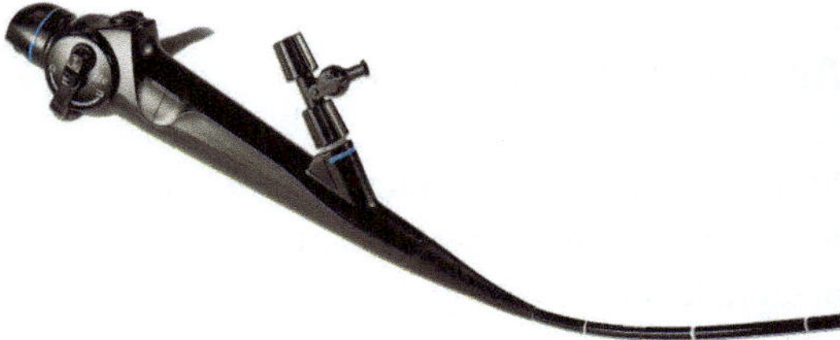

Fig. 4.5 Olympus CYF-V2, Flexible cystoscope

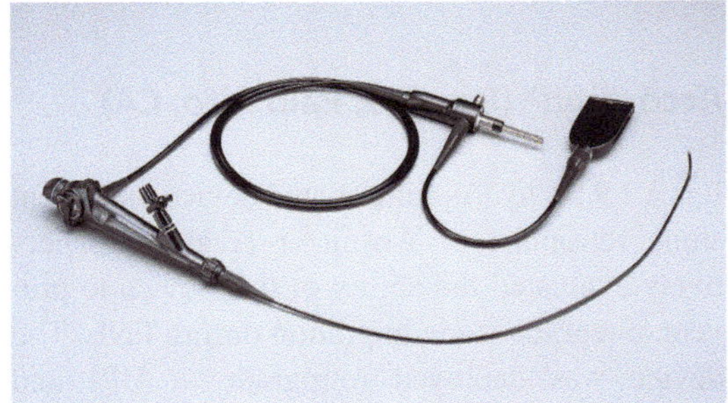

Fig. 4.6 URF-V®, Olympus digital flexible ureteroscope

more amenable location such as the renal pelvis using a basket or grasper. This will allow for easier lithotripsy.

List of Instruments

1. 25 Fr rigid nephroscope
2. Graspers: 2-prong, 3-prong, flexible graspers, stone baskets
3. Flexible cystoscope (Fig. 4.5) and flexible ureteroscope (Fig. 4.6)
4. Lithotripter: Ultrasonic, pneumatic, combined, holmium laser

Case Discussion on Stones in a Horseshoe Kidney

Horseshoe kidney is the most common fusion abnormality of the kidney with an occurrence of 1 in 400 births [45]. This results from abnormal fusion of lower portion of the metanephric blastema resulting in fused lower poles of the kidneys (Figs. 4.7 and 4.8), with the inferior mesenteric artery preventing normal rotation and ascent.

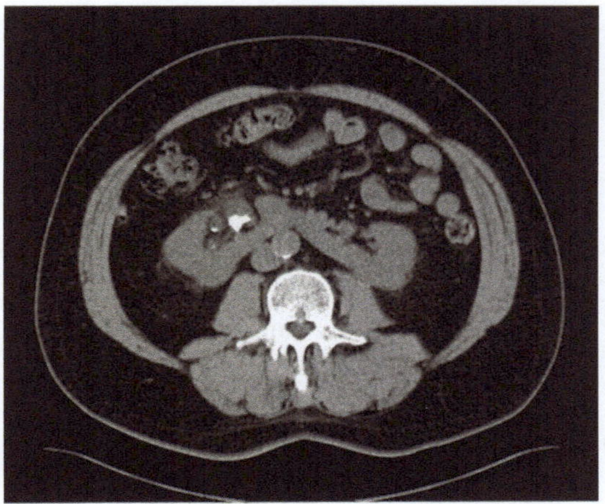

Fig. 4.7 Horse shoe kidney, isthmus in front of great vessels with stones in right moiety

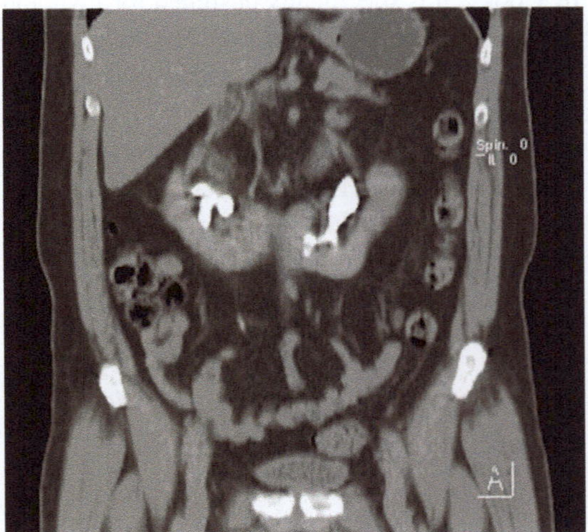

Fig. 4.8 Horseshoe kidney, CT urogram

The pelvi-calyceal system is anteriorly displaced with a high insertion of the ureter. In contrast to normal renal anatomy where all calices are lateral to the renal pelvis and further point laterally, the upper and mid pole calices of horseshoe kidney point posterior, and the lower pole calices point medially and caudally as compared with the renal pelvis (Fig. 4.9). It is important to recognize these features in order to safely obtain access and manage large stones in these kidneys.

These anatomical aberrations result in impaired urinary drainage and urinary stasis predisposing to infections and stone formation. The incidence of stone formation in these kidneys

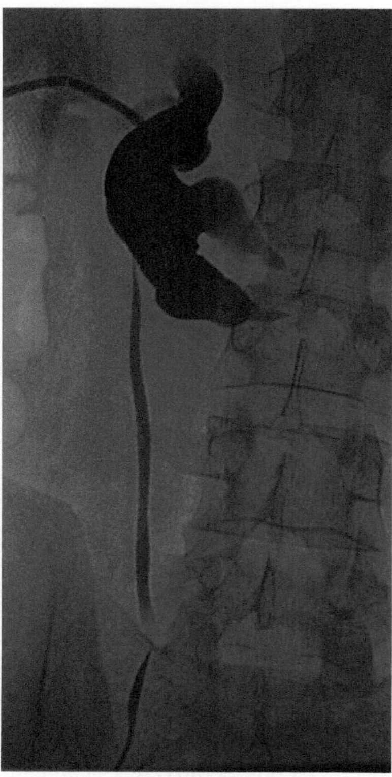

Fig. 4.9 Horse shoe kidney, Antegrade nephrostogram, location of ureter in relation to Pelvicalyceal system

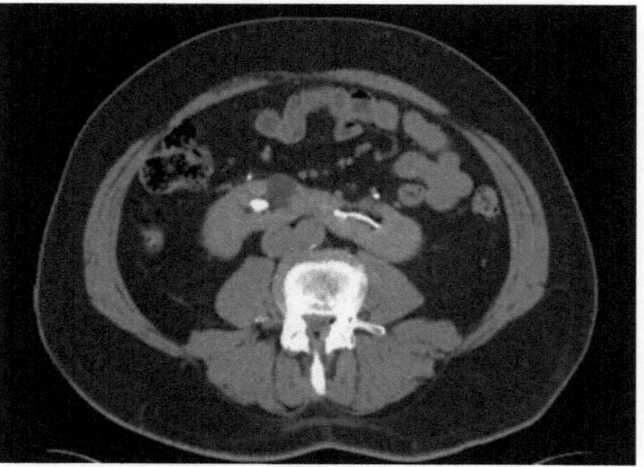

Fig. 4.10 Horseshoe kidney CT urogram, location of ureters in front of isthmus

varies from 20 to 60 % [46]. The most common stone type is calcium oxalate and the most common location is a medial, posterior lower pole calix. Urinary metabolic abnormalities are found in a high percentage of people further predisposing to stone formation [47]. These kidneys also have an abnormal vasculature with accessory arteries entering the renal hilum, and aberrant polar and isthmus arteries originating from the aorta, hypogastric or common iliac arteries. The majority of vessels, except a select few supplying the isthmus, enter the kidney from its ventromedial aspect. A puncture of the posterior or posterior lateral aspect of the kidney will be well away from major renal vessels.

These anatomic alterations represent a challenge to the treatment of renal stones. The modalities of treatment available for stones in horseshoe kidney include PNL, shock wave lithotripsy (SWL) and retrograde ureteroscopy with holmium laser lithotripsy.

SWL is the least invasive treatment option, but poses challenges of stone localization due to the low position of the kidney and superimposition of spine and pelvic bones. High ureteric insertion with stasis and pelvic dilatation may impair stone fragment clearance. It is considered the treatment of choice for small calculi but stone-free rates are less than 40 % for stones larger than 2 cm [48].

Ureteroscopy is hampered by high ureteral insertion, passage in front of isthmus and the acute angulation of the medial and lower pole calices (Fig. 4.10). Flexible ureteroscopy may be an effective, safe treatment for stones less than 2 cm in select horseshoe kidneys with stone-free rates of up to 88.2 % [49].

PNL is considered the treatment of choice for stones greater than 2 cm or SWL failures. Stone-free rates of more than 75 % have been have been reported in various series [50–52].

The optimal site for access is the posterior upper pole (Fig. 4.11). The upper pole is the point closest to skin for a horseshoe kidney (Fig. 4.12), with lower pole calices more anteriorly and medially located. When performing PNL in a horseshoe kidney, longer sheaths and instruments or flexible scopes may be necessary to access the entire collecting system, especially for stones located in lower and medial calices [50–52]. Preoperative CT is useful for selection of the appropriate percutaneous access [53, 54]. Obtaining access through an upper pole calix [54–56], using multiple accesses for stone retrieval

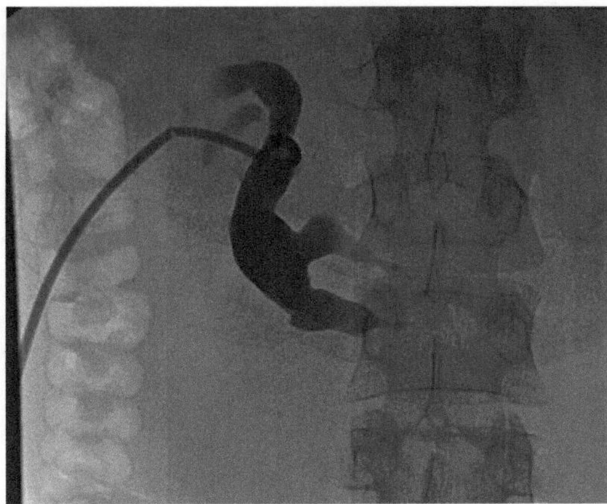

Fig. 4.11 Horse shoe kidney, Antegrade nephrostogram with access via upper pole

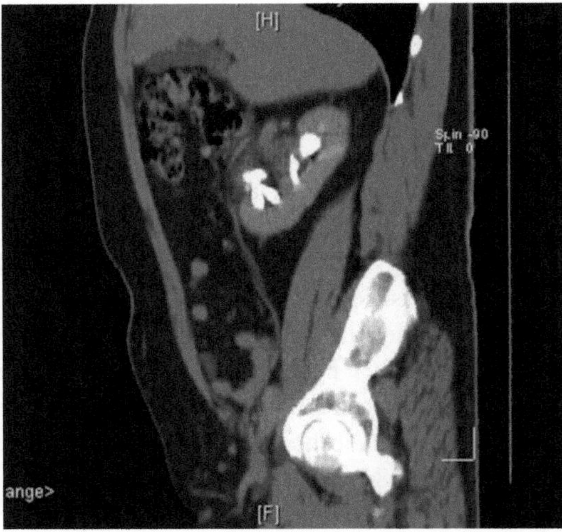

Fig. 4.12 Horse shoe kidney CT urogram, upper pole is much closer to skin than lower pole

[52, 54], flexible scopes [50, 52, 53] and second look nephroscopy [51, 55, 57] may be necessary to obtain higher stone-free rates. Despite these anatomical challenges, PNL in the horseshoe kidney has been shown to be as effective as in normal anatomic kidneys. One study reported no difference in stone clearance rates, operative times, need for auxillary procedures, drop in hemoglobin or overall complication rates between PNL performed in horseshoe kidneys versus normal kidneys. Patients in both groups had similar stone burdens and BMI [58]. Another study found the presence of staghorn stones to be the only factor on logistic regression affecting stone-free rates in patients with horseshoe kidneys. They did not find upper pole access or use of flexible nephroscope as determinant of stone-free rates. Unfortunately due to the rarity of condition there is a lack of randomized controlled trials to evaluate the impact of these factors on stone-related outcomes [59].

The risk of pleural effusion, hemothorax or pneumothorax is low because of the lower position of the kidneys. Even for upper pole access, supra-costal access is unlikely. In a series of 37 PNL in horseshoe kidneys, only one pneumothorax was reported [50].

The anterior position of the kidneys increases the likelihood of a retrorenal colon. This in theory would increase the risk of colonic injury during PNL; however, the risk of colonic injuries reported in various series is low. In three series including multiple patients, the risk of colonic injury was 2 % [50–52]. A preoperative CT scan can help in reducing this complication by better delineating the anatomy, as with normal kidneys.

Ozden and associates retrospectively compared complication rates in horseshoe kidneys versus normal kidneys [58]. Stone burden, operation time, stone-free rates, and auxiliary procedure rates were similar between the groups. The percentages of minor and major complications were also similar.

Percutaneous nephrolithotomy in a horseshoe kidney is a challenging but safe procedure. A thorough knowledge of anatomical disposition, vascular anatomy is essential for the planning of the procedure. The procedure may require extra long sheaths or nephroscopes to gain access to all parts of the kidney. A flexible nephroscope is invariably required to gain access to all the calices. The tools utilized for stone fragmentation and retrieval are the same as for any other PNL. A full range of urological armamentarium including lasers, baskets, and flexible scopes is required to make these patients stone-free. Good quality studies are required to optimize factors leading to improved stone-free rates.

References

1. Mulvaney WP. Attempted disintegration of calculi by ultrasonic vibrations. J Urol. 1953;70(5):704–7.
2. Grocela JA, Dretler SP. Intracorporeal lithotripsy. Instrumentation and development. Urol Clin North Am. 1997;24(1):13–23.
3. LeRoy AJ, Segura JW. Percutaneous ultrasonic lithotripsy. AJR Am J Roentgenol. 1984;143(4):785–8.
4. Pietrow PK, Auge BK, Zhong P, Preminger GM. Clinical efficacy of a combination pneumatic and ultrasonic lithotrite. J Urol. 2003;169:1247–9.
5. Marberger M, Stackl W, Hruby W, Kroiss A. Late sequelae of ultrasonic lithotripsy of renal calculi. J Urol. 1985;133(2):170–3.
6. Terhorst B. The effect of electrohydaulic waves and ultrasound on the urothelium. Urologe A. 1975; 14:41–5.
7. Diri A, Resorlu B, Astarci M, Unsal A, Germiyonoglu C. Tissue effects of intracorporeal tissue techniques during percutaneous nephrolithotomy: comparison of pneumatic and ultrasonic lithotripters on rat bladder. Urol Res. 2012;40(4):409–13.
8. Hofbauer J, Hobarth K, Marberger M. Electrohydraulic versus pneumatic disintegration in the treatment of ureteral stones: A randomized, prospective trial. J Urol. 1995;153(3 Pt 1):623–5.
9. Piergiovanni M, Desgrandchamps F, Cochand-Priollet B, Janssen T, Colomer S, Teillac P, Le Duc A. Ureteral and bladder lesions after ballistic, ultrasonic, electrohydraulic, or laser lithotripsy. J Endourol. 1994;8(4): 293–9.
10. Zhu S, Kourambas J, Munver R, Preminger GM, Zhong P. Quantification of the tip movement of lithotripsy flexible pneumatic probes. J Urol. 2000;164(5):1735–9.
11. Denstedt JD, Eberwein PM, Singh RR. The Swiss lithoclast: A new device for intracorporeal lithotripsy. J Urol. 1992;148(3 Pt 2):1088–90.
12. Haupt G, Pannek J, Herde T, Schulze H, Senge T. The lithovac: A new suction device for the Swiss lithoclast. J Endourol. 1995;9(5):375–7.
13. Zhong P, Preminger GM. In vitro comparison of different modes of intracorporeal shock wave lithotripsy. J Urol. 1995;153:285A.
14. Haupt G, Olschewski R, Hartung S, Senge T. Comparison of laser and ballistic systems by in vitro lithotripsy with a standardized stone model. J Endourol. 1993;7:S62.
15. Murthy PV, Rao HS, Meherwade S, Rao PV, Srivastava A, Sasidharan K. Ureteroscopic lithotripsy using miniendoscope and Swiss lithoclast: experience in 147 cases. J Endourol. 1997;11(5):327–30.
16. Teh CE, Zhong P, Preminger GM. Laboratory and clinical assessment of pneumatically driven intracorporeal lithotripsy. J Endourol. 1998;12(2):162–9.
17. Denstedt JD. Use of Swiss lithoclast for percutaneous nephrolithotripsy. J Endourol. 1993;7(6):477–80.
18. Chew BH, Arsovska O, Lange D, Wright JE, Beiko DT, Ghiculete D, et al. The Canadian StoneBreaker trial: a randomized, multicenter trial comparing the LMA StoneBreaker™ and the Swiss LithoClast® during percutaneous nephrolithotripsy. J Endourol. 2011;25(9):1415–9.
19. Denstedt JD, Razvi HA, Rowe E, Grignon DJ, Eberwein PM. Investigation of the tissue effects of a new device for intracorporeal lithotripsy—the Swiss Lithoclast. J Urol. 1995;153(2):535–7.
20. Vorreuther R, Klotz T, Heidenreich A, Nayal W, Engelmann U. Pneumatic v electrokinetic lithotripsy in treatment of ureteral stones. J Endourol. 1998;12(3):233–6.
21. Wang AJ, Baldwin GT, Gabriel JC, Cocks FH, Goldsmith ZG, Iqbal MW, et al. In-vitro assessment of a new portable ballistic lithotripter with percutaneous and ureteroscopic models. J Endourol. 2012;26(11):1500–5.
22. Watson GM, Wickham JE. Initial experience with a pulsed dye laser for ureteric calculi. Lancet. 1986; 1(8494):1357–8.
23. Dushinski JW, Lingeman JE. High-speed photographic evaluation of holmium laser. J Endourol. 1998;12(2):177–81.
24. Wollin TA, Denstedt JD. The holmium laser in urology. J Clin Laser Med Surg. 1998;16(1):13–20.
25. Sun Y, Gao X, Zhou T, Chen S, Wang L, Xu C, et al. 70 W holmium: yttrium-aluminum-garnet laser in percutaneous nephrolithotomy for staghorn calculi. J Endourol. 2009;23(10):1687–91.
26. Teichman JM, Vassar GJ, Bishoff JT, Bellman GC. Holmium:YAG lithotripsy yields smaller fragments than lithoclast, pulsed dye laser or electrohydraulic lithotripsy. J Urol. 1998;159(1):17–23.
27. Vassar GJ, Teichman JM, Glickman RD. Holmium:YAG lithotripsy efficiency varies with energy density. J Urol. 1998;160(2):471–6.
28. Jou YC, Shen JH, Cheng MC, Lin CT, Chen PC. Percutaneous nephrolithotomy with holmium: yttrium-aluminum-garnet laser and fiber guider—report of 349 cases. Urology. 2005;65(3):454–8.
29. Michel MS, Honeck P, Alken P. New endourologic technology for simultaneous holmium:YAG laser lithotripsy and fragment evacuation for PCNL: ex-vivo comparison to standard ultrasonic lithotripsy. J Endourol. 2008;22(7):1537–9.
30. Zhong P, Tong HL, Cocks FH, Preminger GM. Transient oscillation of cavitation bubbles near stone surface during electrohydraulic lithotripsy. J Endourol. 1997;11(1):55–61.
31. Kim SC, Matlaga BR, Tinmouth WW, Kuo RL, Evan AP, McAteer JA, et al. In vitro assessment of a novel dual probe ultrasonic intracorporeal lithotriptor. J Urol. 2007;177(4):1363–5.
32. Pugh JW, Canales BK. New instrumentation in percutaneous nephrolithotomy. Indian J Urol. 2010;26(3): 389–94.
33. Krambeck AE, Miller NL, Humphreys MR, Nakada SY, Denstedt JD, Razvi H, et al. Randomized controlled, multicentre clinical trial comparing a dual-probe ultrasonic lithotrite with a single-probe lithotrite

for percutaneous ephrolithotomy. BJU Int. 2011;107(5):824–8.
34. Soucy F, Ko R, Denstedt JD, Razvi H. Occupational noise exposure during endourologic procedures. J Endourol. 2008;22(8):1609–11.
35. Auge BK, Lallas CD, Pietrow PK, Zhong P, Preminger GM. In vitro comparison of standard ultrasound and pneumatic lithotrites with a new combination intracorporeal lithotripsy device. Urology. 2002;60(1): 28–32.
36. Hofmann R, Weber J, Heidenreich A, Varga Z, Olbert P. Experimental studies and first clinical experience with a new Lithoclast and ultrasound combination for lithotripsy. Eur Urol. 2002;42(4):376–81.
37. Lehman DS, Hruby GW, Phillips C, Venkatesh R, Best S, Monga M, et al. Prospective randomized comparison of a combined ultrasonic and pneumatic lithotrite with a standard ultrasonic lithotrite for percutaneous nephrolithotomy. J Endourol. 2008; 22(2):285–9.
38. Zhu Z, Xi Q, Wang S, Liu J, Ye Z, Yu X, et al. Percutaneous nephrolithotomy for proximal ureteral calculi with severe hydronephrosis: assessment of different lithotriptors. J Endourol. 2010;24(2):201–5.
39. Louie M, Lowe G, Knudsen BE. Comparison of the lithoclast ultra and cyberwand in a cystolitholapaxy model. In: Proceedings of the Society of Photo-Optical Instrumentation Engineers, 27–31 Jan 2008, San Jose, CA. 6842:684215-1–684214-6.
40. Rané A, Kommu SS, Kandaswamy SV, Rao P, Aron M, Kumar R, et al. Initial clinical evaluation of a new pneumatic intracorporeal lithotripter. BJU Int. 2007;100(3):629–32.
41. Andonian S, Okeke Z, Anidjar M, Smith AD. Digital nephroscopy: the next step. J Endourol. 2008;22(4): 601–2.
42. Hoffman N, Lukasewycz SJ, Canales B, Botnaru A, Slaton JW, Monga M. Percutaneous renal stone extraction: in vitro study of retrieval devices. J Urol. 2004;172(2):559–61.
43. Khanna R, Sarkissian C, Monga M. The roth-net device for percutaneous stone retrieval. J Endourol Part B, Videourology. 2011;25.
44. Wosnitzer M, Xavier K, Gupta M. Novel use of a ureteroscopic stone entrapment device to prevent antegrade stone migration during percutaneous nephrolithotomy. J Endourol. 2009;23:203–7.
45. Decter RM. Renal duplication and fusion anomalies. Pediatr Clin North Am. 1997;44(5):1323–41.
46. Weizer AZ, Silverstein AD, Auge BK, Delvecchio FC, Raj G, Albala DM, et al. Determining the incidence of horseshoe kidney from radiographic data at a single institution. J Urol. 2003;170(5):1722.
47. Raj GV, Auge BK, Assimos D, Preminger GM. Metabolic abnormalities associated with renal calculi in patients with horseshoe kidneys. J Endourol. 2004;18(2):157–61.
48. Stein RJ, Desai MM. Management of urolithiasis in the congenitally abnormal kidney (horseshoe and ectopic). Curr Opin Urol. 2007;17(2):125–31.
49. Molimard B, Al-Qahtani S, Lakmichi A, Sejiny M, Gil-Diez de Medina S, Carpentier X, et al. Flexible ureterorenoscopy with holmium laser in horseshoe kidneys. Urology. 2010;76(6):1334–7.
50. Raj GV, Auge BK, Weizer AZ, Denstedt JD, Watterson JD, Beiko DT, et al. Percutaneous management of calculi within horseshoe kidneys. J Urol. 2003;170(1):48–51.
51. Shokeir AA, El-Nahas AR, Shoma AM, Eraky I, El-Kenawy M, Mokhtar A, et al. Percutaneous nephrolitholomy in treatment of large stones in horseshoe kidneys. Urology. 2004;64(3):426–9.
52. Al-Otaibi K, Hosking DH. Percutaneous stone removal in horseshoe kidneys. J Urol. 1999;162(3 Pt 1):674–7.
53. Lingeman JE, Saw KC. Percutaneous operative procedures in horseshoe kidneys. J Urol. 1999;161:371.
54. Liatsikos EN, Kallidonis P, Stolzenburg JU, Ost M, Keeley F, Traxer O, et al. Percutaneous management of staghorn calculi in horseshoe kidneys: a multi-institutional experience. J Endourol. 2010;24(4):531–6.
55. Miller NL, Matlaga BR, Handa SE, Munch LC, Lingeman JE. The presence of horseshoe kidney does not affect the outcome of percutaneous nephrolithotomy. J Endourol. 2008;22(6):1219–25.
56. Rana AM, Bhojwani JP. Percutaneous nephrolithotomy in renal anomalies of fusion, ectopia, rotation, hypoplasia, and pelvicalyceal aberration: uniformity in heterogeneity. J Endourol. 2009;23(4):609–14.
57. Razvi S, Zaidi Z. Percutaneous nephrolithotomy (PCNL) in horse shoe kidneys. J Pak Med Assoc. 2007;57(5):222–5.
58. Ozden E, Bilen CY, Mercimek MN, Tan B, Sarıkaya S, Sahin A. Horseshoe kidney: does it really have any negative impact on surgical outcomes of percutaneous nephrolithotomy? Urology. 2010;75(5):1049–52.
59. Skolarikos A, Binbay M, Bisas A, Sari E, Bourdoumis A, Tefekli A, et al. Percutaneous nephrolithotomy in horseshoe kidneys: factors affecting stone-free rate. J Urol. 2011;186(5):1894–8.

5 Post-percutaneous Nephrolithotomy Drainage

Michelle Jo Semins and Brian R. Matlaga

Key Take Home Points

1. Post-PCNL drainage tubes have been steadily decreasing in size over the previous decade.
2. Tubeless PCNL is a reasonable modification in a properly selected patient and may help increase patient comfort, decrease hospital stay, and quicken time to recovery.
3. Several hemostatic agents are available for use during a tubeless procedure, but the potential benefits of these agents are not yet clear.

Introduction

The initial report of kidney stone removal through an operatively established nephrostomy tract was in 1941 by Rupel and Brown [1] for anuria from an obstructing calculus. It was over three decades later that the first formal percutaneous nephrolithotomy (PCNL) was performed in 1976 by Fernstrom and Johannson [2]. The benefit of PCNL is that it can clear large and complex stone burdens with great efficiency and it is significantly less invasive than open surgery. PCNL has been increasing in frequency since its introduction, and as surgical technology continues to advance its efficacy and safety profile have markedly increased [3]. Likely due to these factors, the utilization of PCNL has been increasing at a great rate [4].

Standardly, PCNL requires placement of a nephrostomy tube at the procedure's conclusion, which ensures adequate renal drainage. Additionally, the nephrostomy tube also simplifies reaccess to the kidney should there be residual stone requiring a second procedure. Although these advantages are clinically important, the nephrostomy drain can also cause some degree of morbidity and discomfort for the patient.

As PCNL has become more popular and more commonly performed over the recent decades, many modifications have been reported with the goals of minimizing morbidity and pain for the patient as well as shortening the time to full recovery. Among these have been placement of smaller tube sizes, mini-PCNL with smaller incisions and instruments, tubeless with various types of internal drainage, and the totally tubeless technique [5, 6]. Herein, we review the various techniques used to drain the kidney after PCNL.

M.J. Semins, M.D. (✉)
Department of Urology, University of Pittsburgh Medical Center, Pittsburgh, PA, USA
e-mail: mjsemins@gmail.com

B.R. Matlaga, M.D., M.P.H.
Johns Hopkins Medicine, The James Buchanan Brady Urological Institute, Baltimore, MD, USA

The Size of Nephrostomy Tube

Traditionally a large-bore nephrostomy tube was left in place after the standard PCNL to allow for maximal drainage and tamponade bleeding while allowing for easy access if a second procedure

S.Y. Nakada and M.S. Pearle (eds.), *Surgical Management of Urolithiasis: Percutaneous, Shockwave and Ureteroscopy*, DOI 10.1007/978-1-4614-6937-7_5, © Springer Science+Business Media New York 2013

was necessary. Commonly utilized nephrostomy tube sizes range from 5 French all the way up to 32 French. As the surgical technique of PCNL became mature, increasing interest was focused on improving the discomfort associated with the procedure—as a result, surgeons began to examine the use of different drain sizes, to assess for improved tolerance of smaller tubes.

Initially, studies evaluating PCNL performed with varying postoperative nephrostomy sizes were retrospective analyses. Maheshwari et al. [7] compared the use of a 28 French large-bore tube versus a 10 French pigtail catheter and found that those patients with the smaller tube had a significantly lower analgesia requirement and shorter duration of nephrostomy tract leakage after tube removal. Several other nonrandomized trials have compared small-bore tubes (9/10 French) with larger tubes (22 French) and showed that patients with smaller tubes placed had less pain, less analgesia requirement, and a decreased hospital stay [8].

Prospectively performed studies demonstrated similar findings. Liatsikos et al. [9] built on this study and in a prospective fashion evaluated placement of a 24 French reentry malecot tube versus an 18 French catheter with a 7/3 tail stent in a randomized fashion. Quality of life and urgency were similar between groups. The patients with the smaller tube had less pain but in this study there was no assessment of pain until 2 weeks postoperatively. Additionally because of the design of the study, it is unclear whether patient comfort is improved because of the smaller tube or because of bidirectional drainage with the tailless stent in place as well.

Ultimately, randomized controlled trials addressed the question and provided more definitive data. Pietrow et al. [8] evaluated the effect of using a smaller nephrostomy tube for percutaneous drainage after PCNL on postoperative pain in 30 patients in a randomized fashion. Half received a 10 French pigtail catheter while the others had a 22 French Councill-tip catheter placed. There was no difference in hematocrit change and the smaller tube group had significantly less pain by visual analog pain scale at 6 h postoperatively. Pain at 1 and 2 days postoperatively and narcotic usage were also assessed and while there was a trend for benefit with the smaller tube group it was not statistically significant. While there was no increased complication rate, there appeared to be limited usefulness based on this study; however, sample size was small and tube type was different so comparison was imperfect. Desai et al. [10] performed another prospective randomized controlled trial in 30 patients comparing large-bore drainage with a 20 French tube to a small 9 French pigtail tube to antegrade internal stenting. They had strict inclusion criteria with single subcostal access, no residual stones, normal renal function, and an uncomplicated procedure. Nephrostomy tubes were removed at 48 h while stents were removed at 4 weeks. Hospital stay and urinary leak was significantly shorter in the tubeless group but time to discharge was not different between the different tube groups. Analgesic requirement was greater in the larger bore group versus the small tube group and while it was the least in the tubeless group this was not statistically significant. The study group did not report on stent discomfort in the tubeless group.

Types of Drainage Tubes

In addition to different sizes of tubes there are also different types of tubes. Paul et al. [11] nicely reviews the different types of tubes available for post-PCNL drainage and suggests when each one should be placed. They suggest pigtail catheters (5–14 French) with or without a locking mechanism can be placed after a simple PCNL; if the system is delicate or if the procedure is complicated this may not be the ideal tube to use. Balloon retention catheters (12–32 French) can also be used and may allow for better drainage. Possible obstruction with balloon inflation can occur. Malecot tubes are a balloon-less alternative that allows for good drainage and eliminates the risk of obstruction from the self-retaining mechanism of other catheters. They suggest the use of a large-bore reentry tube in complicated renal surgery that allows for reinsertion of the tube after removal if bleeding occurs. Endopyelotomy tubes when antegrade endopyelotomy is also performed and circle nephrostomy tube when prolonged drainage is anticipated as in a calyceal diverticulum are also discussed. Srinivasan et al. [12] also provide a nice review of tube types and their uses which are similar to the previous group's report.

A Brief History of the Evolution of Nephrostomy Drainage

The first report of tubeless PCNL was in 1984 where Wickham et al. [13] reported a totally tubeless procedure in 100 select patients. Two years later in 1986 Winfield et al. [14] reported significant complications in two patients with premature nephrostomy tube removal including serious hemorrhage and significant urinary extravasation requiring stent placement, transfusion, and prolonged hospitalization. Perhaps as a consequence of this report, the standard approach for PCNL became maintenance of the nephrostomy tube for at least 24–48 h [15].

It was a decade later, in 1997, that the tubeless procedure was reintroduced by Bellman et al. Their modification included internal drainage with a stent and their rationale was that with proper drainage of the renal unit, the controlled trauma of a PCNL tract should heal spontaneously [16]. A stent and a Councill catheter were placed in 30 patients with the nephrostomy tube being removed in 2–3 h while only a stent was placed in 20 patients. Those patients who did not have a nephrostomy tube had a decreased hospital stay, lower analgesia requirements, lower overall cost, and a quicker convalescence. Five years later they reported their experience with their first 112 patients undergoing the tubeless procedure for percutaneous renal surgery [17]. In 86 stone patients, over 90 % were stone free with a decreased hospital stay and no external drainage bag. The transfusion rate was 6 %. The disadvantages they noted were prolonged Foley catheter and need for a second procedure to remove the stent. It is important to note that the authors had strict inclusion criteria and only 28 % of their percutaneous procedures over a 5-year period were eligible for the tubeless procedure. Additionally 7 % of these patients did have residual stones though these were all treated successfully with shock wave lithotripsy.

The Tubeless Modifications

Randomized Controlled Trials

Since Bellman and associates reintroduced the tubeless procedure in 1997, a number of randomized control trials have been performed to evaluate it more thoroughly.

Feng et al. [18] looked at various PCNL techniques in 2001 in 30 patients. They evaluated the standard technique with a 22 French nephrostomy tube, the mini-PCNL with a 22 French tube, and the tubeless procedure. Pain scale results were similar but the tubeless group had a shorter hospitalization and less analgesia use. This study was not perfect because although stone burden was reported not to be significantly different it was twice as large (8 cm vs. 4 cm) in the standard tube group. This was also demonstrated in the fact that stone-free rate in this group was only 37.5 % (vs. 62.5 % in the mini-PCNL group and 71.4 % in the tubeless group). Although this study was biased with the standard cohort being more complex, the authors noted decreased cost in the tubeless group.

Desai et al. in 2004 evaluated the outcome of tube size and tubeless as discussed above in a randomized fashion [10]. The tubeless group had a shorter hospital stay and urinary leak was significantly shorter in the tubeless group. They also had less analgesic requirement but this was not statistically significant. This study was a small study of only 30 patients (only ten tubeless patients) with strict inclusion criteria but was one of the first randomized comparisons of tubeless to both large- and small-bore drainage tubes.

Marcovich et al. [19] also performed a randomized study in 2004 comparing different tube sizes with a tubeless procedure. They evaluated 60 patients and found no significant difference between patients with a 24 French reentry tube, an 8 French pigtail catheter, and those with a double J internalized stent. The main limitation of their study was how they defined tubeless because those with an internal stent were still left with a large-bore drainage tube (20 French Councill-tip catheter) removed on the first postoperative day.

A number of investigators from India have investigated tubeless PCNL. There is a large amount of literature regarding post-percutaneous renal surgery drainage out of India. Three randomized controlled trials were all reported in 2008 evaluating the tubeless procedure.

One study included 202 patients using a moderate-sized tube of 16 French versus a 6 French stent [6]. They found a statistically significant difference in postoperative pain as measured by the visual analog scale pain score (59 vs. 31) and analgesia requirement. They also found a lower incidence of urinary leakage from the nephrostomy tube site and a shorter hospital duration (21.8 h vs. 54.2 h). Complete convalescence was 5–7 days for the tubeless group whereas it was 8–10 days for using the standard technique. They found no difference in infection or percent hemoglobin change. Total follow-up for the study was 18 months and CT scan at 1 month revealed all patients to be stone free. In this study location of puncture was not considered. They used suture to close the skin.

Another study out of India in 2008 randomly compared tubeless with stent placement to placement of a small-bore nephrostomy tube of 8 French in 65 patients [20]. They also noted less postoperative pain via the visual analog pain scale, less analgesia requirement, and patients were discharged 9 h earlier. Stone clearance was 87 % in both groups but they only used renal ultrasound and KUB to evaluate patients and considered less than 4 mm residual fragments to be stone free. They too noted no difference in complication rate or hemoglobin drop. One important outcome they evaluated that many groups do not discuss is stent discomfort. The tubeless group had bothersome stent-related symptoms in 39.4 % with 61.5 % of those patients requiring analgesics and/or antispasmodics. They did not measure these outpatient analgesic requirements for these stent symptoms. They also found the duration of perurethral catheter to be longer in the tube group but this was because they waited until urine leakage from the tract stopped (28 h vs. 36 h). Interestingly, one patient with the small-bore tube had pain and required stent placement. They used a pressure dressing at the skin.

One other randomized study from India in 2008 evaluated the difference between a large-bore catheter (22 French) and tubeless in 60 patients [21]. Analgesia requirement, hospital stay, and time to return to normal activity were all significantly less in the tubeless group. The tube group had a 30 min longer operative time suggesting that though the study was randomized the cases with tube placement were more complex. Also, the tubes were removed at 2.5 days but the stents were kept in place for 4.5 weeks. While stent symptoms were not evaluated in this study, one could imagine based on the previous study discussed that this could cause potentially significant distress in the stent group. CT scan was also not done postoperatively in this study.

Tefekli et al. [22] also performed a prospective randomized controlled trial in 2007 and reported benefit in the tubeless group.

Meta-analysis

With more data and literature emerging and many studies including small sample sizes, it can sometimes be difficult to interpret all of this information. For this reason a group from China performed a meta-analysis in 2010 with the existing randomized controlled trials evaluating the tubeless PCNL. This included 14 studies and 776 patients [5]. They subdivided the trials into three groups. There were three studies that compared small-bore tubes (4–10), eight studies that evaluated large-bore tubes (12–24) and two studies that included both sizes versus tubeless. One study included did not report size and was incorporated in with the larger tube group. One limitation of this meta-analysis was that not all of the studies reported all relevant parameters. The authors did find a significant difference in hospital stay but only 11/14 studies reported this information. Additionally the authors did not separate the data by small and large tube groups for this parameter. Postoperative analgesia use was significantly less in the tubeless groups but only four studies were compared. Postoperative pain via the visual analog scale was less in the tubeless group but only five studies were included and there was no difference found between the tubeless and small tube groups. Urine leakage too was significant but also did not show a difference between the tubeless and small-bore groups and only four studies had these data available. In seven studies evaluated, operative time was significantly longer in the large-bore versus the tubeless group. With these operative time results, one has to speculate if there were intrinsic differences between the groups as nephrostomy tube placement should not really take longer than an antegrade stent placement. There were no differences found in stone-free rate (eight studies), postoperative fever (eight studies), or blood transfusion (nine studies). Also, between the small-bore and tubeless groups there were no significant differences found in operative time, postoperative pain, or urine leakage. Again, there were only four studies in the small-bore group.

While this study could not eliminate the intrinsic limitations of the individual studies the results are stronger than the individual studies alone and do support that tubeless PCNL could translate to a shorter hospital stay and less analgesia requirements which could potentially translate to decreased costs and improved quality of care. What most of these studies did not evaluate, however, are stent-related symptoms. Along the same lines, outpatient analgesics and pain was not measured and many studies left the stents in for 4–6 weeks. It is possible that the short inpatient benefits from the tubeless procedure could be reversed with the outpatient disadvantage of stent discomfort, a prolonged requirement for antispasmodics and/or narcotics, and a second procedure to remove the stent. Larger multi-institutional long-term randomized controlled trials that include outpatient evaluations, stent-related symptoms, and the need for an additional procedure are required before definitive conclusions can be made.

Nonrandomized Trials

In addition to randomized trials, many groups have reported their nonrandomized experience with the tubeless procedure [15, 23–25]. Lojananpiwat et al. [26] reported on 37 patients with externalized 6 French ureteral stents placed at the beginning of the procedure and removed at 48 h. Their patients had a significant reduction in length of hospitalization and postoperative analgesia but their average length of hospitalization was still 3.6 days and the majority of their patients (24/37) still required narcotics.

Karami et al. [27] reported on their 5-year experience in 201 patients and found the tubeless procedure to be safe, effective, and economical. Similarly, several other studies have shown good results [28, 29]. One review suggested that a double-J stent may theoretically facilitate small residual stone passage with passive dilation of the ureter [15].

Conservative Modification

While not leaving an externalized drain has been shown to be an effective means of managing post-PCNL drainage, some concerns remain, including adequate hemostasis and need for reaccess for a second-look procedure. One group compared tubeless with internal stenting versus internal stenting with tube placement but early removal on postoperative day 1 if CT imaging showed no complications or recurrent stone disease [30]. This comparison was performed in a prospective randomized controlled fashion and showed equivalent results with regard to analgesic requirement, hospital stay, and change in hemoglobin. They found that the group with early tube removal had a better stone-clearance rate and allowed for reentrance into the system if needed, concluding that it should be considered the standard of care and preserves the advantages offered by the tubeless modification.

Tubeless in Complex PCNL

While the tubeless PCNL has become more popular as many studies have demonstrated its safety and advantage in patient comfort, most surgeons are careful in their selection of patients. Many of the studies discussed had a strict inclusion limiting the tubeless procedure to straightforward, uncomplicated cases.

Recently, as surgeons have become more comfortable with the tubeless procedure and as technology has advanced, expanded criteria have been reported and there is increasing literature of more complex cases being left with internal drainage alone. Some expanded criteria include solitary kidneys, large stone burden, renal insufficiency, multiple access tracts, and supracostal accesses and several groups have reported success in these populations [31–36]. Jou et al. retrospectively reviewed the tubeless procedure in 62 patients with stones greater than 3 cm and found no increase in morbidity as did Falahatkar et al. who achieved an 88 % stone-free rate in 42 staghorn calculi undergoing the tube-free PCNL [37, 38].

Shah et al. [33] retrospectively reported their experience in 72 patients with supracostal access. These patients also showed benefit with earlier discharge by 19 h, decreased postoperative pain via the visual analog pain scale, and less analgesia requirement. Complications and transfusions were comparable between groups. These patients also had their urethral catheter removed sooner, as in the control group they waited for leakage from the tract to stop. This is a limitation to their study because awaiting catheter removal prolonged the control group's hospitalization and also resulted in increased measurement of analgesia. Since these are the main outcome measurements the significance of the differences detected is questionable. They also had one major complication in each group both requiring exploratory surgery. The patient in the study group had a retroperitoneal hematoma and that in control group had a splenic rupture and hemoperitoneum.

Shoma and Elshal [39] performed a prospective randomized controlled trial comparing tubeless to standard PCNL without a strict inclusion criteria. They had negative results in patients with supracostal access and renal insufficiency. They suggest these should be considered contraindications to the tubeless procedure.

Tubeless PCNL has also been investigated in obese patients. Yang and Bellman in 2003 reported their experience in percutaneous renal surgery in 133 patients [40]. Subgroups for analysis consisted of 45 patients with BMI less than 25, 55 patients with BMI 25–30, 28 patients with BMI 30–40, and 5 morbidly obese patients with BMI over 40. Stone removal was the primary goal in 104 patients whereas 29 patients underwent percutaneous antegrade endopyelotomy. Two patients required readmission for low hematocrit and hematuria and one required embolization for a pseudo-aneurysm. All patients requiring transfusion had BMI less than 30 (nine patients). There were no other differences between the groups. Stents were removed at 1 week. While obesity made the case more complex, this group did have exclusion criteria including greater than two accesses, perforation of the collecting system, operative time greater than 2 h, residual stones, significant bleeding, or plan for second-look nephroscopy.

The first case report of bilateral tubeless PCNL was by Weld and Wake [41]. Shah et al. then reported a small retrospective analysis of 20 patients comparing bilateral PCNL to bilateral tubeless PCNL [42]. Results showed less analgesia and a 20 h earlier discharge but this was not statistically significant because of the small sample size. Also, their study was limited because the tubeless group was a more recent cohort so it is unclear whether discharge was sooner because protocols were improved and as a result of less time in the hospital, less analgesia was measured. Additionally, stone burden was much larger in the standard group and there were twice as many patients with staghorn calculi. This was illustrated in operating time as well as the standard group was much longer. Though this was a poor comparative study, it still demonstrated that bilateral tubeless PCNL can be done safely. Other groups have also reported these outcomes [41–43].

Tubeless has also been successfully reported in patients undergoing PCNL in the supine position as reported in 184 patients, spinal anesthesia in 10 patients (65 from 13), and patients with a history of open renal surgery in 25 patients, [44–46]. Lastly, patients with pelvic kidneys have successfully undergone the tubeless procedure laparoscopically assisted [47].

Tubeless in Children

Modifications have not been limited to adults. More groups are extending various techniques to children as well. Salem et al. [48] reported success in 20 children (average age 7.5 years) undergoing the tubeless procedure when comparing their outcomes to ten similar patients undergoing the standard technique with a tube. They found the tubeless group had less pain, shorter hospital stay, and the technique was less "troublesome." They did have to convert to open surgery in one case because of extravasation and inability to access the kidney.

Totally tubeless PCNL has also been investigated in the pediatric population and while some groups showed it was safe and effective with decreased hospital stay and analgesic use, others have not shown a statistically significant benefit [49, 50].

Totally Tubeless PCNL

As technology advances and criteria for tubeless PCNL expands, several groups have reintroduced the totally tubeless procedure without internal or external drainage despite previously reported poor results by Winfield et al. [14]. Crook et al. [51] reported the totally tubeless procedure to be safe and well-tolerated in select patients in his experience with 100 patients over a 10-year period (1996–2006). Istanbullouglu et al. [52] performed a randomized trial in 2009 in 90 patients comparing totally tubeless to standard PCNL and also found it to be safe and effective in properly selected patients. Aghamir et al. [53] also conducted a randomized study in 60 patients evaluating the totally tubeless PCNL in patients with renal anomalies. They found the totally tubeless group to have decreased hospitalization time, analgesia, and return to normal activities. Totally tubeless was also shown to be safe and feasible in supracostal access [54].

Lastly, totally tubeless has also been reported in patients undergoing bilateral PCNL [55]. This group from Turkey in 2009 described their experience with six patients. Hospitalization was 1.8 days with only half of the patients being discharged after 1 day. One patient became anuric postoperatively for 16 h with a significant rise in creatinine requiring urgent bilateral stent placement. The only difference between this patient and the others was a larger hemoglobin decrease of 2.6 with the authors suggesting clot obstruction for this complication.

Types of Internal Drainage

With surgeons more often performing tubeless PCNL with internal drainage, groups have experimented with different types of stents. Double J, externalized stents exiting the urethral meatus, tail stents, and stents with flank tethers have all been used with good results.

Bellman introduced antegrade stent placement in the reverse direction with the tether exiting the flank [56]. He suggested removal in the office at 3–12 days postoperatively. It also may be possible to still reaccess the tract with this type of internal drainage if a second-look procedure is needed [15]. Tethers can also be left on double J stents distally as well.

Tail stents are generally 7/3 French. These were introduced to try to reduce stent symptoms as up to 78 % of stent patients may have urinary symptoms and discomfort affecting daily activities, inability to work, and loss of income as a result [57]. Dunn et al. [58] found reduced symptoms with the 7/3 French stent in a randomized single-blind study. Tethers can be left on tail stents for ease of removal as well but this requires retrograde placement at the beginning or end of the procedure. Yew and Bellman [59] reported this technical enhancement of their modified tubeless procedure and reported low pain scores and minimal stent symptoms. This technique also eliminates the need for office cystoscopy for stent removal. The one concern of leaving an internal catheter with an externalized tether is accidental premature removal.

One study looked at the difference between 6 French double-J stents and externalized 6 French stents in a prospective randomized analysis [60]. The external stent was removed with the Foley catheter on the first postoperative day. While both were found to be feasible, the externalized group reported no stent-related symptoms while 52 % of patients in the double-J group experienced symptoms. The Polaris stent placed in the reverse direction is one other unique type of stent worth mentioning that has been reported for internal drainage post-PCNL [61].

Hemostatic Agents in the Nephrostomy Tract

As tubeless PCNL has become more popular and many studies have shown complication rates to be similar to the standard technique, the main concern remains adequate hemostasis without having the tube to tamponade bleeding. Hemostatic agents have been around since the 1970s in nonurologic disciplines. The FDA defines these agents as materials that assist in hemostasis by accelerating the clotting process of blood [62]. There are liquid and flowable agents that are used to augment the clotting cascade. The liquid agents typically contain fibrinogen and thrombin to help produce a fibrin clot independent of patient factors [62]. The flowable agents typically contain gelatin, which provides a matrix for platelet adhesions and aggregation and when mixed with thrombin aids in clot formation. Unlike the liquid agents, gelatin has no fibrinogen and depends on patient factors to start the reaction that assists in clot formation. Gelatin material also expands upon contact with blood and therefore has an additional pressure effect for hemostasis [62]. Because of these properties and the concern for hemostasis in the tubeless procedure, surgeons began to experiment with these agents in the nephrostomy tract off-label. Choe et al. [62] thoroughly describe all of the different hemostatic agents available and their mechanism of action. Below is a summary of the agents and the studies conducted using them to seal the nephrostomy tract.

Fibrin Glue

Fibrin glue was first used in the urologic discipline for ureteral and renal trauma in the late 1980s and was shown to be safe [63]. Once introduced, the indications for its use expanded and surgeons began to use it in reconstructive surgeries to heal fistulae, simple prostatectomies, and to patch complications and other urologic injuries [64].

The first report of using fibrin glue for hemostasis of a percutaneous nephrostomy tract was also in the late 1980s [65]. It wasn't until 2003, however, that the first larger report was published. In a retrospective review of 43 patients undergoing tubeless PCNL, 20 patients had tisseel placed to seal the tract and were compared to tubeless alone [66]. Hospital stay was shorter in the fibrin group. Analgesia requirement was less but this was not statistically significant. There was no difference in hematocrit drop. Postoperative fevers occurred in 15 % of the fibrin group and one patient developed a wound seroma, all requiring readmissions. Postoperative CT did not reveal any differences between the groups. There were several limitations with this study including the fibrin group being a more recent cohort and thereby possibly having improved protocols. Also because the fibrin patients had a shorter hospital stay, this may account for less analgesia recorded as this was not adjusted for admission time. There were also no validated pain questionnaires used in this study for assessment. Also, fever occurrence in 15 % of patients in the study group suggests that fibrin may cause this reaction; however, the authors state those patients had preexisting UTI.

Noller et al. [67] also successfully reported fibrin sealant in ten kidneys after percutaneous renal stone surgery without complications. These patients were discharged in 1.1 days with an 80 % stone-free rate. None had urinary extravasation on CT scan with IV contrast performed postoperatively.

Shah et al. [68] performed a prospective randomized controlled trial in 2006 in 63 patients comparing tisseel fibrin sealant to tubeless PCNL without the use of a hemostatic agent. They found no difference in hematocrit change or transfusion rate. Patients with tisseel used had less postoperative pain and required less analgesia. They were also discharged 5 h earlier but this was not statistically significant. Only renal ultrasound and KUB were done postoperatively and stone-free status was considered if residual fragments were less than 4 mm. One patient in experimental group had a 6 g/dl hemoglobin drop with retroperitoneal hematoma and septicemia requiring ICU care. This demonstrates despite efforts to prevent bleeding it can still occur. Of note, one potential concern that Uribe discusses in an editorial is the possible lithogenic effects of these agents. No data or reports have illustrated this to date.

Gelatin Matrix

Gelatin is another type of hemostatic agent that has been recently used after percutaneous renal surgery for assistance in clotting. Additionally this type of agent expands upon contact with blood creating an additional compressive effect. Clayman's group describes their technique with floseal and reports its successful use in patients [69, 70]. Comparing it to a 10 French cope loop catheter, there was no difference in postoperative pain or blood loss but there was a trend toward shorter hospitalization but sample size was small. This group chooses to use gelatin because in vitro studies showed fibrin glue congealed when it came into contact with urine causing a thicker mucoid material that did not dissolve after 5 days [71]. Their concern with using fibrin is that it has the potential to cause urinary obstruction. When studying gelatin the same group found that when in contact with human urine the matrix formed a fine suspension of particles. This group of investigators also conducted another study in pigs where they injected floseal or tisseel into the collecting system and at 5 days they found obstruction in 50 % of the pigs [72]. For this reason, they use gelatin and to avoid possible obstruction their technique is to use a 7 French 11.5 mm occlusion balloon in a retrograde fashion extended to the parenchyma (6/7). Patients from their studies did well without obstruction. Bellman also noted in an editorial comment that they realized with further experience that floseal was more superior than fibrin glue and they now use floseal [69].

Aghamir et al. [53] also investigated gelatin in a prospective randomized trial in 20 patients to seal the tract. They found no difference in bleeding or extravasation from the tract. Singh et al. [73] prospectively investigated 50 patients in a randomized fashion using spongostan, an absorbable gelatin tissue hemosealant. They found no difference in hematocrit drop but the study group had a shorter hospital stay ($p = 0.057$), decreased urinary extravasation (1 h vs. 6 h), less analgesia requirement, less pain, and quicker time to return to work. Only ultrasound and KUB/IVP were performed postoperatively. Discharge was 6–8 h earlier. No gross soakage was observed on dressings in either group though mean collections were larger in the gelatin group. One limitation of this study was unbalanced stone size between the groups as burden was significantly larger in the standard group. Despite this mean operative time was 30 min longer in the gelatin group. Stents were kept in place for 4–6 weeks. One potential concern is displacement of the sponge into the collecting system leading to obstruction, but the authors claim complete dissolution of spongostan based on an in vivo study. Based on these results showing limited benefit and a high expense, they conclude gelatin should be used only in cases of persistent visible diffuse hemorrhage despite tamponade.

Summary of Hemostatic Agents

With the goal of these agents being to enhance hemostasis, most of the studies conducted found no change in hematocrit. Given the extra expense and potential complications discussed, these studies do not support the routine clinical use of hemostatic agents in tubeless PCNL. Some authors suggest these agents may be beneficial in robust bleeding but realistically tube placement should be highly considered in these circumstances. Additionally these studies do not show a difference in the degree of urinary extravasation based on imaging and dressing assessment but most studies did not objectively measure this parameter. There may be a benefit, but the literature to date does not illustrate a profound difference to justify this extra expense. Further study is needed in a large multi-institutional prospective randomized trial.

Diathermy Coagulation

While many groups have experimented with agents to promote hemostasis some groups have chosen to use diathermy coagulation for control of bleeding. The benefits of this technique are no potential for viral transmission, unlike the human-based hemostatic agents, less cost than fibrin glue and gelatin matrix, and no possibility of allergic reactions. Concerns are potential destruction of tissue and vascularization leading to inhibition of proper healing of the tract.

Jou et al. [74] reported their experience in 249 patients using spot electrocauterization of bleeding points with an elongated 8 French electrode probe through the working channel along the nephrostomy tract. While there was no difference in operative time, hospital stay or infection rate, they did find a statistically significant transfusion rate 1.2 % versus 6.5 % (control group = 92 pts). They did not report pain assessment or analgesic measurements. A French group also reported success using a rollerball in the tract and good, safe results with use of a 26 French resectoscope [75]. Other investigators report this technique to be simple and effective [76].

Conclusion

As our field continues to advance more modifications of drainage post-PCNL will continue. The above studies show the tubeless procedure may improve patient comfort postoperatively with the avoidance of an external tube. As such, it may reduce hospital stay and analgesic requirement allowing for earlier return to normal activity. Additionally, site leakage may be less also improving patient comfort. Disadvantage of this modification is the need for a second procedure for stent removal at a later date which entails a cost and extra burden for the patient unless the internal drainage is externalized for ease of removal, but this carries the risk of early dislodgement. Additionally, many patients suffer from stent-related symptoms, a parameter not reported by most groups studying the modified procedure. This could theoretically lead to prolonged time to convalescence rather than the reported quicker return to normal activity. Furthermore, the tubeless procedure eliminates the ability to reaccess the tract if residual stone remains. Though ureteroscopy remains an option in these cases, percutaneous nephroscopy through and existing tract may be simpler, but this has not been studied. The totally tubeless procedure eliminates the convenient possibility of both of these options.

Table 5.1 Inclusion criteria for tubeless percutaneous nephrolithotomy

Inclusion criteria
Minimal bleeding at completion of the case
Single-tract procedure
Complete clearance of stone
Small stone burden
Singular stone location
Normal renal function
No perforations
No complications
Healthy, low-risk patients
Unilateral procedure
Operative time less than 3 h

While the tubeless PCNL remains a modification that carries great potential benefit, careful patient selection is still encouraged. While many groups have reported success in complex groups, the potential for risk may outweigh the currently calculated benefit on certain cohorts. We recommend maintaining a strict inclusion criteria when selecting these patients (Table 5.1). Additionally, some patients who have had stents previously and did not tolerate them may do better with a nephrostomy tube rather than internal drainage so patient preference should be discussed as well. Additionally, internal drainage with tube placement and early tube removal, particularly in complex patients, is one option that should be considered as it has shown equivalent results and carried additional benefits, though the existing literature with this technique is limited. Absolute or relative contraindications for the tubeless procedure are shown in Table 5.2.

Lastly, while some groups have reported a significant cost advantage with the tubeless procedure, most groups have not analyzed this

Table 5.2 Absolute/relative contraindications for tubeless percutaneous nephrolithotomy

Staghorn calculi
Solitary kidney
Renal dysfunction
Bilateral procedure
Supracostal access
Multiple accesses
Altered anatomy
Poor hemostasis
Pyonephrosis
Residual stone burden
Suspected infection stones
Perforation of pelvicaliceal system or other collecting system injury
Prolonged OR time
Higher-risk patients

parameter in a sophisticated manner and further study is needed [18]. Bellman et al. [16] reported a 129 % increased procedure cost in the standard tube group but these results need to be verified and extended to the postoperative period.

References

1. Rupel E, Brown R. Nephroscopy with removal of stone following nephrostomy for obstructive calculous anuria. J Urol. 1941;46:177–82.
2. Fernström I, Johannson B. Percutaneous pyelolithotomy: a new extraction technique. Scand J Urol Nephrol. 1976;10(3):257–9.
3. Lingeman JE, Newmark JR, Wong MYC. Classification and management of staghorn calculi. In: Smith AD, editor. Controversies in endourology. Philadelphia: WB Saunders; 1995. p. 136–44.
4. Kerbl K, Rehman J, Landman J, Lee D, Sundaram C, Clayman RV. Current management of urolithiasis: progress or regress? J Endourol. 2002;16(5):281–8.
5. Yuan H, Zheng S, Liu L, Han P, Wang J, Wei Q. The efficacy and safety of tubeless percutaneous nephrolithotomy: a systematic review and meta-analysis. Urol Res. 2011;39(5):401–10.
6. Agrawal MS, Agrawal M, Gupta A, Bansai S, Yadav A, Goyal J. A randomized comparison of tubeless and standard percutaneous nephrolithotomy. J Endourol. 2008;22(3):439–42.
7. Maheshwari PN, Andankar MG, Bansal M. Nephrostomy tube after percutaneous nephrolithotomy: large-bore or pigtail catheter? J Endourol. 2000; 14(9):735–7.
8. Pietrow PK, Auge BK, Lallas CD, Santa-Cruz RW, Newman GE, Albala DM, et al. Pain after percutaneous nephrolithotomy: impact of nephrostomy tube size. J Endourol. 2003;17(6):411–4.
9. Liatsikos EN, Hom D, Dinlenc CZ, Kapoor R, Alexianu M, Yohannes P, et al. Tail stent versus re-entry tube: a randomized comparison after percutaneous stone extraction. Urology. 2002;59(1):15–9.
10. Desai MR, Kukreja RA, Desai MM, Mhaskar SS, Wani KA, Patel SH, et al. A prospective randomized comparison of type of nephrostomy drainage following percutaneous nephrostolithotomy: large bore versus tubeless. J Urol. 2004;172(2):565–7.
11. Paul EM, Marcovich R, Lee BR, Smith AD. Choosing the ideal nephrostomy tube. BJU Int. 2003;92(7): 672–7.
12. Srinivasan AK, Herati A, Okeke Z, Smith AD. Renal drainage after percutaneous nephrolithotomy. J Endourol. 2009;23(10):1743–9.
13. Wickham JE, Miller RA, Kellett MJ, Payne SR. Percutaneous nephrolithotomy: one stage or two? Br J Urol. 1984;56(6):582–5.
14. Winfield HN, Weyman P, Clayman RV. Percutaneous nephrostolithotomy: complications of premature nephrostomy tube removal. J Urol. 1986;136(1): 77–9.
15. Agrawal MS, Agrawal M. Tubeless percutaneous nephrolithotomy. Indian J Urol. 2010;26(1):16–24.
16. Bellman GC, Davidov R, Candela J, Gerspach J, Kurtz S, Stout L. Tubeless percutaneous renal surgery. J Urol. 1997;157(5):1578–82.
17. Limb P, Bellman GC. Tubeless percutaneous renal surgery: review of first 112 patients. Urology. 2002; 59(4):527–31.
18. Feng MI, Tamaddon K, Mikhail A, Kaptein JS, Bellman GC. Prospective randomized study of various techniques of percutaneous nephrolithotomy. Urology. 2001;58(3):345–50.
19. Marcovich R, Jacobson AI, Singh J, Shah D, El-Hakin A, Lee BR, et al. No panacea for drainage after percutaneous nephrolithotomy. J Endourol. 2004; 18(8):743–7.
20. Shah HN, Sodha HS, Khandkar AA, Kharodawala S, Hedge SS, Bansal MB. A randomized trial evaluating type of nephrostomy drainage after percutaneous nephrolithotomy: small bore v tubeless. J Endourol. 2008;22(7):1433–9.
21. Singh I, Singh A, Mittal G. Tubeless percutaneous nephrolithotomy: is it really less morbid? J Endourol. 2008;22(3):427–34.
22. Tefekli A, Altunrende F, Tepeler K, Tas A, Aydin S, Muslumanoglu AY. Tubeless percutaneous nephrolithotomy in selected patients: a prospective randomized comparison. Int Urol Nephrol. 2007;39(1): 57–63.
23. Al-Ba'adani TH, Al-Kohlany KM, Al-Adimi A, Al-Towaitym, Al-Baadani T, Alwan M, et al. Tubeless percutaneous nephrolithotomy: the new gold standard. Int Urol Nephrol. 2007;40(3):603–8.

24. Goh M, Wolf Jr JS. Almost totally tubeless percutaneous renal nephrostolithotomy: further evolution of the technique. J Endourol. 1999;13(3):177–80.
25. Mouracade P, Spie R, Lang H, Jacqmin D, Saussine C. Tubeless percutaneous nephrolithotomy: what about replacing the Double-J stent with a ureteral catheter? J Endourol. 2008;22(2):273–5.
26. Lojanapiwat B, Soonthornphan S, Wudhikarn S. Tubeless percutaneous nephrolithotomy in selected patients. J Endourol. 2001;15(7):711–3.
27. Karami H, Jabbari M, Arbab AH. Tubeless percutaneous nephrolithotomy: 5 years of experience in 201 patients. J Endourol. 2007;21(12):1411–3.
28. Abou-Eiela A, Emran A, Mohsen MA, Reyad I, Bedair AS, Kader MA. Safety and efficacy of tubeless percutaneous renal surgery. J Endourol. 2007;21(9): 977–84.
29. Gupta NP, Kesarwani P, Goel R, Aron M. Tubeless percutaneous nephrolithotomy: a comparative study with standard percutaneous nephrolithotomy. Urol Int. 2005;74(1):58–61.
30. Mishra S, Sabnis RB, Kurien A, Ganpule A, Muthu V, Desai M. Questioning the wisdom of tubeless percutaneous nephrolithotomy (PCNL): a prospective randomized controlled study of early tube removal vs tubeless PCNL. BJU Int. 2010;106(7):1045–8. discussion 1048–9.
31. Shah HN, Kausik VB, Hegde SS, Shah JN, Bansal MB. Tubeless percutaneous nephrolithotomy: a prospective feasibility study and review of previous reports. BJU Int. 2005;96(6):879–83.
32. Sofer M, Beri A, Friedman A, Aviram G, Mabjeesh NJ, Chen J, et al. Extending the application of tubeless percutaneous nephrolithotomy. Urology. 2007;70(3):412–6. discussion 416–7.
33. Shah HN, Hegde SS, Shah JN, Bansal MB. Safety and efficacy of supracostal access in tubeless percutaneous nephrolithotomy. J Endourol. 2006;20(12):1016–21.
34. Sofikerim M, Demirco D, Huri E, Erşekerci E, Karacagil M. Tubeless percutaneous nephrolithotomy: safe even in supracostal access. J Endourol. 2007;21(9):967–72.
35. Rana AM, Mithani S. Tubeless percutaneous nephrolithotomy: call of the day. J Endourol. 2007;21(2): 169–72.
36. Malcolm JB, Derweesh IH, Brightbill EK, Mehrazin R, DiBlasio CJ, Wake RW. Tubeless percutaneous nephrolithotomy for complex renal stone disease: single center experience. Can J Urol. 2008;15(3):4072–6. discussion 4076–7.
37. Jou YC, Cheng MC, Lin CT, Chen PC, Shen JH. Nephrostomy tube-free percutaneous nephrolithotomy for patients with large stones and staghorn stones. Urology. 2006;67(1):30–4.
38. Falahatkar S, Khosropanah I, Roshani A, Neiroomand H, Nikpour S, Nadjafi-Semnani M, et al. Tubeless percutaneous nephrolithotomy for staghorn stones. J Endourol. 2008;22(7):1447–51.
39. Shoma AM, Elshal AM. Nephrostomy tube placement after percutaneous nephrolithotomy: critical evaluation through a prospective randomized study. Urology. 2012;79(4):771–6.
40. Yang RM, Bellman GC. Tubeless percutaneous renal surgery in obese patients. Urology. 2004;63(6): 1036–40. discussion 1040–1.
41. Weld KJ, Wake RW. Simultaneous bilateral tubeless percutaneous nephrolithotomy. Urology. 2000;56(6): 1057.
42. Shah HN, Kausik VB, Hegde SS, Shah JN, Bansal MB. Safety and efficacy of bilateral simultaneous tubeless percutaneous nephrolithotomy. Urology. 2005;66(3):500–4.
43. Gupta NP, Kumar P, Aron M, Goel R. Bilateral simultaneous tubeless percutaneous nephrolithotomy. Int Urol Nephrol. 2003;35(3):313–4.
44. Rana AM, Bhojwani JP, Junejo NN, Das Bhagia S. Tubeless PCNL with patient in supine position: procedure for all seasons? With comprehensive technique. Urology. 2008;71(4):581–5.
45. Singh I, Kumar A, Kumar P. "Ambulatory PCNL" (tubeless PCNL under regional anesthesia)—a preliminary report of 10 cases. Int Urol Nephrol. 2005;37(1):35–7.
46. Shah HN, Mahajan AP, Hegde SS, Bansai M. Tubeless percutaneous nephrolithotomy in patients with previous ipsilateral open renal surgery: a feasibility study with review of literature. J Endourol. 2008;22(1):19–24.
47. Matlaga BR, Kim SC, Watkins SL, Kuo RL, Munch LC, Lingeman JE. Percutaneous nephrolithotomy for ectopic kidneys: over, around, or through. Urology. 2008;67(3):513–7.
48. Salem KH, Morsi HA, Omran A, Daw MA. Tubeless percutaneous nephrolithotomy in children. J Pediatr Urol. 2007;3(3):235–8.
49. Ozturk A, Guven S, Kilinc M, Topbaş E, Piskin M, Arslan M. Totally tubeless percutaneous nephrolithotomy: is it safe and effective in preschool children? J Endourol. 2010;24(12):1935–9.
50. Aghamir SMK, Salavati A, Aloosh M, Farahmand H, Meysamie A, Pourmand G. Feasibility of totally tubeless percutaneous nephrolithotomy under the age of 14 years: a randomized clinical trial. J Endourol. 2012;26(6):621–4.
51. Crook TJ, Lockyer CR, Keoghane SR, Walmsley BH. Totally tubeless percutaneous nephrolithotomy. J Endourol. 2008;22(2):267–71.
52. Istanbulluoglu MO, Ozturk B, Gonen M, Cicek T, Ozkardes H. Effectiveness of totally tubeless percutaneous nephrolithotomy in selected patients: a prospective randomized study. Int Urol Nephrol. 2009;41(3):541–5.
53. Aghamir SM, Mohammadi A, Mosavibahar SH, Meysamie AP. Totally tubeless percutaneous nephrolithotomy in renal anomalies. J Endourol. 2008;22(9): 2131–4.
54. Gonen M, Cicek T, Ozkardeş H. Tubeless and stentless percutaneous nephrolithotomy in patients requiring supracostal access. Urol Int. 2009;82(4):440–3.
55. Istanbulluoglu MO, Ozturk B, Cicek T, Ozkardeş H. Bilateral simultaneous totally tubeless percutaneous nephrolithotomy: preliminary report of six cases. J Endourol. 2009;23(8):1255–7.

56. Shpall AI, Parekh AR, Bellman GC. Modification of tubeless percutaneous nephrolithotomy: antegrade stent with flank tether. Urology. 2006;68:880.
57. Joshi HB, Stainthorpe A, MacDonagh RP, Keeley Jr FX, Timoney AG, Barry MJ. Indwelling ureteral stents: evaluation of symptoms, quality of life, and utility. J Urol. 2003;169(3):1065–9.
58. Dunn MD, Portis AJ, Kahn SA, Yan Y, Shalhav AL, Elbahnasy AM, et al. Clinical effectiveness of new stent design: randomized single-blind comparison of tail and double-pigtail stents. J Endourol. 2000;14(2):195–202.
59. Yew J, Bellman GC. Modified "tubeless" percutaneous nephrolithotomy using a tail-stent. Urology. 2003;62(2):346–9.
60. Gonen M, Ozturk B, Ozkardes H. Double-j stenting compared with one night externalized ureteral catheter placement in tubeless percutaneous nephrolithotomy. J Endourol. 2009;23(1):27–31.
61. Berkman DS, Lee MW, Landman J, Gupta M. Tubeless percutaneous nephrolithotomy (PCNL) with reversed polaris loop stent: reduced postoperative pain and narcotic use. J Endourol. 2008;22(10):2245–9.
62. Choe CH, L'Esperance JO, Auge BK. The use of adjunctive hemostatic agents for tubeless percutaneous nephrolithotomy. J Endourol. 2009;23(10):1733–8.
63. Kram HB, Ocampo HP, Yamaguchi MP, Nathan RC, Shoemaker WC. Fibrin glue in renal and ureteral trauma. Urology. 1989;33(3):215–8.
64. Evans LA, Ferguson KH, Foley JP, Rozanski TA, Morey AF. Fibrin sealant for the management of genitourinary injuries, fistulas, and surgical complications. J Urol. 2003;169(4):1360–2.
65. Pfab R, Ascherl R, Blümel G, Hartung R. Local hemostasis of nephrostomy tract with fibrin adhesive sealing in percutaneous nephrolithotomy. Eur Urol. 1987;13(1–2):118–21.
66. Mikhail AA, Kaptein JS, Bellman GC. Use of fibrin glue in percutaneous nephrolithotomy. Urology. 2003;61(5):910–4.
67. Noller MW, Baughman SM, Morey AF, Auge BK. Fibrin sealant enables tubeless percutaneous stone surgery. J Urol. 2004;172(1):166–9.
68. Shah HN, Hegde S, Shah JN, Mohile PD, Yuvaraja TB, Bansal MB. A prospective, randomized trial evaluating the safety and efficacy of fibrin sealant in tubeless percutaneous nephrolithotomy. J Urol. 2006;176(6 Pt 1):2488–92. discussion 2492–3.
69. Borin JF, Sala LG, Eichel L, McDougall EM, Clayman RV. Tubeless percutaneous nephrolithotomy using hemostatic gelatin matrix. J Endourol. 2005;19(6):614–7. discussion 617.
70. Kaufmann OG, Sountoulides P, Kaplan A, Louie M, McDougall E, Clayman R. Skin treatment and tract closure for tubeless percutaneous nephrolithotomy: University of California, Irvine, technique. J Endourol. 2009;23(10):1739–41.
71. Uribe CA, Eichel L, Khonsari S, Finley DS, Basillote J, Park HK, et al. What happens to hemostatic agents in contact with urine? An in vitro study. J Endourol. 2005;19:312–7.
72. Kim IY, Eichel L, Edwards R, Uribe C, Chou DS, Abdelshehid C, et al. Effects of commonly used hemostatic agents on the porcine collecting system. J Endourol. 2007;21:652.
73. Singh I, Saran RM, Jain M. Does sealing of the tract with absorbable gelatin (Spongostan) facilitate tubeless PCNL? A prospective study. J Endourol. 2008; 22(11):2485–93.
74. Jou YC, Cheng MC, Sheen JH, Lin CT, Chen PC. Electocauterization of bleeding points for percutaneous nephrolithotomy. Urology. 2004;64(3):443–6. discussion 446–7.
75. Mouracade P, Spie R, Lang H, Jacqmin D, Saussine C. "Tubeless" percutaneous nephrolithotomy: a series of 37 cases. Prog Urol. 2007;17(7):1351–4.
76. Aron M, Goel R, Kesarwani PK, Gupta NP. Hemostasis in tubeless PNL: point of technique. Urol Int. 2004;73(3):244–7.

Complications of Percutaneous Nephrolithotomy

6

Shadi Al Ekish, Sammy Elsamra, and Gyan Pareek

Introduction

Since the initial description of "percutaneous pyelolithotomy" by Fernstrom and Johansson in 1976, percutaneous nephrolithotomy (PCNL) has become the standard for the treatment of large renal or proximal ureteral stones [1]. Recently, various versions of the procedure have expanded indications to treat a variety of stone burdens and have rendered open nephrolithotomy as a historic procedure. With shorter procedure times, lower transfusion rates, lower narcotic requirements, shorter hospital stay, faster convalescence, and lower cost, PCNL can be applied to nearly any stone burden or location [2]. Despite overall safety and effectiveness of PCNL for the therapy of renal stones [3], PCNL can still be associated with significant morbidity, especially when complications are monitored in a standardized fashion. One recent study cited a nearly 60 % complication rate [4]. While the majority of these complications are mild, the urologist must be ready to prevent, appropriately identify, and treat any complication that he/she could encounter during or after PCNL.

S. Al Ekish (✉) • G. Pareek
Department of Urology, Rhode Island & The Miriam Hospital, Providence, RI, USA
e-mail: shadiali1@yahoo.com; gyan_pareek@brown.edu

S. Elsamra
Division of Urology, The Warren Alpert Medical School of Brown University, Providence, RI, USA
e-mail: selsamra@gmail.com

The focus of this chapter is to provide the reader with an appreciation for the complications associated with PCNL. A review of recent literature pertaining to the prevention, early identification, and proper management of issues that may arise during or after PCNL will be discussed followed by a case presentation used to highlight lessons learned during this summary.

Classification of Complications and General Outcomes

Standardization of complications in the PCNL literature has been difficult and limited for many reasons. First, PCNL has become an increasingly varied procedure with many different approaches to patient positioning, imaging modality, site of kidney access, method of tract dilation, size of nephroscopes and tubes used, and postprocedure kidney drainage (if any). Clearly this variation makes any type of comparison or standardization of complications and outcomes difficult. Secondly, the literature has only recently reflected the use of a standardized schema for the grading of surgical complications. Several studies have been published reporting on complications of PCNL in large series of patients, but none utilize a standard for the classification of complications, hence making interpretation difficult. The modified Clavien classification of surgical complications is a simple, reproducible, and a comprehensive method and has been the standard most commonly utilized system in urology [5].

S.Y. Nakada and M.S. Pearle (eds.), *Surgical Management of Urolithiasis: Percutaneous, Shockwave and Ureteroscopy*, DOI 10.1007/978-1-4614-6937-7_6, © Springer Science+Business Media New York 2013

Table 6.1 Clavien complication grades

Modified Clavien classification of surgical complications	
Grade	Definition
Grade 1	Any deviation from the normal postoperative course without the need for pharmacological treatment or surgical, endoscopic, and radiologic interventions
	Allowed therapeutic regimens are: drugs as antiemetics, antipyretics, analgesics, diuretics, electrolytes, and physiotherapy. This grade also includes wound infections opened at the bedside
Grade 2	Required pharmacological treatment with drugs other than such allowed for grade 1 complications. Blood transfusions and total parenteral nutrition are also included
Grade 3	Requiring surgical, endoscopic, or radiological intervention
Grade 3a	Intervention not under general anesthesia
Grade 3b	Intervention under general anesthesia
Grade 4	Life-threatening complication (including CNS complications excluding transient ischemic attacks) requiring intensive care (ICU) management
Grade 4a	Single-organ dysfunction (including dialysis)
Grade 4b	Multiorgan dysfunction
Grade 5	Death of patient

Definitions of Clavien complication grades listed in Table 6.1.

Recently, Tefekli et al. sought to report their complications using the modified Clavien classification system. Their single institution case series reviewed 255 complications occurring in 237 of 811 patients who underwent PCNL between 2003 and 2006. They reported an overall complication rate of 29 %. There were 33 grade 1 (4 %), 132 grade 2 (16.3 %), 54 grade 3a (6.6 %), 23 grade 3b (2.8 %), 9 grade 4a (1.1 %), and 3 grade 4b (0.3 %) complications, and 1 death (0.1 %). Most complications were related to bleeding and urine leakage. Grade 2 and 3a complications were significantly more common in patients with complex renal stones, defined as stones with components in both calix and pelvis. Limitations in this study were the retrospective nature of data collection and the imprecise method of discerning simple from complex stones. Further, residual fragments, whether significant or insignificant, were not cited as complications. This may be misleading, as the authors pointed out, as subsequent treatment may qualify as 3a or 3b complication. Further, the single institution data was not stratified by many factors (age, comorbidity, BMI, renal anomalies), possibly influencing the outcome and complication rates [6].

A contemporary report by de la Rosette et al. sought to report complications on PCNLs performed between 1994 and 2007 using the modified Clavien classification. Interestingly, the authors reported data based on their transition from five urologists performing PCNLs to one operating urologist under the auspice of an endourology center with a dedicated team for PCNLs in 2002. While patients in the latter cohort were more likely to be older, on anticoagulation, or with positive urine culture and less likely to have had prior SWL, they exhibited similar distribution of sex, prior PCNL, history of diabetes, stone burden, and history of renal anomalies. In their cohort of 244 patients, their global Clavien complications were grade 0 in 53.7 %, grade 1 in 25.8 %, grade 2 in 16.8 %, grade 3a in 0.4 %, grade 3b in 0.4 %, and grade 4 in 0.4 %. Complication rates decreased after 2002 (with implementation of the dedicated endourology surgeon and team) from 60.3 to 40.9 %. Negative urine culture, smaller stone size, more favorable stone position, balloon dilation as opposed to telescopic dilation, lithotripsy device utilized, and decreased operative time were also associated with decreased complications on univariate analysis. Independent factors on multivariate analysis for complicated outcome were stone size (OR 1.25), type of lithotripsy device (OR 1.35) and incidence of perioperative complications (OR 3.71). The limitation of this single institution study included the retrospective nature, extended study period which allowed for heterogeneity in instruments and techniques.

Table 6.2 Complication rates by different studies

Summary of studies evaluating complications of PCNL using Clavien classification system					
			de la Rosette et al. [10]		
Study		Tefekli et al [6]	Pre-2002	Post-2002	de la Rosette [7]
Number of patients		811	27	104	5,803
Grade 1		4 %	41.2 %	19.9 %	11.1 %
Grade 2		16.3 %	14.7 %	17.6 %	5.3 %
Grade 3	3a	6.6 %	1.4 %	0 %	2.3 %
	3b	2.8 %	0 %	0.6 %	1.3 %
Grade 4	4a	1.1 %	0 %	0.6 %	0.3 %
	4b	0.3 %	0 %	0 %	0.2 %
Grade 5		0.1 %	0 %	0 %	0.03 %
Overall complication rate		29 %	60.3 %	40.9 %	20.53 %

Summarizing all single institution studies is of limited value given the recent changes and issues associated with modern PCNL and with institution-specific capabilities, limitations, and norms of acceptability for their patient populations. With this in mind, the Endourologic Society formed the Clinical Research Office of the Endourologic Society (CROES) in order to provide a central hub for the organization, structure, and facilitation of a global network for endourologic research. Their first mission was to identify indications and outcomes for PCNL from centers worldwide, namely, the PCNL Global Study (PCNLGS).

The PCNLGS was a prospective observational study of over 5,800 patients from over 90 urologic centers from around the world. Patient data was pooled centrally in the CROES where several parameters including outcomes and complications were evaluated. The distribution of scores in modified Clavien grades was: grade 0 (79.5 %), grade I (11.1 %), grade II (5.3 %), grade IIIa (2.3 %), grade IIIb (1.3 %), grade IVa (0.3 %), grade IVb (0.2 %), or grade V (0.03 %). The 30-day stone-free rate was 75.7 %, and 84.5 % of patients did not need additional treatment. Major procedure-related complications included significant bleeding (7.8 %), renal pelvis perforation (3.4 %), and hydrothorax (1.8 %). Blood was transfused in 328 (5.7 %) of patients, and 10.5 % of patients developed a fever of greater than 38.5 °C postoperatively [7]. We have summarized the complication rates by Clavien grade of the studies discussed in Table 6.2. Several subsequent sub-analyses of this case series have focused on the impact of calculus size, patient position during PCNL, and method of tract dilation, among other factors, on PCNL outcome.

Preoperative Evaluation and Special Populations as Risk Factors

A key component to decreasing the risk of surgical complications is proper patient selection. Patient factors and stone factors should help identify those patients who would be benefited most, and potentially harmed least, by PCNL. Patients should have nephrolithiasis appropriate for PCNL, as this treatment is more morbid than both ureteroscopy and shock-wave lithotripsy (discussed elsewhere in the book). Besides obtaining medical clearance from a patient's primary care physician or specialist, such as cardiology, the urologist should be familiar with appropriate basic screening of patients to help minimize postoperative complications.

The urologist should be keen on screening for uncorrected coagulopathy. A thorough personal history screening for any easy bruising or bleeding with routine activities may suggest an underlying (and undiagnosed) coagulopathy, which may prompt further work-up prior to PCNL. Acquired coagulopathy should also be corrected or reversed prior to PCNL as bleeding is one of the most frequent complications encountered.

Aspirin, warfarin, clopidrogel, and nonsteroidal anti-inflammatory medications should be held for 7–10 days prior to the procedure, with direction from the primary care physician or specialist. Further, PT/PTT/INR should be checked preoperatively in those patients who are on warfarin to ensure proper levels prior to procedure. Those patients on anticoagulation medications with shorter half-lives such as dabigatran, lovenox, heparin, or fondaperineux should have their medication held prior to the procedure based on the half life (commonly used is 5–7 half lives) and with the guidance of the patient's primary care physician or a hematologist. The urologist should also be aware of some medications or supplements, not used for the purpose of anticoagulation, that may affect coagulation. Omega-3 fatty acids supplementation (or fish-oil supplements) and certain herbal supplements often affect coagulation and may lead to occult diathesis. They may affect platelet function directly (e.g. Garlic, Ginseng, Ginko Baloba, and Ginger) or interact with the metabolism or function of blood thinning medications [8].

Patients should also be free of any active urinary tract infection prior to PCNL. A preoperative negative urine culture is ideal but a urinary tract infection that is without any signs of systemic inflammatory response which has been treated with antibiotics preoperatively (ideally for 2–3 days) is necessary to prevent sepsis postoperatively.

Adequate radiographic investigation is essential before creating the nephrostomy tract and is of paramount importance to prevent major PCNL related complications. Proper identification of the stone burden allows for the selection of ideal treatment modality, such as ureteroscopy and SWL, which may spare the patient morbidity. Further, proper stone identification will allow for ideal access, which may further minimize morbidity. While plain radiographs and/or ultrasound may suffice, cross-sectional imaging, such as computerized tomography (CT), helps more accurately define stone burden as well as kidney vasculature and nearby structures such as the bowel, liver, and spleen.

Potential preoperative risk factors such as advanced age, renal anomalies, increased body mass index (BMI), and size and character of stone burden are of crucial importance to proper preoperative risk stratification. Additionally, factors beyond patient or stone may impact outcomes as the surgeon's experience has a role in preventing postoperative outcomes.

Operative Volume and Surgeon Experience

Surgeon experience appears to be an important factor in minimizing complications associated with PCNL. In a sub analysis of the CROES PCNLGS, Opondo, sought to compare the complication rate and severity in high-volume versus low-volume institutions [9]. Data from 3,933 patients were included. Patients were excluded if the PCNL was performed in centers with volume less than ten cases per year and in those with history of prior renal surgery. In their study low-volume and high-volume centers were determined as those institutions performing less than and greater than 77 cases per year. Thirteen of 71 centers were identified to be high volume. Higher stone-free rates, lower complication rates, and shorter hospital stays were independently associated with case volume on multivariate analysis. High-volume centers were identified to have lower rates of intraoperative perforation, failed access, or hydrothorax, though statistical significance was identified only in the rate of perforation. Further, reported bleeding, change in hemoglobin, and transfusion rates were all statistically significantly lower in high-volume centers. Interestingly, severity of complications decreased with increasing annual volume until approximately 120 cases, at which point complication severity increased. This volume of cases associated with a nadir in complications coincided with the case volume that yielded peak stone-free rate (both were approximately 120 cases per year). A possible explanation is referral bias, with more complicated cases skewing the results.

The issue of training and learning curves has recently been reviewed by de la Rosette et al. [10]. Cited in their review were studies by Allen et al. [11] and Tanriverdi et al. [12] that evaluated single surgeon competency and excellence by monitoring operating time, fluoroscopic screening time, and radiation dose. The study by Tanriverdi et al. also reviewed stone-free and complication rates. Both studies suggest that significant improvements in operative time and fluoroscopic time are obtained at 60 cases. Excellence was reported by Allen, et al. at 115 cases. However, neither of the studies utilized complications when measuring competency (both papers cited no major complication rates). The latter study reported no improvement in estimated blood loss or transfusion rates with increased volume. As suggested by these reports, experience of all team members in the operating suite may influence (and improve) outcomes and complication rates.

Advanced Patient Age and Comorbidity

Often advanced age is a concern for procedural or postprocedural complications. A recent study sought to compare outcomes and complications of all PCNLs performed between 1997 and 1999. Twenty-eight PCNLs performed on 27 patients over the age of 60 were compared to 178 PCNLs performed on 166 patients younger than 60. Despite a slightly higher rate of staghorn calculi in the elder cohort, stone burden was similar as were stone-free rates. Both cohorts had similar transfusion rates (21 % in the elder and 18 % in the younger cohorts), complication rates, and length of stay. The senior group experienced two renal pelvic perforations managed conservatively (grade 1), four patients had post-op fever without bacteremia (grade 1), and one patient was reported to have high-grade fever and was found to have a urinary tract infection and perinephric hematoma (grade 2) that were treated with antibiotics and conservative therapy [13]. Clearly cited in their methods section was a selection bias of only those "in good general health."

Okeke et al. [14] reviewed the data from the PCNLGS and stratified patients into two groups: those 70 years or greater and those under 70 years of age. A matched analysis was utilized to assess stone-free status of 334 patients in each arm. The data revealed a complication rate of 19.9 % in the elderly versus 6.6 % in the young. Moreover, major complications, defined as Clavien III or IV, were seen in 5.1 % of the elderly versus 0.0 % of the young. The authors did cite that the elderly in their study, as in the general population, did have a greater incidence of comorbidity and anticoagulation use.

While age is an important factor during preoperative risk stratification perhaps it is not as important as comorbidity. Resorlu et al. evaluated 283 patients between 60 and 81 years old for complications post-PCNL. Patients were stratified into three groups based on Charlson Comorbidity Index (CCI) scores of 0, 1, or 2 and greater. Their overall postoperative complication rate was 39 %. The most common complication was hemorrhage requiring transfusion (12 %), resulting in patients with a higher CCI. Life-threatening complications increased from 7.6–12 to 28.6 % as the CCI increased from 0–1 to 2 and greater. The only mortality in the study was noted in a patient with a CCI score of greater than 2. CCI, intraoperative bleeding, and operative time were all independent factors predictive of postoperative complications on multivariate analysis. Based on these findings, those with increased CCI may be offered conservative observation or uretero-renoscopic treatment in order to avoid high complication rates [15].

Influence of Obesity

While BMI has been associated with increased complications and worse outcomes in many different types of surgery, it has not been associated with poorer outcomes or increased complications for PCNL based on several studies [16–18]. Bagrodia et al. [19], identified no increased operative time, need for multiple access, difference in stone-free rates, transfusion requirements, complication rates, second look rates, or length of stay in a series of 200 patients stratified by BMI. These results were echoed recently by Tomaszewski et al. [20] whereby 187 patients stratified by BMI categories (ideal, overweight, obese, and morbidly obese) experienced no difference in stone-free rate, complication rate, hemorrhage, or hospital length of stay. Certainly, anesthetic precautions tailored to airway management in obese patients and appropriate length instruments would be required for obese patients.

Renal Anomalies (Solitary, Malrotated, Ectopic, Horseshoe, and Transplanted Kidneys)

Solitary kidney, as a result of traumatic, surgical, or congenital reasons, presents a unique concern to the urologist planning PCNL. Clearly, the safety cushion of a contralateral kidney is not present and hence any complication compromising the kidney may render the patient anephric and dependent on dialysis. Further, it is likely that those with solitary kidney are likely to have more comorbidities which would place them at higher risk for postoperative complications. This situation was evaluated in the PCNLGS as 189 of 5,745 patients with complete data collection were with solitary kidney [21]. Patients with solitary kidney were similar to their bilateral nephric counterparts in distribution of sex, BMI, and comorbidities other than incidence of coronary artery disease and American Society of Anesthesiologist (ASA) scores, in which mono-kidney patients had higher incidence and scores. Patients with solitary kidney also had higher incidence of nephrostomy drainage and pyelolithotomy. Access sites, location of access (supracostal vs. infracostal), modality of image-guided access, and tract dilation methods were similar in both groups. Those with solitary kidney had lower stone-free rates, higher transfusion rates (particularly in those dilated with telescopic dilators), higher pre- and postoperative serum creatinine levels (though the change was similar to that of the bilateral kidney cohort). Incidence of post-op fevers, perforations, hydrothorax, and failed procedures were similar in both groups.

Anatomic renal anomalies such as renal ectopia and horseshoe kidney carry a theoretical risk for increased stone formation due to urinary stasis from proximal ureteral or ureteropelvic junction distortion from anomalous vasculature or orientation [22]. This has shown to translate to decreased stone clearance in such kidneys after SWL [23]. Hence, PCNL offers the advantage of adequate fragmentation and removal of stone burden. However, should these same anatomic anomalies be a source for concern of increased risk of complication?

Three case series have reviewed their outcomes and complications associated with PCNL in anomalous kidneys. Mosavi-Bahar et al. reported their experience in PCNL on 17 patients with various anomalies (horseshoe kidneys, ectopia, malrotation, and small kidneys). No serious complications were encountered though they reported two pleural injuries that required no further management (grade 1) [24]. In a subsequent series, 48 patients with anomalous kidneys underwent PCNL with 81 % stone-free rate and no major complications (three patients required transfusion—grade 2 and two had perinephric collection—grade 1) [25]. Similar results were expressed by Gupta et al. with three complications noted in 52 renal units (46 patients); two with post-PCNL sepsis (grade 2) and one with pleural injury requiring thoracic tube drainage (grade 3b) [26]. Access to anterior calices was obtained with laparoscopic assistance in some cases. While complications in all three series were minimal, it is clear that these are challenging cases and should be done only by those with substantial experience.

Similar to anomalous kidneys, in their anatomic considerations, are transplanted kidneys. While their superficial pelvic position allows for direct access to the calix, there is the concern for overlying bowel necessitating ultrasonic or CT-guided access placement. Further, issues with immunosuppression intrinsic to the transplantation can result in increased risk of postoperative complications. One series of 13 patients cited no

Table 6.3 Comparison of SFR and complications in stones aggregated by size and character

	Xue et al. [31]			Desai et al. [32]	
	20–30 mm	31–40 mm	41–60 mm	Non-staghorn	Staghorn
Number of patients	1,202	202	44	3,869	1,466
Stone-free rate	90.0 %	83.3 %	84.1 %	82.5 %	56.9 %
Mean operative time	71.3 min	79.5 min	90.8 min	65 min	100 min
Postoperative fever	8.4 %	7.3 %	17.9 %	8.7 %	14.8 %
Transfusion rate	4.4 %	4.4 %	13.3 %	4.5 %	9.0 %
Collecting system perforation	Not listed			2.8 %	4.4 %
Multiple accesses	1.4 %			5 %	16.9 %

intraoperative complications [27]. Three patients however developed sepsis, gastrointestinal bleeding, and herpes esophagitis, all Clavien grade 2, respectively, postoperatively.

History of Prior Renal Surgery

While the influence of prior surgery on an upcoming open or laparoscopic case cannot be overstated, several studies suggest that prior renal surgery may not have a great impact on the outcomes of PCNL or its complications. In 2003, Basiri et al., published their series of 65 patients, with a history of prior open nephrolithotomy, and 117 patients, without a history of prior open nephrolithotomy, who underwent PCNL [28]. There was no difference in stone-free rates, inability to access the collecting system, incidence of postoperative pyelonephritis, or incidence of hemorrhage. However, this study was limited by the fact that the cohorts with history of open nephrolithotomy were more likely to harbor a single stone. A similar study without this limitation, revealed no difference in operating time, postoperative analgesic dose, pain scores, intraoperative or postoperative complication rates in 27 patients with a history of open renal surgery compared to 62 patients without history of prior renal surgery [29].

The effects of shockwave lithotripsy (SWL) on tissue has been examined. In one study, 1,008 patients (230 patients failed SWL), underwent PCNL were reviewed [30]. PCNL performed an average 3.5 months after SWL required similar operative times and fluoroscopic screening times with those PCNLs without a history of prior SWL. However, PCNL performed on those with history of prior failed-SWL, was for significantly smaller stones yielding longer operative and fluoroscopic times per square centimeter of stone. Overall complication and transfusion rates were similar in both cohorts at 26.5 and 9.1 % versus 28.8 and 9.2 %, respectively.

Stone Burden

Stone burden and location clearly influence outcomes and complication rates. Xue et al. [31], evaluated stone characteristics and outcomes in 1,448 patients whose data was collected in the PCNLGS. Patients were stratified by stone size (20–30, 30–40, and 41–60 mm) and location (pelvis or upper, mid, or lower calix). Eighty-three percentage of stones were 20–30 mm and 73 % of stones were located in the renal pelvis. With increasing stone size, the authors observed significantly lower stone-free rates and higher rates of postoperative fever and blood loss requiring transfusion (see Table 6.3). Increased stone size and calyceal location was associated with higher ASA score. Postoperative complications were generally associated more with large calyceal, as opposed to renal pelvic, stones.

Staghorn calculi represent the largest stone burden possible within a kidney. The size and branching of such complex calculi present significant challenges during PCNL that may place the patient at increased risk for complication. A comparison of PCNLs performed on staghorn versus non-staghorn calculi in the PCNLGS confirms that staghorn calculi were associated with lower stone-free rate, longer operative times, higher incidence of positive preoperative urine culture, more bleeding, increased transfusion requirement, increased collecting system perforation, and were more likely to undergo multiple access (see Table 6.3) [32]. PCNLs performed on staghorn calculi were also more likely to undergo upper calix access if a solitary access was chosen. These cases were not more likely to experience hydrothorax or failed procedure compared to non-staghorn calculi.

Multiple percutaneous access sites and the use of a flexible nephroscope are two methods to improve PCNL stone-free rates in renal units with staghorn calculi. Few studies have evaluated the outcomes and complications of multiple percutaneous accesses for staghorn calculi. One study evaluated the outcomes and complications of a range of 2–6 percutaneous access sites (median was three) in 169 renal units treated (149 patients) [33]. Blood transfusion was required in 46 patients (30.8 %), urosepsis 8 patients (5.3 %), hydrothorax 7 patients (4.2 %), hemothorax in 1 patient, angioembolization was performed in 4 patients (2.4 %), and perinephric collection was identified in 1 patient. Excluding those with chronic renal failure and anemia preoperatively who received transfusions beyond POD#2, the authors concluded that there was no increased risk of complication using multiple percutaneous accesses. Certainly, the use of a flexible nephroscope though a single access point may improve access to other calices but is limited by its dependence of laser for lithotripsy or basketing, both of which may be time-consuming. Ultimately, multiple accesses may allow for improvements in operative time and decreased torqueing, through a poor access site, and help mitigate complications from treatment through this type of access.

Intraoperative Risk Factors

Patient Positioning

A subanalysis of the PCNLGS on the impact of patient positioning on PCNL outcomes and complications was published in 2011 [30]. One thousand one hundred and thirty-eight and 4,637 patients underwent PCNL in the supine and prone position, respectively. Patient's demographics were similar, except for a greater proportion of female gender, lower age, and greater rate of SWL in the supine group. Patients who underwent PCNL in the prone position enjoyed greater stone-free rates (77 vs. 70 %) but experienced fever more often (11.1 vs. 7.6 %) and were more likely to require blood transfusion (6.1 vs. 4.3 %). Patients who underwent PCNL in the supine position were more likely to have a failed procedure (2.7 vs. 1.5 %). Perforation and hydrothorax rates were similar in both groups at roughly 3 and 2 %, respectively. In terms of Clavien score both cohorts exhibited roughly 20 % complication rate with Clavien I occurring in 12.1 and 10.8 %, Clavien II occurring in 3.8 and 5.6 %, Clavien III occurring in 2.7 and 3.9 %, and Clavien IV occurring in 0.6 and 0.5 % of supine and prone positioned patients. One mortality was observed in both cohorts. Though not substantiated in PCNLGS analysis, theoretical considerations for supine PCNL include decreased anesthetic or cardiac risk associated with prone positioning (particularly in obese patients or those with decreased cardiac index), decreased hydrostatic pressure and perhaps fewer postoperative fevers, decreased radiation exposure to the surgeon's hands, and spontaneous stone drainage. Further, anatomic studies suggest that splenic or liver injuries are more likely to occur with an upper pole stick in the supine position. Conversely, colonic injury is more likely to occur with a lower pole access in the prone position [34].

Who Gets Access?

Access may be obtained by either the urologist in the operating suite at the time of PCNL or the interventional radiologists in the radiology suite preoperatively. Many centers in the USA rely on the interventional radiologist to obtain the percutaneous renal access, a trend attributed primarily to the lack of percutaneous access training for urologists during residency. Several reports proved the safety and efficacy of PCNL access created by urologists [35, 36].

Watterson et al., compared access obtained by a urologist with that by a radiologist, both cohorts of patients had similar rates of supracostal access, with similar mean access difficulty scores between groups. They concluded that access related complications were less and stone-free rates were improved during urologist acquired percutaneous access [37].

Method of Dilation

PCNL tract dilation can be achieved using several methods, using Alken metal co axial dilators, Amplatz fascial dilators, or balloon dilation systems. Rigid metal dilators are a series of dilators mounted together in a telescopic system. This system is generally utilized in patients with scarring secondary to previous renal surgery or inflammation. Because of the metallic nature of these dilators and difficulty in maintaining accurate depth of dilation, these dilators can induce considerable renal trauma especially when pushing hard against tough fibrous tissues. The Amplatz sequential fascial dilators consist of progressively larger and firm polyurethane dilators. Due to the repeated dilation required, these dilators carry the risk of bleeding each time a dilator is withdrawn. Balloon dilators are the most frequently utilized method of track dilatation and were developed to achieve dilation in a single step eliminating the need for serial dilation. Briefly, the balloon system creates a tract through a less traumatic lateral and radial force rather than shearing action. Studies have found that bleeding and transfusion rates are less with the balloon dilators compared with amplatz fascial dilators [38, 39]. However, Gonen et al., compared balloon dilatation with Amplatz dilation of the nephrostomy tract in a retrospective chart review of 229 patients. They noted no difference in operative time or estimated blood loss [40]. Benway and Nakada published a rebuttal, illustrating that multiple studies have reproducibly demonstrated lower rate of hemorrhagic complications in patient undergoing balloon dilation compared with serial dilation [41].

More recently, the PCNLGS, Yamaguchi et al., concluded that metal coaxial and Amplatz sequential dilators and smaller sheath size are associated with shorter operating times than balloon dilation and larger sheath size. Factors predictive of bleeding complications include stone load, caseload, sheath size, and operating time. One variable observed was that surgeons were reporting the use of coaxial and Amplatz sequential dilators may have had longer experience and, hence, obtained better access compared to those using balloon dilators [42]. Regardless of the tract dilation method used, caution should be taken to dilate the tract only up to the peripheral aspect of the collecting system under radiology guidance.

Radiation Exposure

Recently, radiation exposure has been identified as a modifiable risk factor for subsequent development of malignancy [43]. One recent study by Mancini et al. reviewed the records of 96 patients who underwent PCNL. Increased body mass index, higher stone burden, stone nonbranched configuration, and a greater number of percutaneous access tracts were all associated with increased effective radiation dose. BMI was particularly interesting as it exhibited a dose-related effect. In other words, obese patients with a BMI between 30 and 39.9 kg/m^2 had a more than twofold increase in effective radiation dose, and those with BMI 40 kg/m^2 or greater had a more than threefold increase in effective radiation dose compared to those with normal BMI. In their study, site of stone, site of access, stone composition, and EBL were not associated with effective radiation dose [44].

Tubes Post-op (Tubeless PCNL)

Placement of a temporary percutaneous tube though a dilated nephrostomy tract after PCNL is routinely done for renal drainage, in order to facilitate reentry for second look procedures and to tamponade potential bleeding [45]. Additionally, recent evidence suggests that PCNL may be performed tubeless or without the use of a post procedural tube exiting the flank. In a study examining tubeless PCNL, Bellman et al. demonstrated shorter convalescence, shorter length of stay, and decreased pain as well as significant cost savings without increase in complications [46]. Since that study, many reports have been published demonstrating the feasibility of tubeless PCNL. In a systematic review of 24 studies, 11 of which were randomized controlled studies, postoperative pain scores, analgesic requirements, length of stay, and convalescence time were all significantly shorter in the tubeless population. Stone-free rates and morbidity were similar between the various tubeless PCNL and standard tubed PCNL cohorts. Specifically, measured blood loss and transfusion rates were similar. Hydrothorax incidence was nearly double in the tubed cohort but this was without statistical significance. Similarly postoperative pyrexia and duration of urinary leakage was encountered less in the tubeless cohorts as opposed to the tubed population. At our institution, tubeless PCNL is performed routinely in procedures where the stone burden is less than 1.5 cm and in cases judged intraoperatively to be atraumatic and with good antegrade flow at the end of the procedure.

Intraoperative Complications

Hemorrhage

The kidney is a highly vascular organ, with each kidney receiving 12.5 % of cardiac output. Hemorrhage is one of the most common complications of PCNL. Older reports have cited a post-procedural transfusion rate of up to 34 % [47]. More recently transfusion rates have been lower. In a review of 1,585 PCNLs performed on 1,338 patients, bleeding occurred in 6 % of procedures with only 0.8 % requiring transfusion or angioembolization [48]. In the PCNLGS, bleeding complications were reported in 7.8 % of procedures and transfusions were administered in 5.7 % [4].

Stoller et al. have linked the increased the risk of bleeding requiring blood transfusion during PCNL to the experience of the surgeon and multiple access points. Kidneys with intricate anatomy were associated with an increased risk of renal bleeding [49, 50]. Lam and associates found that the creation of an additional nephrostomy tract in patients treated for staghorn stone decreased transfusion requirements [51]. Patients on anticoagulant or antiplatelet medications were also more likely to experience bleeding [52]. Also, patients with staghorn or large stones, a solitary kidney, and those with DM were associated with increased risk of bleeding during PCNL [53, 54].

Intraoperative bleeding during PCNL may be difficult to manage and may present technical challenges if not appropriately managed. If significant bleeding is encountered, our initial step is to reinsert the 30 Fr dilating balloon utilized to create the tract. With the balloon reinflated, the tamponade effect is carried out over 10 min. If vital signs are appropriate, the balloon is deflated and the site is inspected for continued venous and or arterial bleeding. If bleeding continues to be significant, a 36 Fr Occlusive Kaye tamponade balloon catheter is placed. This specialized nephrostomy tamponade catheter has a dual action; it tamponades the tract and renal parenchyma and drains the kidney, maintaining ureteral access through its 14 Fr internal lumen [55]. In the event of severe bleeding that does not respond to the aforementioned approaches, selective or super selective angioembolization is indicated.

Injury to the Lung and Pleura

Supracostal access through the upper calix provides a straight tract along the long axis of the kidney and is a favored and efficient approach for the treatment of for upper, staghorn, and upper ureteral stones. However, due to the close proximity of the pleura to the kidneys, the supracostal access carries a higher risk for pleural or lung injury resulting in hydrothorax, pneumothorax, hemothorax, or nephropleural fistula.

In a series of 240 patients undergoing 300 percutaneous accesses (33 % supracostal), Munver et al. [56] compared complications associated with supracostal access to those occurring with an infracostal approach. The incidence of complications from the supracostal approach was reported as 16.3 %, with the highest percentage being intrathoracic complications. A higher rate of complications was found when the supra 11th rib access was utilized. These complications included; hemothorax/hydrothorax in 4 %, nephropleural fistula in 2 %, and pneumothorax in 1 % of access tracts. Subsequently, Lojanapiwat et al. [57] reported intrathoracic complication rates of 15.3 % for the supracostal access and 1.4 % for infracostal access. Complications with supracostal access were noted to be reduced by proper positioning of the nephrostomy sheath in the calyceal system during the procedure and by keeping the nephrostomy tube well drained post operatively to minimize urine leakage into the pleura.

Bowel Injury

Bowel injury is an unusual complication during PCNL, reported in approximately 1 % of cases. One predisposing factor, a retrorenal colon, occurs in approximately 0.6 % of patients. The variant anatomy occurs more frequently on the left side near the lower pole of the kidney. Congenital renal anomalies such as horse shoe kidney, ectopia, and fusion anomalies also increase the risk for colonic perforation during PCNL. Anomalies of the colon must be considered in patients with previous gastrointestinal surgery, over distended bowel secondary to chronic constipation or those patients with neurologic impairment. Other scenarios predisposing to possible colonic injury include anterior calyceal access, patients with previous extensive renal surgery [58] and in those patients with musculoskeletal anomalies like kyphoscoliosis [59].

Conservative management may be sufficient in the majority of cases where the perforation is extraperitoneal and the patient does not have peritoneal signs or sepsis. The placement of a Double J® stent should be undertaken and nephrostomy tube should be pulled back into the colon under fluoroscopic guidance to separate the colon from the renal collecting system. A Foley catheter is left in the bladder to maintain low pressure system in the urinary tract. The patient is placed on broad-spectrum antibiotics and given low-residue diet. After 5–7 days, imaging of the colon and/or a retrograde pyelogram is performed. At this point, if no nephrocolic fistula or extravasation is present, the foley catheter is taken out and the colostomy tube is drawn from the colon and kept as a drain for 3 days. If no evidence of fistula is observed at this point, the tube is removed [60, 61]. If the patient has intraperitoneal perforation, sepsis or failed conservative management, open repair with the assistance of a general surgeon should be undertaken.

Duodenal Injury

The second and third parts of the duodenum are located in the retroperitoneal space, anteromedial to the hilum of the right kidney. The duodenum can be injured if a needle, the stiff part of guide wire or a dilator is advanced too deeply during establishment of the nephrostomy access or during the procedure. There are a few cases reported in the literature, usually diagnosed when nephroduodenal communication is demonstrated on an intraoperative or postoperative nephrostogram [62, 63]. Exploratory laparotomy is required in most cases, especially if the patient has peritonitis or sepsis or if the perforation is large. Conservative management has been reported. Bowel rest is achieved with total parenteral nutrition and nasogastric suction, broad spectrum antibiotics are administered with conservative management of the nephrostomy tube. An upper gastrointestinal series and nephrostogram are performed 2 weeks later to assure fistula closure [62].

Spleen, Liver, and Gall Bladder Injury

Hepatic and splenic injuries during PCNL are uncommon due to the cephalic location of these organs in the abdomen. Patients with hepatosplenomegaly or those with an access above the 11th rib (especially if undertaken during inspiration) are at greater risk. A CT scan should be performed in organomegaly cases to assess the possibility of a safe tract and to help with the placement of the nephrostomy tube [64]. Splenic injury during left PCNL is potentially fatal due to massive bleeding and consequent hypovolemic shock. The majority of patients will require exploration and splenectomy. In select hemodynamically stable patients, nonoperative management may be considered [65, 66].

Liver injury is much less common than splenic injury. While the majority of patient with splenic injury require open surgery; most of the patients with liver injuries can be successfully managed conservatively. Postoperative watchful monitoring of the patient with serial physical examinations, hematocrit measurements, and imaging (CT scan) will dictate the type of management. Gallbladder injury during PCNL has been reported in several case studies [67–69]. Patient with previous abdominal surgeries are at increased risk. Due to high mortality associated with biliary peritonitis, early recognition and treatment with cholecystectomy and peritoneal lavage are often necessary.

Hypothermia

Core body temperature have been noted to fall 2 °C on average during PCNL [70]. Accurate monitoring of core body temperature with an esophageal probe is indicated. Hypothermia can be caused by large areas of exposed body surface, use of room temperature irrigant, prolonged operative time, vasodilatation secondary to general anesthesia, and, low ambient temperature. If not corrected intraoperatively, hypothermia can lead to coagulopathy and platelet dysfunction, impaired drug clearance, and postoperative shivering causing increased oxygen demand leading to an increased risk of myocardial infarction and arrhythmia [65]. Therefore, it is important to use blankets and/or warming devices and warmed irrigant during the procedure. While perhaps uncomfortable for the surgeon, warm ambient room temperature may mitigate complications.

Injury to the Collecting System and Fluid Extravasation

Fluid extravasation occurs when there is a tear in the pelvicalyceal system or the access sheath is malpositioned outside the kidney. A properly placed access sheath will prevent significant extravasation from the renal access site. Perforation of the collecting system should be suspected if retroperitoneal fat is visualized or in case of abdominal and flank distension during the procedure. Normal saline should be utilized as the irrigation fluid to avoid electrolyte imbalance, hemolysis, and minimize adverse consequences of extravasation. The surgeon should monitor the amount of irrigant utilized. If there is a discrepancy in the inflow-outflow fluid amount of more than 500 ml, then the procedure should be terminated. Extravasation increases the chance of stone fragment migration outside the collecting system with a reported rate of 1 % [71]. Pursuing of these stone fragments will enlarge the perforation and is not recommended; however, the patient should be informed of the migrated stones to avoid mismanagement in the future.

Small amount of extravastion is of nonclinical significance and resolve with nephrostomy tube drainage alone. Clinically significant retroperitoneal or intraperitoneal extravasation occur in fewer than 1 % of cases [72]. Patient may experience persistent ileus, fever, abdominal distension, and respiratory compromise. Diuretics, image-guided drainage, and open surgical drainage are treatment options in these scenarios.

Nerve Injuries

Neuropraxia may result if the patient is improperly padded and/or positioned. Particular care should be paid to neutral cervical position during the rotation of a patient into and out of the prone position as cervical neuropraxias may result. The surgeon should guide and be actively involved in the patient positioning to prevent position-related nerve injuries by ensuring that all of the pressure points are well protected. Brachial plexus injury, shoulder dislocation, and other peripheral nerve damage have been reported during PCNL. A neurology consultation should be obtained if nerve injury is suspected. Most cases resolve within a few days with the help of physical therapy.

Air Embolism

A vascular air embolism during PCNL is a rare complication and may occur when the carbon dioxide is used to opacify the collecting system or during reversal of airflow during ultrasonic lithotripsy [73]. Clinical signs include sudden hypotension, hypoxemia, tachycardia, and circulatory arrest. A machinery-type murmur (classically termed mill-wheel murmur) can be auscultated over the heart.

Therapy includes immediate cessation of the procedure and placement of large-bore nephrostomy tube. Additionally, the patient is placed in a left lateral decubitus with the head down to trap air in the right atrium which can be aspirated utilizing the central venous access line.

Ureteral Avulsion

Ureteral avulsion represents one of the catastrophic complications following PCNL. Fortunately it is extremely rare and usually the result of overly forceful manipulation of a large or impacted calculus that has been engaged in a basket [74]. The basket should always be withdrawn under direct vision. Such a complication mandates open surgical repair. Safety wires are crucial to avoid ureteral avulsion and should be confirmed to be in proper placement at the onset of the procedure.

Immediate Postoperative Complications

Fever and Sepsis

Preoperative urine culture should be performed routinely for patients undergoing PCNL, Antibiotic therapy for patients with a UTI is generally started at least 1 week prior the procedure. It is recommended to obtain a repeat culture to confirm a sterile urine before the planned surgery. Post procedure antibiotics for 7 days are advised for patients with struvite stone because of the difficulty in clearing bacteruria in these patients.

Postoperative septicemia has been reported to occur in 0.6–1.5 % of patients undergoing PCNL [46,75,78]. Patients develop postoperative fever must be monitored closely for signs of sepsis. Early identification and treatment with antibiotics and large amounts of supportive intravenous fluids, optimal renal drainage, and electrolyte control improves chances for survival.

If pus is encountered during establishing the PCNL access, sample must be taken for analysis and culture. A percutaneous tube is left in the kidney and broad spectrum antibiotic therapy is begun. The procedure is delayed until sterile urine can be demonstrated.

Several studies have evaluated the phenomenon of fever post-PCNL. One paper suggested that those patients pyrexia greater than 38 °C who were hemodynamically stable and with negative preoperative urine culture may have spiked due to nonbacteriologic reasons [76]. More recently, a prospective study evaluated 204 PCNLs performed in 198 patients over a 2-year period [77]. Twenty (9.8 %) patients developed systemic inflammatory response (SIRS) postoperatively, six of whom required intensive care. Preoperative urine culture obtained from the urinary bladder had poor concordance with renal pelvic urine or stone culture obtained on the day of surgery. Multiple access tracts and stone size greater than 10 cm^2 were significant on multivariate analysis for predicting postoperative SIRS. One study found decreased incidence of positive renal pelvic urine and stone culture, SIRS, and endotoxemia in patients with large stone burden or hydronephrosis who were instructed to ingest nitrofurantoin for 1 week prior to surgery [78]. Similar results were seen in another study evaluating ciprofloxacin administration for 1 week prior to PCNL [79]. The PCNLGS also addressed this matter in a report by Gutierrez et al. in which 550 of 5,313 (10.4 %) patients had documented fever postoperatively [80]. Of those with negative preoperative urine culture, 8.8 % developed fever versus 18.2 % of those with positive preoperative urine culture. Positive preoperative urine culture, staghorn calculus, preoperative nephrostomy, lower patient age, and history of diabetes increased the risk of postoperative fever.

Death

Postoperative mortality following PCNL is extremely rare in the contemporary medicine. Old series reported rates varied between 0.1 and 0.3 % [74]. The two major causes of death are myocardial infarction and pulmonary embolism Careful preoperative assessment to identify patients at risk is of paramount importance.

Investigations should include chest X-ray and electrocardiogram and cardiac stress test in patient with risk factors. Sequential compressive devices and early ambulation after the procedure are recommended for every patient undergoing PCNL. Patients at risk of DVT should be given subcutaneous heparin pre procedure.

In case of postoperative DVT with an immature nephrostomy tract, the administration of anticoagulant places the patient at high risk of bleeding. Therefore, an inferior vena cava filter may be considered to prevent the propagation of the thrombus to the lung.

Delayed Complications

Delayed Hemorrhage

Delayed postoperative bleeding requiring intervention and occurs in about 1 % of all PCNL patients. The most common etiology is an arteriovenous fistula or pseudoaneurysm. One study found that stone size was a major predictor for delayed bleeding [81]. Presentation may occur in the postoperative period, at the time of percutaneous nephrostomy tube removal, or several days to weeks later [82, 83].

The patient may present with gross hematuria, dizziness, or shock. Supportive care with IV fluid resuscitation and, if needed, blood transfusion should be initiated. Manual pressure can be applied to the nephrostomy site and if the bleeding is refractory interventional radiology should be consulted for angiography. If the nephrostomy tract is still stented, dilation of a balloon during angiography may help reveal bleeding that would be refractory to tamponade. Selective angiographic embolization is usually successful in this situation. Infrequently, partial or total nephrectomy may be necessary.

Nephrocutaneous Fistula

Nephrocutaneous fistulas after PCNL are unusual. Prolonged drainage from the nephrostomy is usually caused by distal obstruction due to unrecognized stone, ureteral edema, blood clot, infundibular stenosis, or stricture. Typically, resolving the distal pathology is sufficient for closure.

Stricture

The ureteropelvic junction and the proximal ureter are the most susceptible ureteral segments to develop strictures [84]. Strictures develop secondary to intense inflammatory reaction induced by impacted stone or due to surgical manipulation for stone extraction. There are no cases of strictures reported in the contemporary literature following PCNL [33]. However, old series showed an incidence of about 0.2 % [71]. Most cases can be managed by endourological means. Extensive strictures may warrant open repair.

Infundibular Stenosis

In 2002, Parsons et al. reviewed their cases of acquired infundibular stenosis (IS) following PCNL and found that 5 of 223 (2 %) of patients developed IS. The stenosis was most commonly found in the area of the previous PCNL and in some cases up to 1 year after the procedure. The factors contributing to IS were prolonged operative time, a large stone burden requiring multiple percutaneous procedures, and extended postoperative nephrostomy tube drainage. Symptomatic cases were managed by endourologic means. In most cases, only observation was required [85].

Perinephric Hematoma, Urinoma, and Abscess

Perinephric hematomas occur in nearly one-third of patients undergoing PCNL [86]. Perinephric hematoma is usually of little clinical significance. However, if the patient becomes unstable and has a low hematocrit with clear voided urine and nephrostomy tube output, a significant perinephric hematoma should be suspected. Immediate abdominal CT scan should be done to confirm the diagnosis. If conservative managements fails, angioembolization of the bleeding vessels should be attempted, followed by drainage of the collection. In few cases, open surgical exploration may be necessary.

Perinephric urinoma is a rare condition result from a tear in the collecting system with subsequent urine extravasation around the kidney and distal obstruction secondary to stone, blood clot, or ureteral wall edema. Antegrade nephrostogram at the end of the procedure or at the time of nephrostomy tube is important to look for extravasation and distal flow obstruction. Stent placement is required to allow urinoma resolution. Ultrasound-guided percutaneous drainage is necessary in case if conservative management fails.

Case Discussion

GO is a 50-year-old healthy gentleman with a 1.5 cm right renal pelvic stone (Fig. 6.1), who elected to proceed with a PCNL. Preoperative laboratory evaluation was normal. As is customary at our institution, renal access was obtained on the day of surgery by interventional radiology. The patient arrived to the operating room with a Kumpe catheter left above the 12th rib with access to the superior pole calix (Fig. 6.2). Dilation of this tract ensued, initially with a 8–10 Fr obturator/sheath dilator and then with a Bard

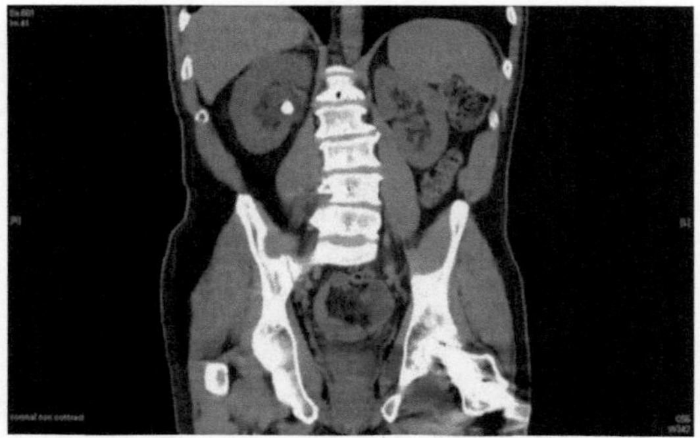

Fig. 6.1 Nonenhanced abdominal-pelvic CT showing a right renal pelvic stone

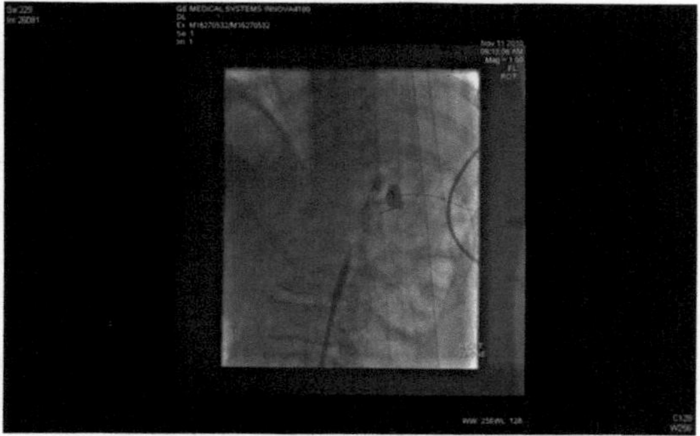

Fig 6.2 An abdominal radiograph showing Kumpe catheter above the 12th rib with access to the superior pole calix

X-Force Balloon dilator to 30 Fr once two wires were through (Fig. 6.3). A 30 Fr renal access sheath was placed over the stiffened balloon, which was then deflated and removed allowing for nephroscopy through the sheath. The stone was adequately fragmented and removed. Flexible nephroscopy and antegrade nephrostogram after lithotomy revealed no residual fragments or extravasation. The renal sheath was removed and a 5 Fr Pollack catheter was left as a safety for access postoperatively. A chest X-ray postoperatively revealed atelectasis without any effusion. On postoperative day #2 the patient experienced an acute desaturation episode and a chest X-ray revealed a large right pleural effusion (Fig. 6.4). Patient underwent a thoracentesis and antegrade nephrostogram. Antegrade nephrostogram revealed a fistula tract, confirming nephropleural fistula and, in the same setting, a

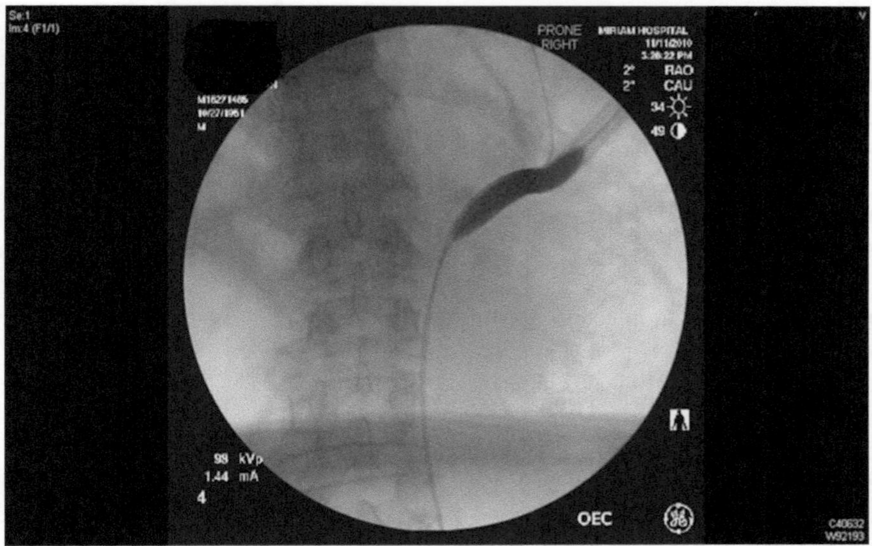

Fig 6.3 A radiograph image demonstrating balloon dilatation of the nephrostomy tract

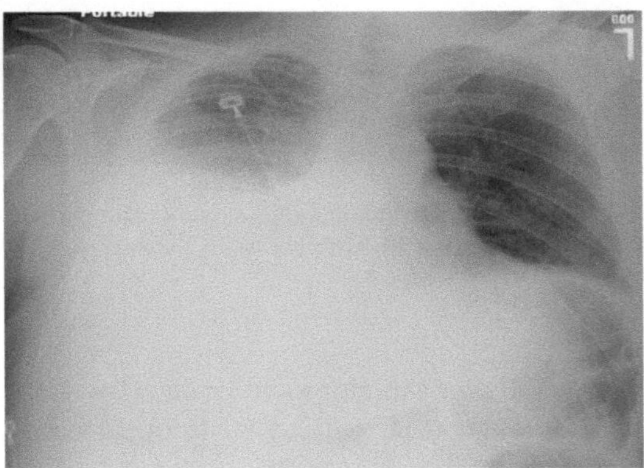

Fig. 6.4 Chest X-ray revealing a large right pleural effusion

JJ ureteral stent was placed in an antegrade fashion to promote drainage of urine down the ureter (Fig. 6.5). In an effort to prevent reflux of urine a Foley catheter was left in place. Aspirated fluid exhibited an elevated creatinine and further confirmed the diagnosis. A 10-Fr pigtail chest tube was ultimately placed and drained nearly 1 L of urine from the patient's thorax. The patient was monitored with chest X-rays and subsequently had his chest-tube removed followed by his Foley catheter and JJ ureteral stent.

There are several points worthy of mention during the review of this case. First, should interventional radiology place the access, clear communication of ideal access should be held prior to the arrival of the patient. Perhaps this complication may have been averted had the access been a mid or lower pole site. Second, the clinician must have a heightened index of suspicion of pleural effusion with or without fistula should the patient develop respiratory symptoms, especially if the access obtained and dilated was supracostal. Third, after prompt recognition, maximal urinary drainage down the ureter can be promoted with the placement of a JJ stent and a Foley catheter. Certainly, removal of any tubes within the original tract is necessary. Further, thoracic drainage is therapeutic of the effusion but also diagnostic of any further drainage. When the thoracic drain fails to drain further, it suggests that urine is no longer being shunted to the thorax. However, the clinician must discern cure of effusion from loculation of fluid in another compartment away from the thoracic drain as the reason for lack of drainage from the thoracic drain. Hence, chest X-ray or CT chest would beneficial in ruling out other sites of pleural effusion inaccessible to the drain prior to removal of the chest tube.

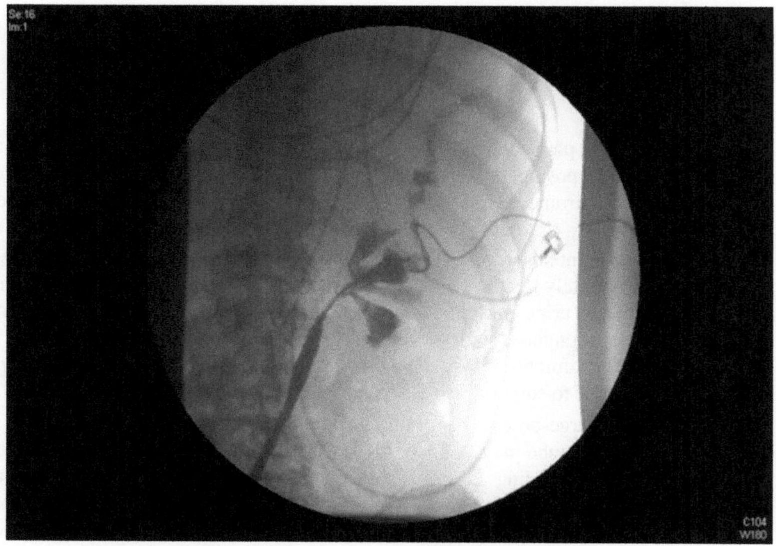

Fig. 6.5 Antegrade nephrostogram showing nephropleural fistula

Appendix 1: Prevention, Identification, and Treatment of Complications of PCNL

	Preventative measures	Identification	Treatment
Intraoperative complications			
Bleeding	Solitary kidney, supracostal access, multiple access at high risk; unideal access at high risk as it may predispose to excessive torqueing	Poor visualization	Tamponade with renal access sheath, if red-out place Kaye tamponade reentry balloon or other large caliber Foley
Collecting system perforation	Avoid excessive pressure with ultrasonic or pneumatic lithotripsy device, ensure there is appropriate visualization and appreciation for anatomy during use of lithotripsy device	Direct visualization of injury or intraoperative antegrade nephrostogram revealing extravasation	Appropriate prolonged decompression of renal pelvis with indwelling JJ ureteral stent vs. PCNU
Colonic injury	Preoperative imaging with CT; prone position may decrease risk for bowel perforation	Stool or gas per PCN, opacification of colon during antegrade nephrostogram	Abort procedure, do not dilate tract (if not already done) withdrawal of PCN to colonic lumen
Liver or splenic injury	Preoperative imaging with CT if hepatomegaly or splenomegaly suspected Laparoscopic access to the collecting system	Excessive blood loss, hemodynamic instability, and severe abdominal pain	Intravenous fluid support and blood transfusion Conservative vs. exploration

(continued)

(continued)

	Preventative measures	Identification	Treatment
Postoperative complications			
Fever	Appropriate pain control and activity postoperatively, incentive spirometry	Routine vital check	Obtain cultures and chest X-ray if indicated, encourage incentive spirometry and ambulation, abx as indicated
Urosepsis	Ensure patient has negative or appropriately treated preoperative urine culture, consider prophylaxis with cipro or nitrofurantoin for 1 week prior to surgery	Consider sending urine and stone culture when patient has large stone or history of recurrent infections	Culture-based antibiotics, ICU setting if patient condition requires
Bleeding	Leaving a large-bore nephrostomy tube may not improve bleeding	Persistent drainage of bloody urine from nephrostomy tube, monitor hgb/hct	Transfuse as indicated, consider ongoing drainage, if persistent anemia consider angiography with or without concurrent access tract dilation to identify if bleeding is venous or arterial
Pulmonary			
Pleural effusion	Avoid supracostal access. Chest intraoperative fluoroscopy	Intraoperative fluoroscopy of costophrenic angle post lithotomy, CXR for any pulmonary symptoms (SOB, desaturation, etc.)	Conservative if small and asymptomatic Thoracostomy tube if large and symptomatic
Nephro-pleural fistula	Avoid supracostal access	Persistent drainage from the thoracostomy tube placed for hydrothorax Nephrostogram Retrograde pyelogram	Thoracostomy tube and ureteral stent
Persistent drainage from percutaneous site	Nephrostogram before removing the nephrostomy tube to make sure that there is no distal ureteral obstruction due to stone fragments or blood clots	Prolonged urinary leakage from the nephrostomy tube site	Ureteral stent and antibiotics

Appendix 2: Percutaneous Nephrilithotomy Complications Rate in Different Major Studies

	de la Rosette [7]	Duvdevani et al. [48]	Tefekli et al. [6]
Number of procedures	5,803	1,585	811
No complications	85.50 %	88.50 %	71.00 %
Fever (temp. > 38.5)	10.50 %	Unknown	2.80 %
Urosepsis	Unknown	1.30 %	0.30 %
Significant bleeding	7.80 %	6.00 %	Unknown
Requiring transfusion	5.70 %	0.80 %	10.90 %
Renal pelvis perforation	3.40 %	1.80 %	1.10 %
Hydrothorax	1.80 %	1.00 %	
Failure to complete procedure	1.70 %	Unknown	0.20 %
Pyelocutaneous fistula	Unknown	0.13 %	Unknown
Colonic perforation	Unknown	0.06 %	0.3 % (neighboring organ injury)
Bladder rupture	Unknown	0.06 %	Unknown

References

1. Fernström I, Johansson B. Percutaneous pyelolithotomy. A new extraction technique. Scand J Urol Nephrol. 1976;10(3):257–9.
2. Snyder JA, Smith AD. Staghorn calculi: percutaneous extraction versus anatrophic nephrolithotomy. J Urol. 1986;136(2):351–4.
3. Preminger GM, Assimos DG, Lingeman JE, Nakada SY, Pearle MS, Wolf JS, et al. Chapter 1: AUA guideline on management of staghorn calculi: diagnosis and treatment recommendations. J Urol. 2005;173(6): 1991–2000.
4. de la Rosette JJ, Zuazu JR, Tsakiris P, Elsakka AM, Zudaire JJ, Laguna MP, et al. Prognostic factors and percutaneous nephrolithotomy morbidity: a multivariate analysis of a contemporary series using the Clavien classification. J Urol. 2008;180(6):2489–93.
5. Dindo D, Demartines N, Clavien PA. Classification of surgical complications: a new proposal with evaluation in a cohort of 6336 patients and results of a survey. Ann Surg. 2004;240(2):205–13.
6. Tefekli A, Ali Karadag M, Tepeler K, Sari E, Berberoglu Y, Baykal M, et al. Classification of percutaneous nephrolithotomy complications using the modified Clavien grading system: looking for a standard. Eur Urol. 2008;53(1):184–90.
7. de la Rosette JJ, Assimos D, Desai M, Gutierrez J, Lingeman J, Scarpa R, et al. The Clinical Research Office of the Endourological Society Percutaneous Nephrolithotomy Global Study: indications, complications, and outcomes in 5803 patients. J Endourol. 2011;25(1):11–7.
8. Stanger MJ, Thompson LA, Young AJ, Lieberman HR. Anticoagulant activity of select dietary supplements. Nutr Rev. 2012;70(2):107–17.
9. Opondo D, Tefekli A, Esen T, Labate G, Sangam K, De Lisa A, et al. Impact of case volumes on the outcomes of percutaneous nephrolithotomy. Eur Urol. 2012;62(6):1181–7.
10. de la Rosette JJ, Laguna MP, Rassweiler JJ, Conort P. Training in percutaneous nephrolithotomy – a critical review. Eur Urol. 2008;54(5):994–1001.
11. Allen D, O'Brien T, Tiptaft R, Glass J. Defining the learning curve for percutaneous nephrolithotomy. J Endourol. 2005;19(3):279–82.
12. Tanriverdi O, Boylu U, Kendirci M, Kadihasanoglu M, Horasanli K, Miroglu C. The learning curve in the training of percutaneous nephrolithotomy. Eur Urol. 2007;52(1):206–11.
13. Sahin A, Atsü N, Erdem E, Oner S, Bilen C, Bakkaloğlu M, et al. Percutaneous nephrolithotomy in patients aged 60 years or older. J Endourol. 2001;15(5):489–91.
14. Okeke Z, Smith AD, Labate G, D'Addessi A, Venkatesh R, Assimos D, et al. Prospective comparison of outcomes of percutaneous nephrolithotomy in elderly patients versus younger patients. J Endourol. 2012;26(8):996–1001.
15. Resorlu B, Diri A, Atmaca AF, Tuygun C, Oztuna D, Bozkurt OF, et al. Can we avoid percutaneous nephrolithotomy in high-risk elderly patients using the Charlson comorbidity index? Urology. 2012;79(5): 1042–7.
16. Carson 3rd CC, Danneberger JE, Weinerth JL. Percutaneous lithotripsy in morbid obesity. J Urol. 1988;139(2):243–5.
17. El-Assmy AM, Shokeir AA, El-Nahas AR, Shoma AM, Eraky I, El-Kenawy MR, et al. Outcome of percutaneous nephrolithotomy: effect of body mass index. Eur Urol. 2007;52(1):199–204.
18. Koo BC, Burtt G, Burgess NA. Percutaneous stone surgery in the obese: outcome stratified according to body mass index. BJU Int. 2004;93(9):1296–9.
19. Bagrodia A, Gupta A, Raman JD, Bensalah K, Pearle MS, Lotan Y. Impact of body mass index on cost and clinical outcomes after percutaneous nephrostolithotomy. Urology. 2008;72(4):756–60.
20. Tomaszewski JJ, Smaldone MC, Schuster T, Jackman SV, Averch TD. Outcomes of percutaneous nephrolithotomy stratified by body mass index. J Endourol. 2010;24(4):547–50.
21. Bucuras V, Gopalakrishnam G, Wolf JS Jr, Sun Y, Bianchi G, Erdogru T, et al. The Clinical Research Office of the Endourological Society Percutaneous Nephrolithotomy Global Study: nephrolithotomy in 189 patients with solitary kidneys. J Endourol. 2012;26(4):336–41.
22. Husmann DA, Miliner DS, Segura JW. Ureteropelvic junction obstruction with a simultaneous renal calculus: long-term followup. J Urol. 1995;153: 1399–402.
23. Tunc L, Tokgoz H, Tan MO, Kupeli B, Karaoglan U, Bozkirli I. Stones in anomalous kidneys: results of treatment by shock wave lithotripsy in 150 patients. Int J Urol. 2004;11(10):831–6.
24. Mosavi-Bahar SH, Amirzargar MA, Rahnavardi M, Moghaddam SM, Babbolhavaeji H, Amirhasani S. Percutaneous nephrolithotomy in patients with kidney malformations. J Endourol. 2007;21(5):520–4.
25. Rana AM, Bhojwani JP. Percutaneous nephrolithotomy in renal anomalies of fusion, ectopia, rotation, hypoplasia, and pelvicalyceal aberration: uniformity in heterogeneity. J Endourol. 2009;23(4):609–14.
26. Gupta NP, Mishra S, Seth A, Anand A. Percutaneous nephrolithotomy in abnormal kidneys: single-center experience. Urology. 2009;73(4):710–4.
27. Krambeck AE, Leroy AJ, Patterson DE, Gettman MT. Percutaneous nephrolithotomy success in the transplant kidney. J Urol. 2008;180(6):2545–9.
28. Basiri A, Karrami H, Moghaddam SM, Shadpour P. Percutaneous nephrolithotomy in patients with or without a history of open nephrolithotomy. J Endourol. 2003;17(4):213–6.
29. Sofikerim M, Demirci D, Gülmez I, Karacagil M. Does previous open nephrolithotomy affect the outcome of percutaneous nephrolithotomy? J Endourol. 2007;21(4):401–3.
30. Yuruk E, Tefekli A, Sari E, Karadag MA, Tepeler A, Binbay M, et al. Does previous extracorporeal shock

wave lithotripsy affect the performance and outcome of percutaneous nephrolithotomy? J Urol. 2009; 182(5):2534–5.

31. Xue W, Pacik D, Boellaard W, Breda A, Botoca M, Rassweiler J, et al. Management of single large non-staghorn renal stones in the CROES PCNL global study. J Urol. 2012;187(4):1293–7.
32. Desai M, De Lisa A, Turna B, Rioja J, Walfridsson H, D'Addessi A, et al. The clinical research office of the endourological society percutaneous nephrolithotomy global study: staghorn versus nonstaghorn stones. J Endourol. 2011;25(8):1263–8.
33. Singla M, Srivastava A, Kapoor R, Gupta N, Ansari MS, Dubey D, et al. Aggressive approach to staghorn calculi-safety and efficacy of multiple tracts percutaneous nephrolithotomy. Urology. 2008;71(6):1039–42.
34. Duty B, Okhunov Z, Smith A, Okeke Z. The debate over percutaneous nephrolithotomy positioning: a comprehensive review. J Urol. 2011;186(1):20–5.
35. Tomaszewski JJ, Ortiz TD, Gayed BA, Smaldone MC, Jackman SV, Averch TD. Renal access by urologist or radiologist during percutaneous nephrolithotomy. J Endourol. 2010;24(11):1733–7.
36. Wang KJ, Jiang LH, Wang L, Li H. 356 Urologist versus radiologist for percutaneous nephrolithotomy access under fluoroscopic guidance: a systematic review. Eur Urol. 2010;9(2):135.
37. Watterson JD, Soon S, Jana K. Access related complications during percutaneous nephrolithotomy: urology versus radiology at a single academic institution. J Urol. 2006;176(1):142–5.
38. Safak M, Gögüş C, Soygür T. Nephrostomy tract dilation using a balloon dilator in percutaneous renal surgery: experience with 95 cases and comparison with the fascial dilator system. Urol Int. 2003;71(4):382–4.
39. Davidoff R, Bellman GC. Influence of technique of percutaneous tract creation on incidence of renal hemorrhage. J Urol. 1997;157(4):1229–31.
40. Gönen M, Istanbulluoglu OM, Cicek T, Ozturk B, Ozkardes H. Balloon dilatation versus Amplatz dilatation for nephrostomy tract dilatation. J Endourol. 2008;22:901–4.
41. Benway BM, Nakada SY. Balloon dilation of nephrostomy tracts. J Endourol. 2008;22(9):1875–6.
42. Yamaguchi A, Skolarikos A, Buchholz NP, Chomón GB, Grasso M, Saba P, et al. Operating times and bleeding complications in percutaneous nephrolithotomy: a comparison of tract dilation methodsin 5537 patients in the Clinical Research Office of the Endourological Society Percutaneous Nephrolithotomy Global Study. J Endourol. 2011;25(6):933–9.
43. Berrington de González A, Mahesh M, Kim KP, Bhargavan M, Lewis R, Mettler F, et al. Projected cancer risks from computed tomographic scans performed in the United States in 2007. Arch Intern Med. 2009;169(22):2071–7.
44. Berrington de González A, Mahesh M, Kim KP, Bhargavan M, Lewis R, et al. Factors affecting patient radiation exposure during percutaneous nephrolithotomy. J Urol. 2010;184(6):2373–7.
45. Amer T, Ahmed K, Bultitude M. Standard versus tubeless percutaneous nephrolithotomy: a systematic review. Urol Int. 2012;88(4):373–82.
46. Bellman C, Davidoff R, Candela J, Gerspach J, Kurtz S, Stout L. Tubeless percutaneous renal surgery. J Urol. 1997;157(5):1578–82.
47. Stoller ML, Wolf Jr JS, St Lezin MA. Estimated blood loss and transfusion rates associated with percutaneous nephrolithotomy. J Urol. 1994;152(6 Pt 1):1977–81.
48. Duvdevani M, Razvi H, Sofer M, Beiko DT, Nott L, Chew BH, et al. Third prize: contemporary percutaneous nephrolithotripsy: 1585 procedures in 1338 consecutive patients. J Endourol. 2007;21(8):824–9.
49. Sampaio FJB. Surgical anatomy of the kidney. In: Smith AD, Badlani GH, Kavoussi LR, editors. Smith's textbook of endourology. St Louis: Quality Medical Publishing; 1996. p. 153–84.
50. Martin X, Murat FJ, Feitosa LC, Rouvière O, Lyonnet D, Gelet A, et al. Severe bleeding after nephrolithotomy: results of hyperselective embolization. Eur Urol. 2000;37(2):136–9.
51. Lam HS, Lingeman JE, Mosbaugh PG, Steele RE, Knapp PM, Scott JW, et al. Evolution of the technique of combination therapy for staghorn calculi: a decreasing role for extracorporeal shock wave lithotripsy. J Urol. 1992;148(3 Pt 2):1058–62.
52. Dore B, Conort P, Irani J, Amiel J, Ferriere JM, Glemain P, et al. Percutaneous nephrolithotomy (PCNL) in subjects over the age of 70: a multicentre retrospective study of 210 cases. Prog Urol. 2004;14: 1140–5.
53. Turna B, Nazli O, Demiryoguran S, Mammadov R, Cal C. Percutaneous nephrolithotomy: variables that influence hemorrhage. Urology. 2007;69(4):603–7.
54. El-Nahas AR, Shokeir AA, El-Assmy AM, Mohsen T, Shoma AM, Eraky I, et al. Postpercutaneous nephrolithotomy extensive hemorrhage: a study of risk factors. J Urol. 2007;177(2):576–9.
55. Kerbl K, Picus DD, Clayman RV. Clinical experience with the Kaye nephrostomy tamponade catheter. Eur Urol. 1994;25(2):94–8.
56. Munver R, Delvecchio FC, Newman GE, Preminger GM. Critical analysis of supracostal access for percutaneous renal surgery. J Urol. 2001;166(4):1242–6.
57. Lojanapiwat B, Prasopsuk S. Upper-pole access for percutaneous nephrolithotomy: comparison of supracostal and infracostal approaches. J Endourol. 2006; 20(7):491–4.
58. Hopper KD, Sherman JI, Williams MD, Ghaed N. The variable anteroposterior position of the retropertoneal colon to the kidneys. Invest Radiol. 1987;22(4): 298–302.
59. Hadar H, Gadoth N. Positional relations of colon and kidney determined by perirenal fat. AJR Am J Roentgenol. 1984;143(4):773–6.

60. Neustein P, Barbaric ZL, Kaufman JJ. Nephrocolic fistula: a complication of percutaneous nephrostolithotomy. J Urol. 1986;135(3):571–3.
61. Appel R, Musmanno MC, Knight JG. Nephrocolic fistula complicating percutaneous nephrostolithotomy. J Urol. 1988;140(5):1007–8.
62. Culkin DJ, Wheeler Jr JS, Canning JR. Nephro-duodenal fistula: a complication of percutaneous nephrolithotomy. J Urol. 1985;134(3):528–30.
63. Kumar A, Banerjee GK, Tewari A, Srivastava A. Isolated duodenal injury during relook percutaneous nephrolithotomy. Br J Urol. 1994;74(3):382–3.
64. Hopper KD, Yakes WF. The posterior intercostal approach for percutaneous renal procedures: risk of puncturing the lung, spleen, and liver as determined by CT. AJR Am J Roentgenol. 1990;154(1):115–7.
65. Kondás J, Szentgyörgyi E, Váczi L, Kiss A. Splenic injury: a rare complication of percutaneous nephrolithotomy. Int Urol Nephrol. 1994;(4)26:399–404.
66. Thomas AA, Pierce G, Walsh RM, Sands M, Noble M. Splenic injury during percutaneous nephrolithotomy. JSLS. 2009;13(2):233–6.
67. Kontothanassis D, Bissas A. Biliary peritonitis complicating percutaneous nephrostomy. Int Urol Nephrol. 1997;29(5):529–31.
68. Saxby MF. Biliary peritonitis following percutaneous nephrolithotomy. Br J Urol. 1996;77(3):465–6.
69. Fisher MB, Bianco Jr F, Carlin AM, Triest JA. Biliary peritonitis complicating percutaneous nephrolithomy requiring laparoscopic cholecystectomy. J Urol. 2004;171(2 Pt 1):791–2.
70. Roberts S, Bolton DM, Stoller ML. Hypothermia associated with percutaneous nephrolithotomy. Urology. 1994;44(6):832–5.
71. Lee WJ, Smith AD, Cubelli V, Badlani GH, Lewin B, Vernace F, et al. Complications of percutaneous nephrolithotomy. AJR Am J Roentgenol. 1987;148(1):177–80.
72. Lingeman JE, Coury TA, Newman DM, Kahnoski RJ, Mertz JH, Mosbaugh PG, et al. Comparison of results and morbidity of percutaneous nephrostolithotomy and extracorporeal shock wave lithotripsy. J Urol. 1987;138(3):485–90.
73. Cadeddu JA, Arrindell D, Moore RG. Near fatal air embolism during percutaneous nephrostomy placement. J Urol. 1997;158(4):1519.
74. Segura JW, Patterson DE, LeRoy AJ, Williams HJ Jr, Barrett DM, Benson RC Jr, et al. Percutaneous removal of kidney stones: review of 1,000 cases. J Urol. 1985;134(6):1077–81.
75. Lang EK. Percutaneous nephrostolithotomy and lithotripsy: a multi-institutional survey of complications. Radiology. 1987;162(1 Pt 1):25–30.
76. Cadeddu JA, Chen R, Bishoff J, Micali S, Kumar A, Moore RG, et al. Clinical significance of fever after percutaneous nephrolithotomy. Urology. 1998;52(1):48–50.
77. Korets R, Graversen JA, Kates M, Mues AC, Gupta M. Post-percutaneous nephrolithotomy systemic inflammatory response: a prospective analysis of preoperative urine, renal pelvic urine and stone cultures. J Urol. 2011;186(5):1899–903.
78. Bag S, Kumar S, Taneja N, Sharma V, Mandal AK, Singh SK. One week of nitrofurantoin before percutaneous nephrolithotomy significantly reduces upper tract infection and urosepsis: a prospective controlled study. Urology. 2011;77(1):45–9.
79. Mariappan P, Smith G, Moussa SA, Tolley DA. One week of ciprofloxacin before percutaneous nephrolithotomy significantly reduces upper tract infection and urosepsis: a prospective controlled study. BJU Int. 2006;98(5):1075–9.
80. Gutierrez J, Smith A, Geavlete P, Shah H, Kural AR, de Sio M, et al. Urinary tract infections and post-operative fever in percutaneous nephrolithotomy. World J Urol. 2012. [Epub ahead of print].
81. Srivastava A, Singh KJ, Suri A. Vascular complications after percutaneous nephrolithotomy: are there any predictive factors? Urology. 2005;66(1):38–40.
82. Patterson DE, Segura JW, LeRoy AJ, Benson RC Jr, May G. The etiology and treatment of delayed bleeding following percutaneous lithotripsy. J Urol. 1985;133(3):447–51.
83. Sacha K, Szewczyk W, Bar K. Massive haemorrhage presenting as a complication after percutaneous nephrolithotomy. Int Urol Nephrol. 1996;28(3):315–8.
84. Roth RA, Beckmann CF. Complications of extracorporeal shock-wave lithotripsy and percutaneous nephrolithotomy. Urol Clin North Am. 1988;15(2):155–66.
85. Parsons JK, Jarrett TW, Lancini V, Kavoussi LR. Infundibular stenosis after percutaneous nephrolithotomy. J Urol. 2002;167(1):35–8.
86. Chichakli R, Krause R, Voelzke B, Turk T. Incidence of perinephric hematoma after percutaneous nephrolithotomy. J Endourol. 2008;22(6):1227–32.

7 Ureteroscopic Access: Sheaths, Balloons, and Wireless Approaches

Sara L. Best

Introduction

Since the first ureteroscopy performed by Hugh Hampton Young in 1912 with a pediatric cystoscope [1], there has been extensive technological advancement in the equipment available for endoscopic evaluation and management of the ureter and upper urinary tract. The ureteroscopes themselves have become smaller in diameter and improvements in optics have substantially enhanced visualization. Today's actively deflectable flexible scopes are able to reach most locations within the upper tract to target urinary calculi and tumors found there.

There are a variety of methods in which these ureteroscopes can be passed into the ureter and collecting system. In this chapter, we will review several options for ureteroscopic access, including methods to dilate the ureter should this be necessary.

Initial Steps for Ureteroscopic Access

In preparing to perform ureteroscopy, a variety of wires should be available to gain access to the ureter, since most of the tools used during ureteroscopy (catheters, balloons, dilators, sheaths, and scopes) are passed over these wires in the Seldinger technique [2].

Guidewire Placement

In general, the first step of most ureteroscopic procedures is the retrograde placement of a floppy-tipped guidewire through the ureteral orifice, up through the ureteral lumen to coil in the renal pelvis or one of the calices. Prior to placing this wire, consideration should be given to performing a retrograde pyelogram to map out the ureteral and renal anatomy and guide wire-positioning. The guidewire is then typically passed through the ureteral orifice under cystoscopic and fluoroscopic guidance, such that the distal portion of the wire extends out the patient's urethra.

The choice of guidewire depends on the indication for surgery and the anticipated anatomy. In most cases, a standard PTFE-coated guidewire measuring 0.035 in. or 0.038 in. in diameter can be used as the initial access wire. However, in the setting of obstruction, such as the presence of a ureteral stone, a standard guidewire may not readily bypass the area of obstruction and other access techniques may be helpful. In these cases, a hydrophilic "glidewire" may bypass the obstruction more easily. Once a hydrophilic wire has passed beyond the stone or other lesion, a 5 Fr open-ended ureteral catheter can be passed over it and the wire exchanged for a more secure standard guidewire.

S.L. Best, M.D. (✉)
Department of Urology, University of Wisconsin School of Medicine and Public Health, Madison, WI, USA
e-mail: best@urology.wisc.edu

S.Y. Nakada and M.S. Pearle (eds.), *Surgical Management of Urolithiasis: Percutaneous, Shockwave and Ureteroscopy*, DOI 10.1007/978-1-4614-6937-7_7,

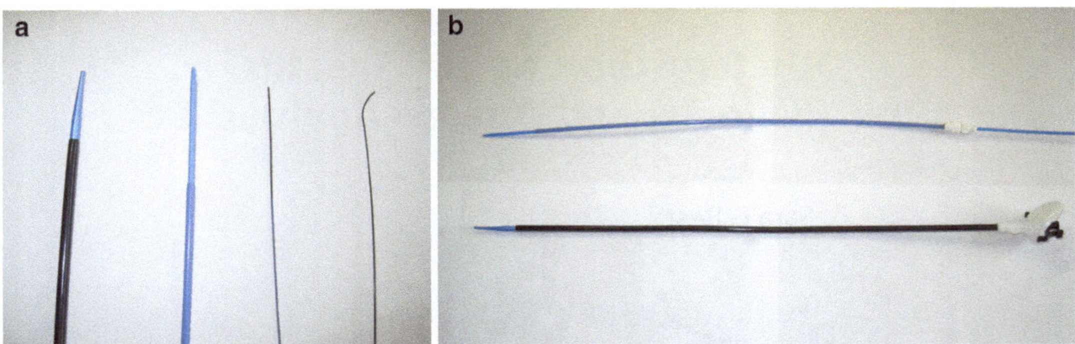

Fig. 7.1 (**a**, from *left* to *right*) Ureteral access sheath, with the inner obturator being *lighter blue* in color; 2-piece 8/10 Fr ureteral dilator; 0.035-in. hybrid wire, a PTFE-coated (*blue*) with a hydrophilic floppy tip (*black*); angled hydrophilic "glidewire." (**b**) 2-piece 8/10 Fr ureteral dilator (*top*). To dilate the ureter, both components are passed together over the working wire. A second wire can then be added by removing the 8 Fr portion (*lighter blue*). A ureteral access sheath (*bottom*) also consists of two parts, both of which are inserted together over the working wire. The inner obturator (*light blue*) is then removed to allow insertion of the ureteroscope

Some surgeons prefer to use a combination wire, such as the Sensor™ (Boston Scientific, Natick, MA) wire, which consists of a standard PTFE-coated wire with the floppy portion being composed of a hydrophilic material (Fig. 7.1).

If difficulty persists despite use of a hydrophilic wire, there are additional techniques that can be used to achieve wire placement. A 5 Fr ureteral catheter can be passed under fluoroscopic guidance over the wire to a position just below the stone or area of difficulty. At this point, the wire can be temporarily removed from the catheter lumen and contrast instilled through the catheter to further define the anatomy (this process can also, in the case of a ureteral stone, sometimes be enough to move the stone sufficiently that a wire can "sneak" past it more easily). A hydrophilic wire, either straight or with a curved/angled end (Fig. 7.1), can then be re-advanced through the ureteral catheter. In some cases, the use of the ureteral catheter straightens the ureter enough to change the angle of the wire tip, improving the odds of bypassing the obstructing lesion.

Finally, should these techniques fail, a "last resort option" in some cases can be to place the safety wire under direct ureteroscopic vision. This option may be best suited to the treatment of impacted stones in the distal ureter, where the ureteral wall is thicker and a semirigid ureteroscope can more safely be advanced into the ureter under direct guidance. Once the stone is visualized with the scope, a guidewire can be passed through the working channel and be directed around the stone at a favorable-appearing location.

Ureteroscope Placement

Once a safety wire has been coiled in the renal collecting system, the next step depends on the indication for the procedure and the type of ureteroscope that will be used.

Many modern semirigid ureteroscopes, with their narrow tips measuring 4.0–7.2 Fr, can be passed into the ureter alongside the safety wire without any more formal dilation of the ureteral orifice. If there is any resistance to scope advancement, the procedure should be halted and a method of ureteral dilation employed, as described below.

For most flexible ureteroscopic procedures, both a safety wire and a second working wire will be needed. This second wire can be added by passing a dual-lumen 10 Fr catheter over the safety wire under fluoroscopic guidance and then inserting the second wire through the open lumen. Another instrument available for this task in a paired 8/10 Fr dilator set, where the 8 Fr portion functions as an obturator, tapered to the size of a wire (Fig. 7.1). This 8 Fr portion can then be removed once the set has been passed over the safety wire and a second wire advanced through the 10 Fr component before it, too, is removed. This technique often provides

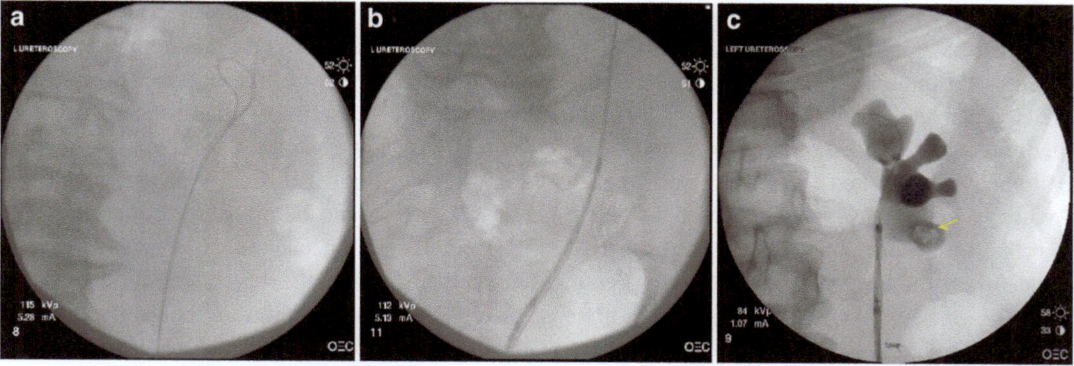

Fig. 7.2 Ureteroscopic insertion using the Seldinger technique. First, two wires (a "working" wire and a "safety" wire) are passed under fluoroscopic and cystoscopic guidance to curl in the renal pelvis (**a**). The flexible ureteroscope is then backloaded onto the working wire and passed into the ureter under fluoroscopic visualization, while holding tension on the wire (**b**). Once the scope is advanced all the way into the renal pelvis (**c**), the working wire can be removed, freeing up the working channel in the scope. A retrograde pyelogram here shows the position of the wire and ureteroscope, as well as a lower pole calculus (*arrow*)

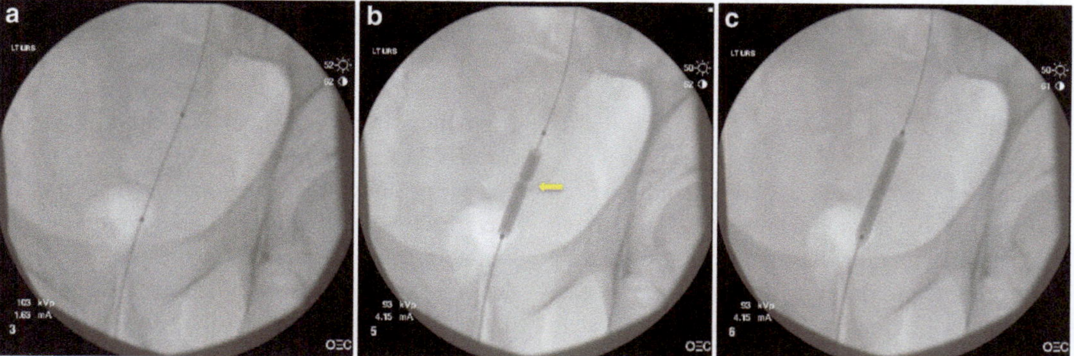

Fig. 7.3 Fluoroscopic images of a ureteral balloon dilator, passed over a working wire. The radio-opaque markers that designate the inflatable segment of the balloon can be easily seen on the pre-inflation image (**a**). Once the balloon is in good position in the distal ureter, it is slowly inflated with half-strength contrast medium, using a pressure syringe (**b**). As the balloon is inflated, often a "waist" will appear (*arrow*), corresponding with a tight spot in the ureter. This waist usually disappears upon full inflation of the balloon (**c**), even at low pressures

sufficient dilation to permit passage of a modern flexible ureteroscope into the ureter. At this point, a flexible ureteroscope can be backloaded over the working wire and advanced under fluoroscopic guidance into the desired location in the ureter or renal pelvis (Fig. 7.2).

Balloon Dilation

Should advancement of the ureteroscope fail, the most common site for the scope to "hang up" is the ureteral orifice/intramural tunnel. One easy modification that can sometimes overcome this is rotating the scope 180° so that the beveled tip faces anteriorly and then gently trying to advance the scope again. If this does not work, dilation of the distal ureter can be accomplished with a balloon dilator. The inflatable portion of these balloons is typically 4–10 cm in length and, while numerous diameters are available, a 12–15 Fr balloon diameter is typically appropriate for this task. These balloons have radio-opaque markers at the proximal and distal ends, which can be used to position the balloon over the working wire using fluoroscopy (Fig. 7.3). Direct visualization of the balloon position can also be accomplished by backloading a cystoscope over the wire first. This can be useful in order to make sure that the ureteral orifice itself is dilated.

Once the balloon is in position in the distal ureter, it can be inflated with half-strength contrast medium using a pressure gauge syringe. Each balloon comes marked with its pressure capacity (typically 17–20 atm.), beyond which the balloon is prone to rupture, but rarely is it necessary to inflate to the maximal pressure. Often, a pressure of 5–7 atm. will suffice to dilate the ureter. Balloon inflation should take place under fluoroscopic guidance and be conducted slowly so that the surgeon can see if a "waist" appears, suggesting a narrow or tight place in the ureter (Fig. 7.3). This waist will often disappear quickly even at low pressure. The balloon can then be deflated and removed, leaving the working wire in place so that the ureteroscope can be advanced over it into the ureter.

"Wireless" Approaches

As has been described, a wire extending from the renal pelvis, down the ureter and out through the patient's urethra, has multiple uses during ureteroscopy, providing a working wire to pass instruments Seldinger-style or to place a stent should the procedure need to be aborted. However, in some cases, the urologist may find this wire obtrusive. For example, the passage of a safety wire at the start of a diagnostic ureteroscopy may disturb a ureteral lesion or "scuff" the ureteral mucosa, impairing the surgeon's ability to identify malignancy. The urologist can avoid these visual inaccuracies by considering careful direct visualization of the distal ureter with a semirigid ureteroscope passed *without* a safety wire. Once the distal ureter has been examined, the position the scope tip can be noted fluoroscopically and a working wire passed through the ureteroscope only as far as the rigid scope has examined, such that none of the unvisualized mucosa is exposed to potential wire trauma. Then, the semirigid scope can be removed, leaving the wire in position, and a flexible ureteroscope passed over the wire into the ureter. The wire can then be removed and the scope carefully advanced up the ureter under direct vision. While this approach allows the urothelial lining of the ureter and collecting system to be visualized without the influence of wire trauma, if resistance to scope passage or any other technical difficulty is encountered, a safety wire should be inserted through the ureteroscope working channel to minimize risk to the ureter. Similarly, after successful endoscopy is completed, consideration should be given to passing a safety wire into the renal pelvis under direct vision through the ureteroscope, before the scope is backed out of the ureter. This way, if any ureteral perforation is noted on pullback ureteroscopy, a stent can easily be placed.

Similarly, a wireless approach may be useful during the ureteroscopic lithotripsy of calyceal stones, if the wire is found to be obtrusive. A working wire is used to advance the ureterscope all the way into the renal pelvis via standard Seldinger-technique. The wire is then removed from the working channel and lithotripsy performed. In this approach, as long as the scope is kept at or above the ureteropelvic junction, the ureteroscope itself functions like a safety wire, maintaining access across the ureter. After lithotripsy is complete, the wire is reinserted through the working channel to coil in the upper tract under direct vision and the scope is backed out, leaving the wire in place to facilitate stent placement if needed. This technique has been reported by several authors with no ureteral perforations or avulsions [3, 4].

Ureteral Access Sheath

Another approach to ureteroscopic access involves the use of a ureteral access sheath. These disposable devices, available from several manufacturers, typically consist of two components, the kink-resistant sheath itself and an inner obturator that tapers to the diameter of the working wire and functions to dilate the ureter during sheath insertion (Fig. 7.1). These devices are available in a variety of diameters from 10/12 to 14/16 Fr, with the first number describing the inner diameter of the sheath and the second number, the outer diameter. They are also available in lengths from 20 to 55 cm to accommodate variations in patient body habitus and surgical indication.

Clinical Utility

There are several potential advantages provided by a ureteral access sheath. Several authors have reported the use of a 12/14 Fr or larger diameter sheath to minimize the rise in intrarenal pressures while maximizing irrigation flow, which can improve visualization [5–7]. Sheaths are also useful if the surgeon plans multiple passages of the scope up and down the ureter, such as extracting stone fragments. Use of an access sheath in these cases makes repeated scope passage much easier and likely safer [8]. Finally, some surgeons performing ureteroscopic biopsy of lesions such as upper tract transitional cell carcinoma find that use of a sheath preserves specimen integrity, since the sheath keeps the ureter walls from "scraping" the specimen off the biopsy forceps [9]. A summary of the findings of several studies reporting the use of ureteral access sheaths can be found in Table 7.1.

Technique

Ureteroscopy using an access sheath begins with the retrograde placement of two wires into the renal pelvis. The working wire should be an extra-stiff wire to minimize the risk that the wire will buckle and allow the obturator tip to perforate the ureter. The access sheath should be thoroughly dampened with saline or water to make sure the hydrophilic coating is adequately lubricious. It is then passed over the working wire under fluoroscopic guidance, leaving the safety wire secured in place, next to the sheath. It is possible to perforate the ureter during sheath advancement, so the surgeon should take careful note of any resistance met during placement. After the sheath is positioned, the obturator and working wire are removed, completing sheath deployment.

In some cases, sheath deployment is not possible. Potential causes for this are buckling of the sheath (typically in males), small ureteral caliber, or obstruction from stricture, stone, or other cause. The surgeon should be alert for these possibilities and not try to force the sheath. If the surgeon does not suspect obstruction, consideration can be given to first trying to pass just the smaller caliber internal, obturator portion of the device. This may gently dilate the ureter and allow the combined sheath/obturator to advance successfully on repassage. If the sheath still does not advance as far as desired but is deployed at least into the distal ureter, the sheath can be left in position and the obturator/wire removed to allow ureteroscopic inspection of the area causing resistance. This will allow the surgeon to see if there is an obstructing stone or stricture present. In some cases, deployment of the sheath only as far as the distal or mid-ureter is sufficient to the task at hand and the procedure can proceed. If not, sheath placement can be abandoned and one of the other ureteroscopic access techniques can be used or a stent placed to allow passive ureteral dilation and repeat attempt after a few days.

Upon completion of the planned ureteroscopic task (lithotripsy, biopsy, etc.), the ureter should be carefully inspected for any possible tears as the scope is removed from the upper tract. The sheath should be simultaneously extracted as the scope is withdrawn, such that the entire ureter is directly visualized. If ureteral injury is identified, a stent should be left for several weeks postoperatively, depending on the degree of injury. Even if no injury is seen, temporary placement of a ureteral stent should be strongly considered after access sheath deployment, as some authors have reported a significant number of patients experiencing colic if none is left [10].

Summary

Reduced ureteroscope caliber and better optics have broadened the range of suitable tasks for modern ureteroscopes. The urologist should develop comfort with a variety of ureteral access techniques to maximize success in a wide range of clinical situations.

Table 7.1 Summary of findings from several investigations reporting outcomes using ureteral access sheaths

Study	Number of procedures	Mean stone size (mm)	Inability to pass sheath	Stone fragments extracted?	Definition of "stone-free"	Stone-free rate	Imaging type	Mean follow-up	Complications
L'Esperance et al. [11]	256 total 173 UAS 83 no UAS	8.7 7.3 (p=0.07)	10 %	No	No stones seen	79 % 67 % (p=0.042)	IVU, CT if contrast allergy	NR (methods report imaging routinely obtained 2 months post-op)	NR
Delvecchio et al. [12]	71 UAS	10.7	NR	Yes	No stones seen	77.4 %	IVU vs. CT	332 days	1.4 % stricture
Kourambas et al. [8]	62 total 30 UAS 32 no UAS	13.7 10.1 (p=0.272)	0 % (but balloon dilation required in 2/30)	NR	NR	78.9 % 85.7 % (p=0.78)	IVU vs. CT	3 months	No strictures UAS group UTI (1) Urinary retention (1) Deep vein thrombosis (1) Return to OR for stent (1) No UAS group Stent migration (1)
Gorin et al. [9]	85 (ureteroscopic biopsies)	NA	2.4 %	NA	NA	Sufficient tissue 90.4 %	NR	NR	None (specifically reported no strictures)

NR not reported, *NA* not applicable, *UAS* ureteral access sheath, *IVU* intravenous urography

References

1. Young HH, McKay RW. Congenital valvular obstruction of the prostatic urethra. Surg Gynecol Obstet. 1929;48:509–12.
2. Seldinger SI. Catheter replacement of the needle in percutaneous arteriography; a new technique. Acta Radiol. 1953;39(5):368–76.
3. Dickstein RJ, Kreshover JE, Babayan RK, Wang DS. Is a safety wire necessary during routine flexible ureteroscopy? J Endourol. 2010;24(10):1589–92.
4. Patel SR, McLaren ID, Nakada SY. The ureteroscope as a safety wire for ureteronephroscopy. J Endourol. 2012;26(4):351–4.
5. Auge BK, Pietrow PK, Lallas CD, Raj GV, Santa-Cruz RW, Preminger GM. Ureteral access sheath provides protection against elevated renal pressures during routine flexible ureteroscopic stone manipulation. J Endourol. 2004;18(1):33–6.
6. Ng YH, Somani BK, Dennison A, Kate SG, Nabi G, Brown S. Irrigant flow and intrarenal pressure during flexible ureteroscopy: the effect of different access sheaths, working channel instruments, and hydrostatic pressure. J Endourol. 2010;24(12):1915–20.
7. Rehman J, Monga M, Landman J, Lee DI, Felfela T, Condradie MC, et al. Characterization of intrapelvic pressure during ureteropyeloscopy with ureteral access sheaths. Urology. 2003;61(4):713–8.
8. Kourambas J, Byrne RR, Preminger GM. Does a ureteral access sheath facilitate ureteroscopy? J Urol. 2001;165(3):789–93.
9. Gorin MA, Santos Cortes JA, Kyle CC, Carey RI, Bird VG. Initial clinical experience with use of ureteral access sheaths in the diagnosis and treatment of upper tract urothelial carcinoma. Urology. 2011;78(3): 523–7.
10. Rapoport D, Perks AE, Teichman JM. Ureteral access sheath use and stenting in ureteroscopy: effect on unplanned emergency room visits and cost. J Endourol. 2007;21(9):993–7.
11. L'esperance JO, Ekeruo WO, Scales CD Jr, Marguet CG, Springhart WP, Maloney ME, et al. Effect of ureteral access sheath on stone-free rates in patients undergoing ureteroscopic management of renal calculi. Urology. 2005;66(2):252–5.
12. Delvecchio FC, Auge BK, Brizuela RM, Weizer AZ, Silverstein AD, Lallas CD, et al. Assessment of stricture formation with the ureteral access sheath. Urology. 2003;61(3):518–22. discussion 522.

Ureteroscopy for Ureteral Stones: Case Discussion of Impacted Stone

8

Devon Snow-Lisy and Manoj Monga

Technological advances have led to remarkable improvements in the outcomes after ureteroscopy (URS) for ureteral stones. A landmark systematic review and comprehensive analysis of outcomes in 2007 by the American Urological Association (AUA) and European Association of Urology (EAU) showed that URS favorably compares to shock wave lithotripsy (SWL) for all stone locations. URS for distal ureteral stones yielded a 94 % stone-free rate which decreased only slightly to 78–79 % for large (>10 mm), mid, or proximal ureteral stones [1]. After medical expulsive therapy, URS has also been shown to be the most cost-effective therapy for all ureteral stones [2]. Notably, prospective randomized trials comparing shock wave lithotripsy (SWL) to semirigid URS for either proximal or distal ureteral stones showed lower costs and statistically significantly higher initial stone-free rates with URS [3, 4]. With a continuous trend towards innovation and improvement of endoscopic devices, one can expect that the efficacy and use of URS for the treatment of ureteral stones will only rise. This chapter provides an outline of the technical approach to URS for ureteral stones. We begin with the importance of preoperative counseling, followed by an overall management algorithm, description of surgical equipment, an intraoperative algorithm, and then finish with the postoperative management and recommended follow-up. At the conclusion of the chapter the treatment of a patient with a large impacted proximal ureteral stone will be discussed.

D. Snow-Lisy, M.D. • M. Monga, M.D. (✉)
Department of Urology, Glickman Urologic and Kidney Institute, The Cleveland Clinic, 9500 Euclid Ave Q10-1, Cleveland, OH 44195, USA
e-mail: mongam@ccf.org

Technique

After the diagnosis of ureteral stone is obtained, treatment begins in the clinic with preoperative counseling and obtaining informed consent.

Preoperative Counseling

Because there are multiple potential treatments for ureteral stones, preoperative counseling is vitally important. Discussion begins with what procedures would be indicated and what outcomes that a particular patient could expect. Discussion can cover observation with medical expulsive therapy, URS, and SWL depending on patient and stone factors as delineated in this general management algorithm (Fig. 8.1). At times, if a large intrarenal stone burden (>15 mm) is present, in addition to the ureteral calculus, an antegrade percutaneous approach may be discussed.

Observation with Medical Expulsive Therapy

Observation with medical expulsive therapy is only appropriate for patients with well-controlled

S.Y. Nakada and M.S. Pearle (eds.), *Surgical Management of Urolithiasis: Percutaneous, Shockwave and Ureteroscopy*, DOI 10.1007/978-1-4614-6937-7_8, © Springer Science+Business Media New York 2013

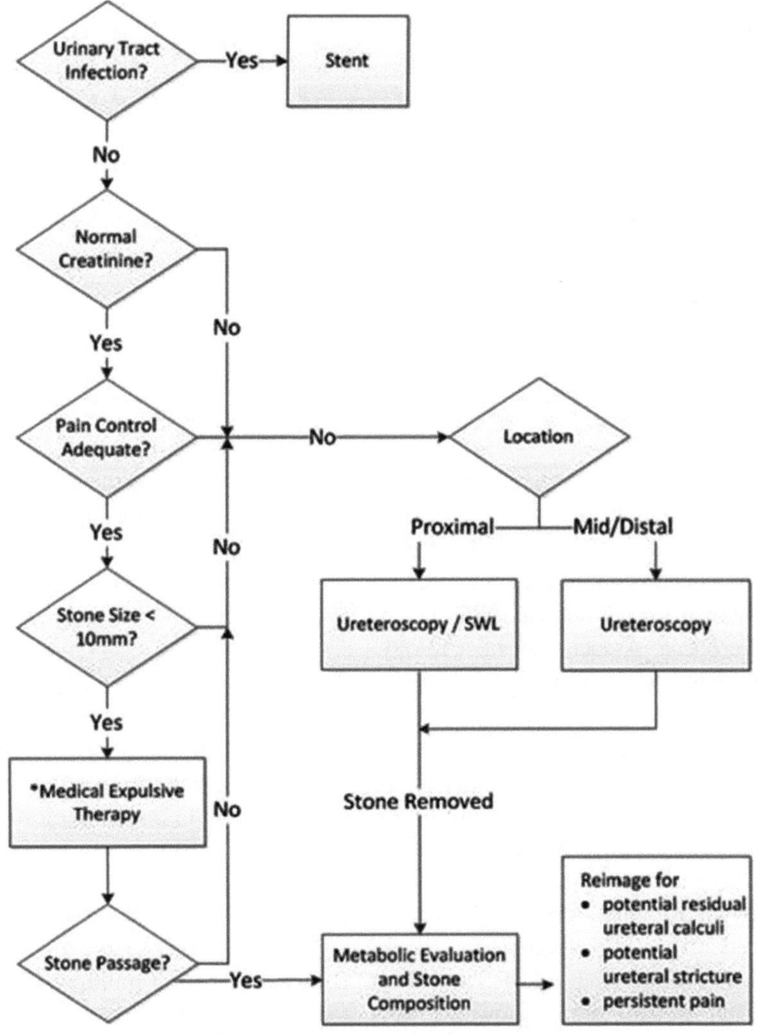

Fig. 8.1 General management pathway for urolithiasis

pain, a sterile urinary tract, stones less than 10 mm, and no renal insufficiency [1]. Analgesia and importantly alpha blockers, if not contraindicated, are prescribed. Alpha blockers increase the likelihood of stone passage (by approximately 40 %) and decrease the pain associated with spontaneous passage [5]. It is important to ensure the patient knows if they elect observation they can decide to undergo further treatment in the future. We recommend education regarding the likelihood of stone passage which is dependent on many patient factors including stone size, history of previous stone passage, and stone location. As a general guideline 68 % of stones ≤5 mm are likely to spontaneously pass, however this decreases to 47 % for stones greater than 5 mm but less than or equal to 10 mm [1]. Another important variable for patient decision-making is the time it takes for the stone to pass and the percentage of patients who ultimately decide to undergo intervention. Both these factors increase with larger stone size; one study showed that 50 % of patients with stones greater than 4 mm took on average 22 days to spontaneously pass their stones, while the remaining required surgical intervention (Fig. 8.2) [6].

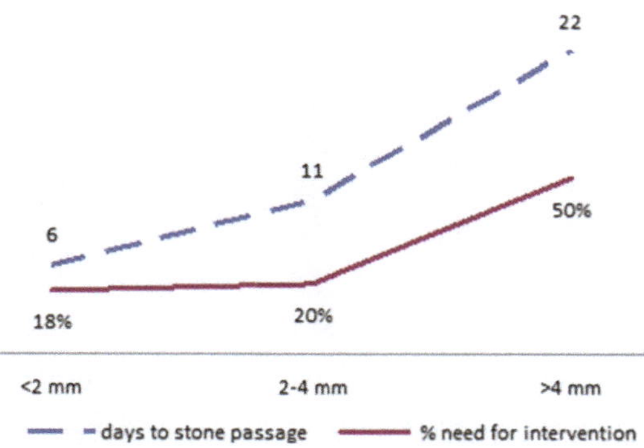

Fig. 8.2 Results of observation and medical expulsive therapy. Numbers of days to stone passage and rates of intervention increase with increasing size. Intervention is required in 50 % of stones greater than 4 mm. These stones take on average 22 days to pass spontaneously [6]

Ureteral Stent

For patients with obstruction and pyelonephritis or acute renal failure due to obstruction, ureteral stent placement (or percutaneous nephrostomy) is indicated for emergent decompression [1, 7]. While alpha-blockers may be utilized to address ureteral stent discomfort, their impact on stone passage after stent placement has not been studied [8]. Early intervention (ureteral stent or ureteroscopy) may be considered for patients with a solitary kidney or transplant kidney.

Shock Wave Lithotripsy

In general, a patient with a stone <15 mm is a suitable candidate for SWL; however patients with larger stones are more likely to need a secondary procedure. Up to 30 % of patients needed a secondary procedure for proximal ureteral stones measuring over 10 mm [1]. Prognostic factors for ureteral calculi include the Hounsfield Units (HU) of the stone, as HU over 1,000 indicate a lower chance of success with SWL [9]. A skin-to-stone distance over 9.2 cm on CT scan also decreases the efficacy of SWL for proximal ureteral calculi [10]. On multivariate analysis for ureteral and renal calculi, both HU >900 and skin-to-stone distance >11 cm separately predicted failure (odds ratio: 2) [11]. A scoring system predicting the likelihood of stone-free status after SWL for proximal ureteral stones incorporated three factors; stone volume less than 0.2 cm^3, mean stone density less than 593 HU, and skin-to-stone distance less than 9.2 cm. The stone-free rate for patients having 0, 1, 2, and 3 factors was 17.9 %, 48.4 %, 73.3 %, and 100 %, respectively (linear-by-linear association test 22.83, $p<0.001$) [10]. Lastly, for most patients with cystine stones, SWL is not recommended given reduced efficacy [12]. Routine stenting is not recommended prior to SWL [13, 14].

Ureteroscopy

While more invasive than SWL, Ureteroscopy (URS) does yield significantly greater stone-free rates for the majority of stone stratifications and is appropriate for stones of any size [15]. Anesthesia requirements for this modality are greater than with SWL and can vary from intravenous sedation to general anesthesia depending on stone location, stone size, and patient factors [16]. URS is preferred for patients in whom SWL is contraindicated or ill-advised, including patients with a skin-to-stone distance greater than 10 cm, stones with high HU, or in patients in whom cessation of anticoagulants is considered unsafe [17–19]. Ureteroscopy may also be considered first line therapy during pregnancy [20]. After uncomplicated ureteroscopy, routine ureteral stenting is optional [15, 21]. Indications for ureteral stenting after ureteroscopy will be discussed in the following section. Comparison of success rates between URS and SWL are shown in Fig. 8.3 [1]. In general, we recommend SWL under sedation for proximal ureteral calculi <1 cm in size, and URS for larger proximal ureteral calculi, or calculi in the mid- or distal ureter.

Percutaneous Nephrolithotripsy

This treatment is useful for large stones over 15 mm in size with significant hydronephrosis, and in patients with urinary diversions or transplant kidneys. This approach may also be preferred in patients who present with a ureteral

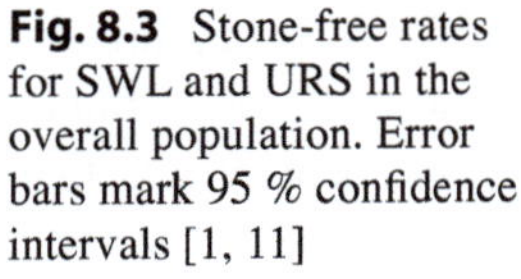

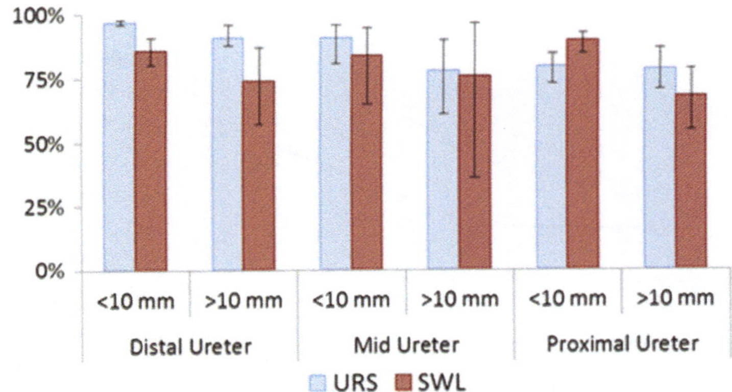

Fig. 8.3 Stone-free rates for SWL and URS in the overall population. Error bars mark 95 % confidence intervals [1, 11]

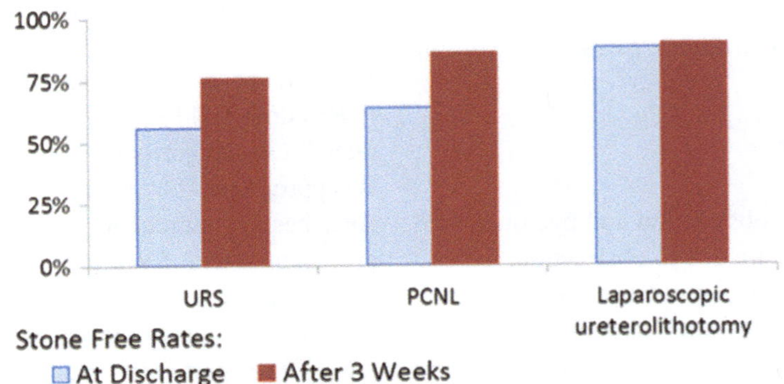

Fig. 8.4 Stone-free rates. Success rates after URS, PCNL, and laparoscopic ureterolithotomy for proximal ureteral stones greater than or equal to 15 mm [26]. One major limitation to this study is that ureteroscopy was only performed with a semirigid ureteroscope. Without using a flexible ureteroscope, which facilitates extraction of small fragments that may have moved to the renal pelvis/lower pole, one would expect stone-free rates to be lower

calculus and a large intrarenal stone burden that would best be addressed with percutaneous removal. Prior failed ureteroscopy and a suspicion of significant impaction due to long-standing obstruction are other relative indications for consideration of an antegrade approach. Typically in these patients we would perform prone ureteroscopy, and consent the patient for the possibility of converting to an antegrade approach under the same anesthetic. A randomized trial compared percutaneous antegrade versus retrograde use of semirigid ureteroscope for laser lithotripsy in the treatment of proximal ureteral stones >10 mm. Antegrade percutaneous semirigid URS showed significantly increased stone-free rates at discharge as compared to retrograde semirigid URS (95.3 % versus 79.5 % $p=0.027$) [22]. Published stone-free rates for percutaneous antegrade removal of proximal ureteral stones >15 mm range from 76 to 100 % [15, 22–26].

Laparoscopic Ureterolithotomy

This procedure has been reported to have stone-free rates ranging from 76 to 98 % [15]. Success rates were compared between URS, Percutaneous Nephrolithotripsy (PCNL), and laparoscopic ureterolithotomy for large (≥5 mm) proximal ureteral stones in a randomized clinical trial (Fig. 8.4) [26]. The authors concluded that ureteroscopy had a more favorable complication profile and success rates were not significantly different between the three groups.

Informed Consent

After description and discussion of the likelihood of success with each procedure, we recommend discussing the risks and benefits of the potential treatments with the patient (Fig. 8.5). After this discussion the patient is encouraged to make a decision based upon their own needs weighing the relative importance of the invasiveness, success rates, and risks associated with each procedure.

Observation/Medical Expulsive Therapy

Risks of this therapy include pain, associated drug side effects (opioids, alpha-blockers), potential decrease in renal function (with prolonged untreated obstruction), and potential need for emergent intervention. We counsel the patients that if the stone does not pass within 4–6 weeks it would be advisable to proceed with intervention. We also counsel that outcomes with SWL may be superior with early intervention rather than following a period of observation as the stone may move to an unfavorable position (more anterior and inferior) or the degree of impaction may increase. A randomized prospective study of 160 patients with proximal ureteral stones has demonstrated that SWL within 48-h of onset of pain decreases the need for re-treatment or secondary procedures and decreases the time to stone clearance [27]. Lastly, we counsel patients on the potential need for reimaging prior to intervention after a period of observation. Though we emphasize the need to strain the urine to monitor for stone passage, other investigators have reported that the risk of a negative ureteroscopy if repeat imaging is not performed is 10 %—this risk is higher (16 %) for distal ureteral calculi and >50 % for stones ≤2 mm in size [28].

	SWL	URS
Sepsis	3%	2%
Steinstrasse	5%	0%
Stricture	0%	2%
Ureteral Injury	2%	4%
UTI	4%	4%

Fig. 8.5 Meta-analysis of complication rates after SWL and ureteroscopy (URS) [1]

Shock Wave Lithotripsy

There is a 1 in 1,000 risk of a serious bleed requiring either hospitalization or transfusion. This risk is highest in patients >65 years old and in those with uncontrolled hypertension [29, 30]. The risk of Steinstrasse is less than 5 % for stones smaller than 1 cm, but increases exponentially with the larger sizes [31]. The risk of septicemia (3 in 100) can be decreased by preoperative treatment with appropriate antibiotics [15, 32].

Ureteroscopy

The most common injury is to the ureter, with a 4 in 100 risk of minor injury requiring a stent for 2–3 weeks and a 1 in 1,000 risk of severe ureteral injury requiring major surgery for repair. Long-term complications include the potential for stricture and are less than 1 in 1,000 [15, 23, 33]. The risk of urinary tract infection after ureteroscopy in an uncomplicated patient with appropriate antibiotic prophylaxis is about 4 in 100 [15, 34]. In patients with a solitary kidney, renal insufficiency, a large residual stone burden, use of a ureteral access sheath, or if there was ureteral injury, a ureteral stent will need to be placed [23].

Ureteral Stent

Most patients (8 in 10) will have lower urinary tract symptoms with ureteral stent placement [35]. Complications include stent migration, infection, stent encrustation, and malfunction, but can generally be avoided with timely removal of the stent (typically 5–7 days after uncomplicated URS) [15].

Percutaneous Nephrolithotripsy

Risks associated with this procedure include lung injury (1 %), significant bleeding requiring blood transfusion (5 %) or embolization (1 %), septicemia (1 %), and rare injury to other organs (colon) and need for secondary procedure [36–38]. If a patient has only a ureteral calculus, often a middle calyceal access will provide adequate access down the ureter while decreasing the risk of bleeding and pulmonary complications [39].

Laparoscopic Ureterolithotomy

The most common complication includes a urine leak (1 in 6 patients) [26]. Risks include need to convert to open procedure (1 in 30) or those associated with laparoscopic surgery in general which include vascular, bowel, and ureteral injuries (1 in 100) [40].

Operative Management

For the description of the procedure the general name of the equipment will be used. Please refer to Fig. 8.6 for a list of the specific ancillary instrumentation that the authors currently utilize. In this section, we will describe the equipment, set-up, preoperative antibiotic recommendation, and a step-by-step guideline for treating a ureteral stone by URS.

Equipment

Guidewires

Guidewires vary with regard to coatings, core material, diameter (most commonly 0.035, 0.038″), tip length, tip stiffness, distal-end stiffness, and tip shape (straight, angled, J curved). The lubricity (slipperiness when wet) of a guidewire can be helpful when negotiating obstruction but also can lead to inadvertent loss of access [41, 42]. There are three general guidewires that are regularly used.

- The working wire/safety wire.
- The lubricious wire for passage across obstacles.
- The rigid wire for ureteral access sheath placement and placement of large caliber ureteral stents.

The Boston Scientific's Sensor 0.035″ guidewire is our standard working wire; combining a hydrophilic tip with a stiffer shaft. However, the Sensor wire is not as lubricious as the Boston Scientific's Glidewire, nor is it as stiff as a Boston Scientific's Amplatz Super Stiff guidewire. The Glidewire has a superior safety profile with regards to risk of perforation and is therefore used if faced with significant impaction [42]. In contrast, the Amplatz superstiff is used to place the ureteral access sheath as it is least likely to buckle [43].

Open before case:	In the room:
20Fr Storz rigid cystoscope with 30° lens	5Fr Open ended catheter
0.035" Boston Scientific Sensor guidewire (straight tip)	0.035" Boston Scientific Glidewire guidewire (straight and angled)
Boston Scientific Single Action Pumping System	Sterile Radiopaque Contrast
Gyrus-ACMI ABP adapter	Cook KMP angled catheter and torque device
Wolf DOC semi-rigid ureteroscope 2.4/4Fr	Wolf "needle" semi-rigid ureteroscope 4.5Fr
0.035" Boston Scientific Amplatz Super Stiff guidewire	Cook Ascend AQ dilation balloon
Cook Flexor Sheath 35 cm for women; 45 cm for men (14/16Fr if stented; 12/14Fr if non-stented)	Cook Flexor Sheath 9/11.5Fr
Wolf Viper flexible ureteroscope	Storz Flex-X2 flexible ureteroscope
Sacred Heart Halo 1.5Fr basket	Cook N-Compass 2.4Fr basket
Bard Optima stent	Coherent Lumenis Holmium laser
16Fr urethral catheter	Boston Scientific laser fiber

Fig. 8.6 Recommended equipment for URS. We recommend opening all equipment in the *left hand column* prior to the start of the procedure. Equipment that should be kept "on hold" in the room in case of difficulty can be found in the *right hand column*

Catheters

A 5-French (Fr) open-ended catheter may be needed to exchange wires if significant obstruction is encountered. This catheter also allows for instillation of radio-opaque contrast which can delineate the anatomy in this setting. Torque catheters (Cook KMP) may be helpful to navigate tortuous ureters. A Cook Dual-lumen catheter (6–10 Fr) may be helpful for placement of a second guidewire.

Ureteral Access Sheaths

Sheaths have been shown to reduce operative time, improve flow rates and visibility due to improved drainage of irrigation, reduce ureteral injury with large stones, as well as increase stone-free rates [44–47]. In addition, it has been proposed that the use of a ureteral access sheath decreases the need for repairs of the flexible ureteroscope [48]. For these reasons we recommend the routine placement of ureteral access sheaths for flexible ureteroscopy except in the cases of small easily basketable stones (≤4 mm). We do not utilize an access sheath for semirigid URS [44, 49]. Ureteral access sheaths should be placed over a rigid wire. Both the Cook Flexor and Gyrus-ACMI Uropass access sheaths have been shown to be superior with regards to kinking, however the Cook Flexor is least likely to buckle with increased axial force [50–52]. A 35 cm length sheath is utilized in women, while a 45 cm sheath is utilized in men. In a pre-stented ureter, a 14/16 Fr sheath can generally be utilized while in an un-stented patient a 12/14 Fr sheath will be appropriate. In pediatric patients or for those in whom resistance is met with a 12/14 Fr sheath, a 9/11.5 Fr sheath may prove successful.

Ureteral Balloon Dilators

Balloon dilators are recommended for dilation of a tight ureteral orifice or stricture that compromises access with a ureteroscope or ureteral access sheath. These are used as a second line since they are associated with increased postoperative pain [44]. We recommend using the Cook Ascend AQ Ureteral Dilation Balloon Catheter because it was noted to have the least variability in ability to dilate across a wide range of constrictive forces [53]. These tools should be used with caution, as often the ureter will "split" in response to high inflation pressures.

Intracorporeal Lithotripters

While there are many different types of lithotripters (mechanical, electrohydraulic, pneumatic, laser, and ultrasonic) the current gold standard for use in URS is the holmium:YAG laser lithotripter [54]. Laser lithotripsy is especially effective as the thin and flexible fibers can be used in flexible ureteroscopes and cause limited ureteral damage since energy propagation is limited by irrigation water [55, 56]. Because studies have shown greater durability and efficiency with 365 μm laser fibers, these are recommended for use in semirigid ureteroscopes. The 200 μm laser fibers are recommended for use with flexible ureteroscopes since they only minimally reduce the maneuverability of the device [57–59].

Ureteral Occluding Devices

These devices are used to prevent stone migration and there have been a variety of designs to accomplish this goal. Such devices include the Boston Scientific Stone Cone, the Cook NTrap, the Boston Scientific Back-stop, the Xenolith Xen-X and the PercSys Accordion [60–62]. These devices can be distinguished based on the stiffness of their tip (stiffest is the Cook Ntrap), their ability to prevent stone migration, and the forces and attempts required to navigate past a point of obstruction [63]. These devices have greatest utility if used in conjunction with pneumatic lithotripsy [64]. With intermittent and judicious irrigation and the use of holmium laser lithotripsy, the risk of stone migration is minimized. We consider utilizing a ureteral occlusion device for large ureteral calculi (>1 cm) with significant associated hydronephrosis, where the likelihood of stone migration will be higher, and retrieval of fragments from a distended collecting system will be more challenging.

Stone Retrieval Devices

Nitinol-based stone baskets have demonstrated excellent retrieval, release, and flexibility leading to their routine use with flexible scopes [65, 66]. It is beyond the scope of this chapter to discuss every basket design but it is worthy of note that tip-less baskets have been demonstrated to be superior both in stone retrieval as well as in reducing the risk of tissue perforation [66, 67]. We recommend different retrieval devices depending on the clinical situation. The Sacred Heart Halo basket is recommended for general use, while the Cook N-Compass with its weaved net configuration is most useful for removing multiple stone fragments [68]. While useful in the kidney for adherent stones, the Cook N-Circle 1.5 Fr basket does not have significant radial dilation forces, which we believe makes it less useful for extracting ureteral stones [53, 69].

Semirigid Ureteroscopes

We utilize a 6 Fr Wolf Dual-Channel semirigid ureteroscope, though a 4.5 Fr Wolf "needle" scope is kept on hand for pediatrics or a tight ureteral orifice. Olympus Gyrus—ACMI, Storz, Stryker, and Wolf all produce a variety of semirigid ureteroscopes. These semirigid ureteroscopes vary based upon angle of the eyepiece (straight/angled), optics (fiber optic/digital), field and angle of view, scope diameter and length, sheath construction, tip style, and number and size of working channels. In contrast to flexible ureteroscopy, a higher density of fiber optic bundles can be incorporated into the design of the semirigid ureteroscope yielding good image quality with fiber optics [70]. When comparing the only digital semirigid ureteroscope available (Olympus Endoeye) to a traditional Storz semirigid ureteroscope, one group found the digital optics to be superior but noted that the larger diameter tip (12 Fr) of the Olympus Endoeye limited the maneuverability and utility of the scope [71]. Like flexible ureteroscopes, semirigid scopes are fragile instruments that are susceptible to damage. Careful handling and caution intraoperatively is important, as most repairs needed are due to excessive force/torquing of the scope (66 %) with laser damage and improper handling accounting for much of the remaining damage [72]. Semirigid ureteroscopes are most useful for distal ureteral stones where flexible ureteroscopes are difficult to use because of buckling into the bladder [73].

Flexible Ureteroscopes

Advances in the technology of flexible ureteroscopes have certainly increased the utility of URS in the treatment of ureteral stones. These fragile scopes now have active deflection over 270° with newer scopes (Dur8-E/Flexvision Y-500/Viper) including lever mechanisms to either increase unidirectional or allow for bidirectional deflection [74]. Other advances include adding in an additional channel (Wolf Cobra), which allows for simultaneous basket and laser fiber utilization: which is most useful for stabilizing stones while performing laser lithotripsy [75]. Unfortunately flexible ureteroscopes are delicate and repairs costly; one group reported repairs to cost $418.19 per use [76]. The majority of repairs for flexible ureteroscopes are to the internal working channel (52 %) [72]. This damage is caused by extreme deflection while using an instrument in the working channel, instrument insertion/extraction, or use of the laser in the distal working channel [72]. By emphasizing careful handling of the scope by the surgeon and careful handling with proper sterilization techniques by ancillary staff, repair costs have been shown to be reduced by up to $300 per use [76]. The Wolf Viper has demonstrated superior optical quality, illumination and maneuverability in vitro and in a calyceal model as compared to the multiple other flexible ureteroscopes (Stryker FlexVision U-500, Storz Flex-X2, Olympus XURF-P5, Olympus URF-P3, ACMI DUR-8 Elite) [77, 78]. In contrast to semirigid ureteroscopes, digital imaging has been widely incorporated into the newer flexible ureteroscopes. A comparison of digital (Olympus URF-V) to fiberoptic flexible ureteroscopes showed that, despite being larger, the digital scope had improved maneuverability and active deflection [79]. Digital imaging also improved color reproducibility, depth of field, and resolution by 2.25–3.15 times [80].

Endo-Irrigation Systems

These systems are necessary for dilating the ureter and for vision during procedures. As placement of baskets, wires, or laser fibers significantly decrease the flow through the scope, pressure irrigation is often required [81]. Active hand-pump systems decrease the total amount of irrigant fluid utilized and decrease stone migration as irrigant pressure can be judiciously utilized [82]. Alternatively, pressurized irrigation up to 300 mmHg can be utilized, with low intrarenal pelvic pressures maintained if a ureteral access sheath is utilized [45].

Set Up

It is recommended that video and C-arm monitors be placed on one side of the patient along with the irrigation, light source, and lithotrite generator. The C-arm is then on the opposite side. This simplifies viewing for the surgeon, decreasing cervical strain if a flat-panel monitor is positioned at eye level directly beside the C-arm monitor. We recommend normal saline irrigant with a hand pump endo-irrigation system to minimize the total volume of irrigant and the pressure utilized [83]. The equipment that is necessary for URS is opened on the working table with the remainder "on hold" in the room. The procedure proceeds in a step wise fashion with ureteral orifice cannulation, placement of a safety wire, insertion of the ureteroscope with ureteral access sheath dilation in certain cases, stone fragmentation and extraction followed by ureteral stent insertion when necessary (Fig. 8.7).

Preoperative Antibiotics

Current AUA guidelines recommend appropriate antibiotics based upon urine culture prior to intervention (urine dipstick is sufficient in uncomplicated cases) [15, 84, 85]. For prophylactic antibiotics a randomized controlled trial demonstrated decreased postoperative bacteriuria with a single oral dose of levofloxacin, with another showing equivalence between a single dose of oral ciprofloxacin and a one-time dose of intravenous cefazolin [86, 87].

Surgical Procedure

Ureteral Orifice Cannulation

After induction of anesthesia and intravenous antibiotics, the patient is positioned in dorsal lithotomy. The legs are carefully padded and the treatment leg is placed in slight extension to reduce the risk of compartment syndrome [88]. Pneumatic compression boots are used to help prevent deep vein thrombosis [89]. Fluoroscopic equipment is necessary and should be available by the initiation of the procedure. Pulsed fluoroscopy may decrease the intraoperative radiation exposure to patient and personnel [90].

After the patient is prepped and draped, a full examination of the bladder is performed with cystoscopy and the appropriate ureteral orifice is cannulated with a general working wire. If the ureteral orifice is unable to be cannulated due to poor visualization or angle from a large prostate, large cystocele, or other reason, then flexible cystoscopy with cannulation may be attempted. Alternatives include using a 70° lens with Albarran deflecting bridge [91]. Methylene blue or indigo carmine may be administered in cases where identification of the ureteral orifice is challenging. If the ureteral orifice is unable to be cannulated due to an impacted intramural ureteral stone then attempts should be made to cannulate the orifice with a lubricious wire. If cannulation of the ureteral orifice is successful then the glidewire is exchanged for a working guidewire using a 5 Fr open-ended ureteral catheter. If cannulation is unsuccessful, then a Collins knife can be used to perform a ureteral meatotomy. After incising the ureteral orifice, the tip of the Collins knife is used to "tease" the impacted intramural stone out of the ureter. If this technique is utilized, the surgeon should evaluate the need to place a ureteral stent postoperatively by visual inspection of the caliber of the distal ureter with a semirigid ureteroscope. Typically following a ureteral meatotomy and stone extraction, a ureteral stent is not required.

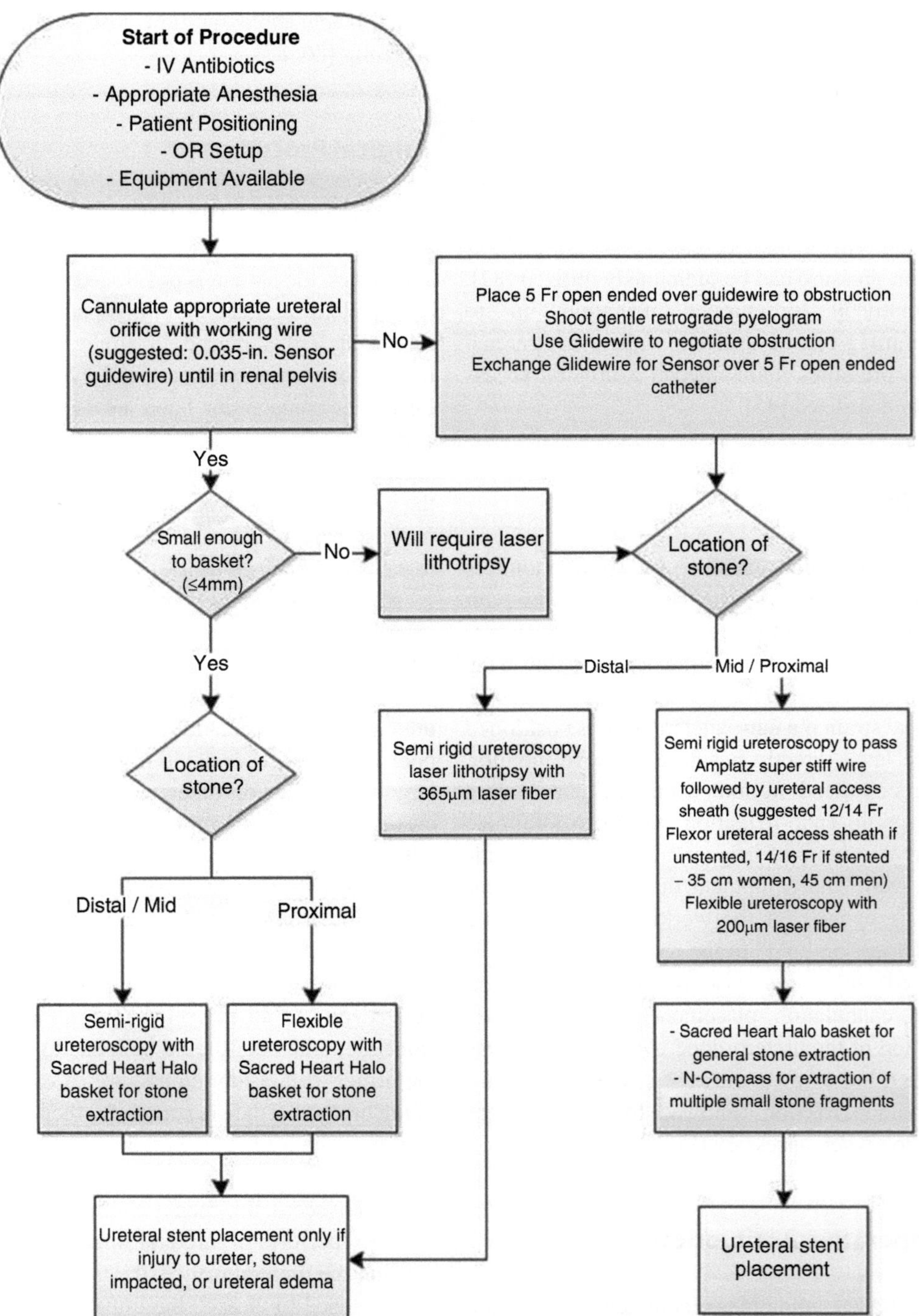

Fig. 8.7 General algorithm of URS for a ureteral stone

Placement of Safety Wire

Once the ureteral orifice is successfully cannulated, the working wire is advanced under fluoroscopic guidance to the renal pelvis, if possible. If the working wire is unable to be advanced into the renal pelvis, this is the first sign of an impacted stone and a 5 Fr open-ended ureteral catheter should be placed over the wire to the point of obstruction. After removal of the guidewire, a gentle retrograde pyelogram is performed to delineate the anatomy. If a blind ending obstruction is seen on retrograde pyelogram, it is likely that guidewire placement will be challenging. At this point we recommend using a well-lubricated lubricious wire placed through the 5 Fr open-ended catheter to the point of obstruction. With the lubricious wire, the surgeon attempts to negotiate the obstruction under fluoroscopic guidance. If a straight tipped lubricious wire is not successful, or if an acute angle is seen on retrograde ureterogram, then an angled-tipped lubricious wire and a torque device may be used to direct the wire and facilitate maneuverability. Once the lubricious wire is advanced past the obstruction, it should be exchanged for a safety wire using a 5 Fr open-ended catheter.

If access cannot be obtained with this method then advancement of a semirigid ureteroscope alongside the partially placed wire up to the level of the obstruction may be attempted. If this is successful, placement of the wire is attempted under direct vision. If necessary, laser lithotripsy of the stone to facilitate passage of the lubricious wire may be attempted. If the ureteroscope is unable to pass due to a ureteral stricture or narrow ureteral orifice, passage of a Wolf needle scope or a flexible ureteroscope may be attempted. Dilation without a safety wire in place is strongly discouraged. If a safety wire is unable to be advanced into the renal pelvis, stone extraction is similarly discouraged. If a safety wire is unable to be placed into the renal pelvis despite maximal attempts, retrograde ureteroscopy is abandoned. At this point, consideration should be given to placement of a nephrostomy tube with subsequent antegrade ureteroscopy.

Ureteroscope Insertion

Once a safety wire is placed, the semirigid ureteroscope is advanced to passively dilate the distal ureter and evaluate the distal ureter for calculi or other pathology. If the surgeon cannot cannulate the ureteral orifice with either the ureteroscope or a coaxial dilator, a rigid wire is inserted through the working channel of the ureteroscope into the ureteral orifice and used as a "filiform" then the scope is rotated until it lies between the general working wire and the rigid wire. This maneuver leads to the two wires acting like a "railroad track" which tents the ureter and allows the scope to be passed along the track. If this maneuver is not successful, then balloon dilation (recommended using a 20 atm. 5 mm × 4 cm balloon) of the ureteral orifice can be performed.

Once the ureteroscope has reached the limit to which it can be advanced, a superstiff wire is placed through the working channel under direct vision. Once the tip is coiled in the renal pelvis, the semirigid ureteroscope is removed and the superstiff is utilized for placement of the ureteral access sheath. Alternatively, if the known calculus is localized to the proximal ureter on preoperative imaging, a dual-lumen catheter or 8/10 Fr coaxial dilator can be used to place the rigid wire. Stones ≤4 mm without signs of impaction on imaging are often amenable to simple basketing and therefore for these stones we do not recommend placing a rigid wire or ureteral access sheath.

A 12/14 Fr ureteral access sheath (14/16 Fr if previously stented; 35 cm in women, and 45 cm in men) is advanced over the rigid wire to the level of the stone. The rigid wire is then removed, leaving the initial guidewire as a safety outside the lumen of the access sheath. Of note, a ureteral access sheath would not be recommended for distal stones given propensity for the sheath to fall out/buckle in the bladder, and these stones are treated expeditiously with a semirigid ureteroscope [44, 49]. The ureteral access sheath is placed with a gentle "jiggling" axial force; taking care not to twist the sheath while advancing or place excessive force. If resistance is encountered, the sheath is removed and ureter dilated with the inner dilator only. If resistance persists then the options are to utilize a smaller caliber sheath, perform ureteroscopy without an access sheath (advancing the ureteroscope over a wire), balloon dilate the ureter and then place the sheath, or place a ureteral stent and attempt staged ureteroscopy in 2 weeks. Generally when using a hand pump irrigator, a ureteral access sheath and an anticipated operating time of less than 1 h, drainage of the bladder with a urethral catheter is unnecessary [47].

Stone Fragmentation/Extraction

We recommend routinely using the semirigid ureteroscope and then, if necessary, switching out to a flexible scope, primarily for proximal ureteral stones in men. Once the stone has been visualized, if it is smaller than the ureter and relatively smooth, then primary basket extraction under direct vision may be performed [92]. For the majority of cases the stone will need to be fragmented. This is commonly performed with the holmium:YAG laser lithotripter. A 200 μm fiber is used in flexible ureteroscopes and a 365 μm fiber in semirigid ureteroscopes. Initial settings for the laser should be 0.8 J and 8 Hertz (Hz). We increase Hz until the stone is adequately fragmenting. The stone fragments are then extracted using a variety of tip-less Nitinol baskets until there are no fragments that are larger than the safety wire (which is 0.035″ in diameter). Please see "Stone retrieval devices" for a description of the different baskets. In patients who have undergone ureteral dilation (ureteral access sheath placement or balloon dilation) a ureteral stent is left for 5–7 days. For individuals with complicated ureteroscopy, namely ureteral injury with perforation, or an impacted ureteral stone, a ureteral stent is placed for 10–14 days. In patients with stones requiring a simple basketing procedure without any of the above factors, a ureteral stent can safely be forgone [93]. An alpha blocker is prescribed to decrease ureteral stent associated symptoms [8].

Complications

Complications can be minimized by careful patient selection, appropriate preparation of the necessary instrumentation and a systematic methodical technique. Though others have proposed the elimination of a safety guidewire, we recommend it's routine use as a "safety net" for stent placement in the event of iatrogenic injury [94]. It is important to emphasize that those who advocate ureteroscopy without a wire, utilize a technique of "dusting the stone" without active fragment extraction [94]. If basketing of stone fragments is a component of the procedure, then a guidewire must be in place.

Infectious Complications

Infectious complications can be minimized with the use of a single-dose prophylaxis as prescribed by the AUA Best Practices statement. If a complication arises, the patient is treated conservatively with antibiotics and supportive care. It is important to leave a urethral catheter in place in a patient who is febrile after instrumentation and stent placement to optimize drainage. If the patient's temperature and leukocytosis do not respond to appropriate antibiotic therapy then ultrasonography is recommended as an initial imaging modality.

Ureteral Injury

Minor ureteral injuries including bleeding, mucosal tears, or perforation can be managed with ureteral stent placement. Blind basketing of a stone is not recommended due to risk of ureteral avulsion. Another cause of ureteral avulsion appears to be caused by undue force placed on a semirigid ureteroscope even without attempted stone removal, which results in a two-point ureteral avulsion [95]. In the situation of an impacted ureteroscope, one group suggests increasing the irrigation pressure and/or performing a rectal/vaginal exam to push the UVJ and distal ureteral segment upward while rotating and gently removing the ureteroscope [33]. Alternatively, one can attempt injection of lubricant through the working channel or alongside the ureteroscope using an additional open-ended catheter. Major ureteral injuries including avulsion or intussusception will require either open or laparoscopic surgical repair with the type depending on the location of the injury.

Ureteral Stricture

Ureteral stricture is a late complication of ureteral injury and should be monitored for in patients with difficult stones, history of multiple procedures, or radiation therapy (see postoperative imaging) [33, 96].

Hematuria

Conservative management is effective for most minor hematuria and consists of increasing fluid intake, diuresis with lasix if appropriate and minimizing anticoagulation. For major hematuria that obscures the endoscopic view, the ureteroscopy should be aborted and a double J stent along with a large bore or three-way urethral catheter placed. With significant hematuria the patient is then admitted for hemodynamic monitoring and observation for potential clot retention.

Retained Stent

The key to avoiding this complication is prevention; timely stent removal to avoid stent encrustration. The approach to the retained ureteral stent should be dictated by the degree of encrustration of the proximal coil—significant encrustration will require a percutaneous approach, while mild encrustration may be managed by a retrograde approach with the adjunct of shockwave lithotripsy. The degree of encrustration of the proximal coil as characterized by computerized tomography is predictive of the need for multiple interventions [96, 97].

Results

Successful URS for ureteral stone depends on the size of the stone as well as the location, with rates varying from 78 % for large mid ureteral stones to 97 % for small distal stones (Fig. 8.8) [1]. Patients with large (>10 mm) stones have lower stone-free rates after first ureteroscopy and are more likely to undergo additional ureteroscopic procedures (1.02 distal, 1.07 proximal) [1]. Interestingly these patients are also less likely to require a secondary or alternative procedure. This potentially reflects the safety and efficacy of second look ureteroscopy in the pre-stented patient. Other factors that may have led to a lower secondary and adjunctive procedure rate in these patients include selection or reporting bias because large (>10 mm) stones represented only 24 % of the total reported cases (387 out of 1,604) and many studies did not report cystoscopy and stent removal as an adjunctive procedure [1].

Postoperative Management

Standard postoperative management includes routine analgesic medications. If a ureteral stent has been placed, alpha blocker medications can be prescribed to help alleviate the frequency, urgency, and pain associated with ureteral stenting [8]. Other adjunctive therapies that have been investigated but not evaluated for cost-effectiveness, include ketorolac-loaded ureteral stents and injection of Botulinum toxin into the peri-ureteral area [98, 99]. Both prospective randomized trials failed to show differences in main endpoints (unscheduled physician contact, early stent removal, or symptom score) but did show a decrease in narcotic use with intervention as determined by pill counts [98, 99]. Interestingly

Stone location	Size of stone (mm)	Stone-free percentage after first ureteroscopy (95% CI)	# of URS performed	# of secondary procedures	# of adjunctive procedures
Distal Ureter	<10	97% (96-98)	1.01	0.05	0.88
	>10	91% (88-96)	1.02	0.14	1
Mid Ureter	<10	91% (81-96)	1	0.34	1.14
	>10	78% (61-90)	1	0.31	0.20
Proximal Ureter	<10	80% (73-85)	1	0.39	0.52
	>10	79% (71-87)	1.07	0.13	0.21

Fig. 8.8 Meta-analysis of results after ureteroscopy including stone-free rates and procedure counts [1]. Secondary procedures describe the need for alternative stone removal methods including open, laparoscopic, and/or percutaneous stone removal procedures. Adjunctive procedures were most commonly cystoscopy and stent removal, but also include procedures related to complications from the initial procedure

a prospective, randomized, double-blinded placebo-controlled trial comparing extended release oxybutynin and phenazopyridine failed to show a difference in bother score between the treatment groups and placebo [100].

Postoperative Imaging

In the interest of reducing the cumulative effect of radiation exposure and reducing healthcare costs, selective postoperative imaging has been evaluated. Evidence shows that selective initial postoperative imaging does not miss ureteral strictures if routine imaging is only performed in patients who had intraoperative ureteral balloon dilation, an impacted stone, intraoperative ureteral mucosal perforation, or recurrent renal colic after uncomplicated URS [101]. Others recommend routine surveillance imaging after ureteroscopy, reporting that up to 2.9 % of patients postoperatively will have silent obstruction [102]. Imaging after a complicated ureteroscopy should be performed 2–3 weeks after stent removal and can consist of ultrasound or nuclear MAG 3 scan. If obstruction is shown, then a CT scan should be obtained to assess for residual or intramural stones. If obstruction is confirmed, the patient should be counseled regarding endoscopic versus robotic/laparoscopic repairs depending on the length and location of the stricture. In general, we counsel patients of a 60–70 % long-term success rate with an endoscopic approach for appropriately chosen strictures (<1 cm) versus a 95 % success rate with the robotic/laparoscopic approach [103, 104].

Five Key Take-Home Points

- Review all images personally and have them available in the operating room at the time of surgery.
- Provide evidence-based preoperative counseling to the patient. This should include the risks and outcomes of all potential procedures.
- Preparation of instrumentation and equipment along with careful positioning reduces complications and operative time.
- Ureteroscopy can be simplified to a general step-by-step technique. We emphasize the importance of a safety wire, an operative plan, and utilizing the therapeutic option of placing a stent and coming back to remove the stone another day.
- Selective imaging is necessary postoperatively. An emphasis should be placed on preventative care to decrease the risk of stone recurrence.

Case Discussion

A 45-year-old female is referred with a month of left flank pain which she rates a 3/10. She initially presented to an outside emergency department with flank pain 3 months ago and was diagnosed with a left sided 1.2 cm proximal ureteral stone on CT scan. She underwent placement of a double J stent followed by SWL therapy at that time. The stent was removed at follow-up 1 week post-op from SWL as the patient had significant stent related symptoms and a KUB at that time showed significant fragmentation of the proximal ureteral stone. One month postoperatively after a repeat CT scan showed new hydronephrosis and persistence of her ureteral stone, she was referred to you for further treatment.

The patient has a 7-year history of nephrolithiasis having passed eight stones of uncertain size and composition. She has not had a metabolic evaluation.

PMH: insomnia, nephrolithiasis, and hypertension

PSH: C section, tubal ligation, and right knee arthroscopy

Family history: hypertension and colon cancer

Social history: former smoker, occasional alcohol, and no drug use

ROS: otherwise negative

Physical Examination: obese mildly uncomfortable woman

CT scan demonstrated a 13×5×6 mm proximal ureteral stone (Fig. 8.9).

The patient was then counseled regarding the following options including:

- Observation and medical expulsive therapy
  - Risks in this case include stone growth, stone movement, pain, potential decrease in renal function from long-standing

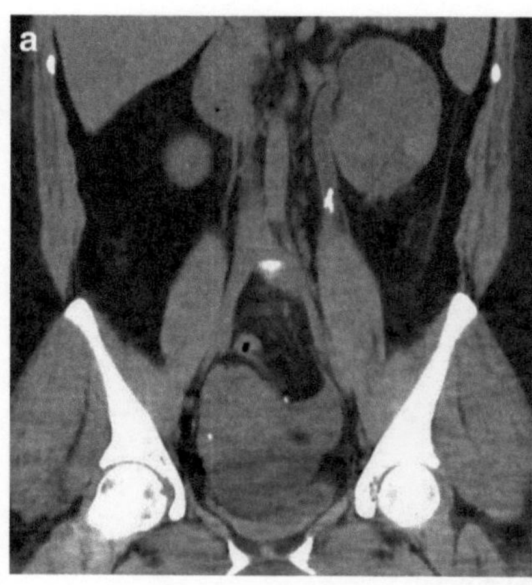

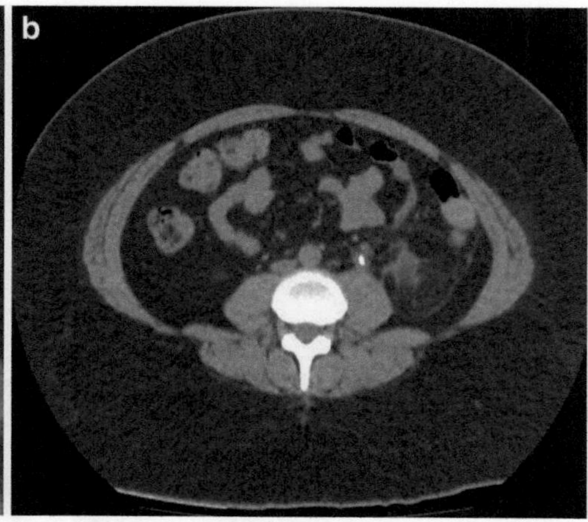

Fig. 8.9 CT scan showing potentially impacted left ureteral stone. A noncontrast CT scan with coronal (**a**) and axial (**b**) cuts shows a large subcapsular hematoma of the left kidney posteriorly measuring up to 9.6 cm following shockwave lithotripsy for a large renal pelvis stone. The patient has moderate hydronephrosis, and left ureteral dilation up to the level of an irregular stone in the proximal ureter (L3) measuring 5×6 mm in greatest cross-sectional diameter and 1.3-cm in craniocaudal diameter. The skin-to-stone distance was measured at 15.6 cm and stone density 1,132 HU

hydronephrosis, and poor chance of spontaneous stone passage (<5 %).

- SWL
  - Risks of urinary tract infection (1 in 25), bleeding (1 in 1,000 with severe bleed), and the need for spontaneous passage/secondary procedure of residual fragments.
  - This therapy was not recommended because of
    - Skin-to-stone distance of 17 cm significantly decreasing success rates [17].
    - Unfavorable Hounsfield units (1,132 HU) [9].
    - Presence of a preexisting subcapsular hematoma.
- URS
  - Risks of urinary tract infection (1 in 25), ureteral injury (1 in 300 with severe injury requiring major surgery), and the potential morbidity from placement of ureteral stent.
  - We estimate her likelihood of success at 80 % stone-free rate with 20 % of patients needing a secondary procedure to clear residual fragments.
- PCNL
  - Risks of urinary tract infection, lung injury (1 in 100), transfusion (1 in 10), embolization (1 in 50), injury to other organs, and need for secondary procedure. In this patient's case, this procedure may be complicated by the preexisting subcapsular hematoma.
  - We estimate the likelihood of success at 95 % stone-free rate.

Risk of stricture was discussed with the patient due to the concern for an impacted stone. Based on the discussion, the patient opted to undergo a URS for the treatment of her stones.

In the operating room under general anesthesia the left ureteral orifice was cannulated with a 0.035″ Boston Scientific Sensor guidewire. The guidewire could not be advanced past the site of obstruction. A 5 Fr open-ended catheter was advanced over the working wire which was then removed and a retrograde pyelogram performed with 3 cm^3 of diluted contrast (Fig. 8.10).

Given confirmation of the suspicion of an impacted ureteral stone, a straight tipped 0.035″ Boston Scientific Glidewire was used to negotiate past the site of obstruction (Fig. 8.11). The 5 Fr open-ended catheter was then advanced over the Glidewire into the collecting system and the Glidewire exchanged for the Sensor wire. If this maneuver had not been successful we would have performed semirigid URS to the level of impaction with laser lithotripsy of the stone and

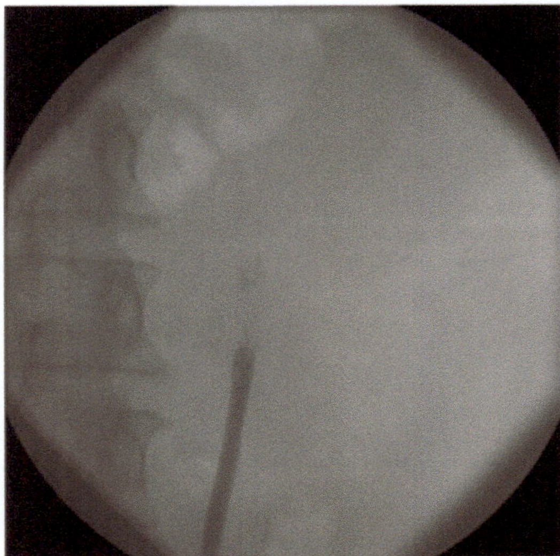

Fig. 8.10 Retrograde pyelogram showing impacted ureteral stone. The retrograde pyelogram demonstrated a blind ending ureter at the position of the proximal ureteral stone—no contrast was noted to pass the stone

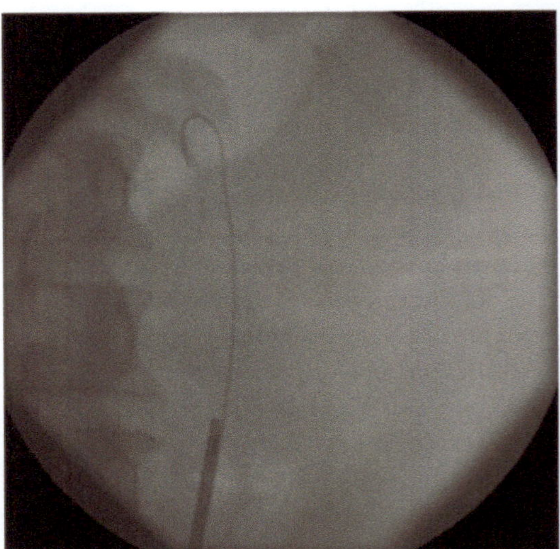

Fig. 8.11 Fluoroscopy of the safety wire coiled in the collecting system

passage of a wire under direct visualization. It is not recommended to basket the stone without a safety wire in place. If this had been unsuccessful then a percutaneous nephrostomy tube would have been placed with plans for subsequent antegrade ureteroscopy given failure of less-invasive means [105].

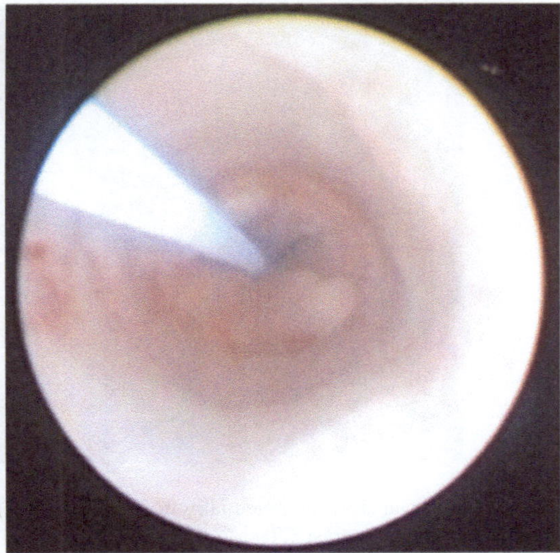

Fig. 8.12 Visualization of reactive polyps and impaction

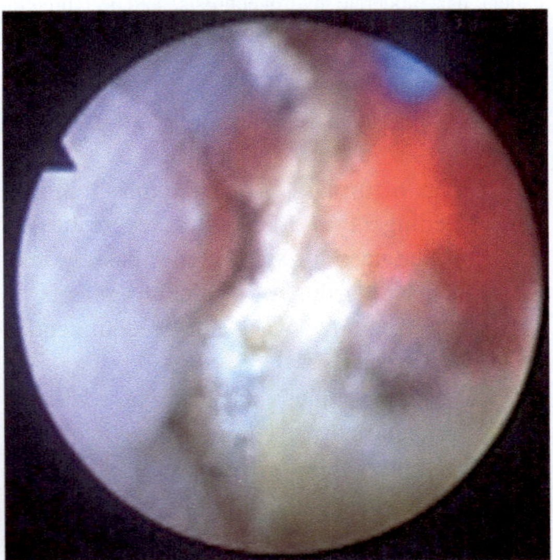

Fig. 8.13 Stone fragmentation with holmium laser. Vision partially obscured by urothelial reaction

After a safety wire was in place, a Wolf 6/7.5 Fr semirigid ureteroscope was advanced to the level of the stone. Significant reactive polyps and impaction were identified distal to the stone (Fig. 8.12).

The ureteroscope was advanced past this area with care. A 15 mm ureteral stone was identified. The stone was fragmented with a 365 μm laser fiber with the laser lithotripter settings at 0.8 J and 8 Hz (Fig. 8.13).

A 1.5 Fr Sacred Heart Halo Basket was then used to remove several fragments, after which a Super Stiff guidewire was advanced into the collecting system under endoscopic and fluoroscopic guidance. At this point a 12/14 Fr Cook Flexor Sheath was advanced to the level of the stone and flexible ureteroscopy performed to facilitate expeditious extraction of the multiple fragments (Fig. 8.14).

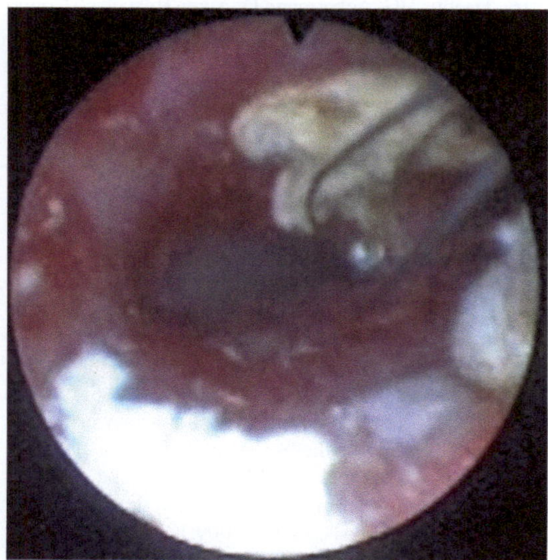

Fig. 8.14 Stone extraction with basket

Due to significant edema and polypoid reaction at the level of the extracted stone, a ureteral stent was placed. Two days postoperatively patient had significant pain and underwent a CT scan without contrast at an outside hospital emergency department which demonstrated persistent hydronephrosis and good stent position. Two weeks postoperatively she had her stent removed and at 4 weeks postoperatively she underwent a diuretic nuclear scan to assess for ureteral stricture (Fig. 8.15). This showed a decrease in function of the left kidney without obstruction. The stones were 60 % calcium phosphate and 30 % calcium oxalate monohydrate stones. Her 24 h urine profile showed a 1.42 L volume with other parameters in the normal ranges. The patient was educated regarding increasing fluid intake and a stone-specific diet.

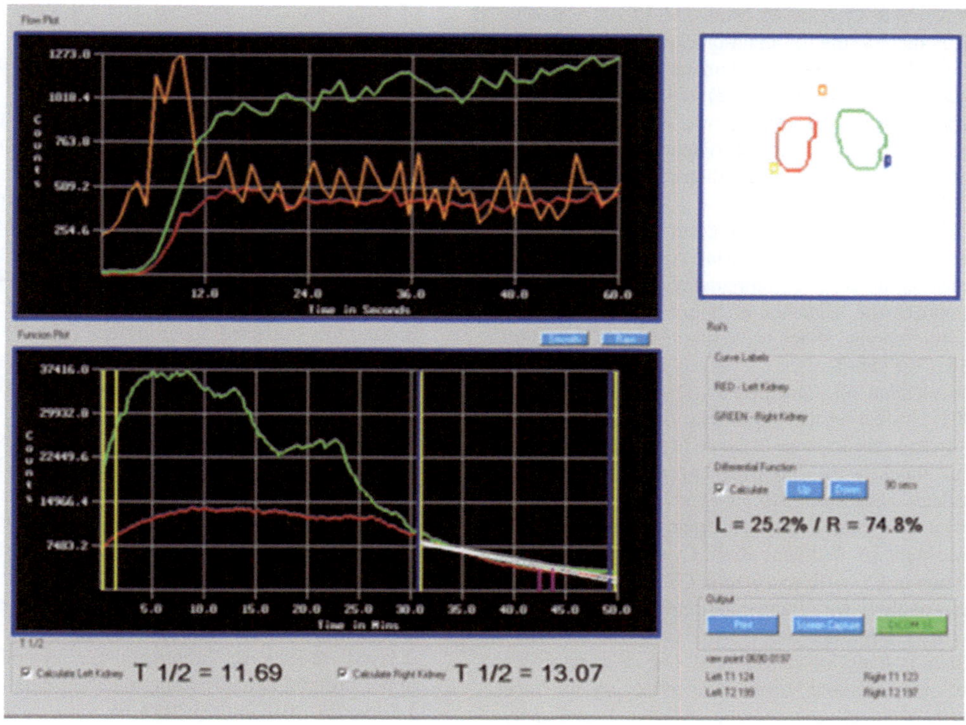

Fig. 8.15 Four week postoperative nuclear diuretic renal scan. Nuclear diuretic renal scan demonstrated a T½ of 11.69 min and 25.2 % function on the left; indicative of decreased function with no obstruction

References

1. Preminger GM, Tiselius HG, Assimos DG, et al. 2007 Guideline for the management of ureteral calculi. Eur Urol. 2007;52(6):1610–31.
2. Lotan Y, Gettman MT, Roehrborn CG, Cadeddu JA, Pearle MS. Management of ureteral calculi: a cost comparison and decision making analysis. J Urol. 2002;167(4):1621–9.
3. Salem HK. A prospective randomized study comparing shock wave lithotripsy and semirigid ureteroscopy for the management of proximal ureteral calculi. Urology. 2009;74(6):1216–21.
4. Verze P, Imbimbo C, Cancelmo G, et al. Extracorporeal shockwave lithotripsy vs. ureteroscopy as first-line therapy for patients with single, distal ureteric stones: a prospective randomized study. BJU Int. 2010;106(11):1748–52.
5. Parsons JK, Hergan LA, Sakamoto K, Lakin C. Efficacy of alpha-blockers for the treatment of ureteral stones. J Urol. 2007;177(3):983–7.
6. Miller OF, Kane CJ. Time to stone passage for observed ureteral calculi: a guide for patient education. J Urol. 1999;162(3 Pt 1):688–90. discussion 690–1.
7. Pearle MS, Pierce HL, Miller GL, et al. Optimal method of urgent decompression of the collecting system for obstruction and infection due to ureteral calculi. J Urol. 1998;160(4):1260–4.
8. Yakoubi R, Lemdani M, Monga M, Villers A, Koenig P. Is there a role for alpha-blockers in ureteral stent related symptoms? A systematic review and meta-analysis. J Urol. 2011;186(3):928–34.
9. Kacker R, Zhoa L, Macejko A, et al. Radiographic parameters on noncontrast computerized tomography predictive of shock wave lithotripsy success. J Urol. 2008;179:1866–71.
10. Ng CF, Siu DY, Wong A, Goggins W, Chan ES, Wong KT. Development of a scoring system from noncontrast computerized tomography measurements to improve the selection of upper ureteral stone for extracorporeal shock wave lithotripsy. J Urol. 2009; 181(3):1151–7.
11. Wiesenthal JG, Ghiculete D, D'A Honey RJ, Pace KT. Evaluating the importance of mean stone density and skin-to-stone distance in predicting successful shock wave lithotripsy of renal and ureteric calculi. Urol Res. 2010;38(4):307–13.
12. Kim SC, Burns EK, Lingeman JE, Paterson RF, McAteer JA, Williams JC Jr. Cystine calculi: correlation of CT-visible structure, CT number, and stone morphology with fragmentation by shock wave lithotripsy. Urol Res. 2007;35(6):319–24.
13. Shen P, Jiang M, Yang J, et al. Use of ureteral stent in extracorporeal shock wave lithotripsy for upper urinary calculi: a systematic review and meta-analysis. J Urol. 2011;186(4):1328–35.
14. Ghoneim IA, El-Ghoneimy MN, El-Nagger AE, Hammoud KM, El-Gammal MY, Morsi AA. Extracorporeal shock wave lithotripsy in impacted upper ureteral stones: a prospective randomized comparison between stented and non-stented techniques. Urology. 2010;75(1):45–50.
15. Preminger GM, Tiselius HG, Assimos DG, et al. 2007 guideline for the management of ureteral calculi. J Urol. 2007;178(6):2418–34.
16. Tiselius HG, Ackermann D, Alken P, Buck C, Conort P, Gallucci M. Guidelines on urolithiasis. Eur Urol. 2001;40(4):362–71.
17. Park BH, Choi H, Kim JB, Chang YS. Analyzing the effect of distance from skin to stone by computed tomography scan on the extracorporeal shock wave lithotripsy stone-free rate of renal stones. Korean J Urol. 2012;53(1):40–3.
18. Ouzaid I, Al-Qahtani S, Dominique S, et al. A 970 Hounsfield units (HU) threshold of kidney stone density on non-contrast computed tomography (NCCT) improves patients' selection for extracorporeal shockwave lithotripsy (ESWL): evidence from a prospective study. BJU Int. 2012;110(11 PtB):E438–42.
19. Watterson JD, Girvan AR, Cook AJ, et al. Safety and efficacy of holmium:YAG laser lithotripsy in patients with bleeding diatheses. J Urol. 2002;168(2):442–5.
20. Semins MJ, Trock BJ, Matlaga BR. The safety of ureteroscopy during pregnancy: a systematic review and meta-analysis. J Urol. 2009;181(1):139–43.
21. Tang L, Gao X, Xu B, et al. Placement of ureteral stent after uncomplicated ureteroscopy: do we really need it? Urology. 2011;78(6):1248–56.
22. Sun X, Xia S, Lu J, Liu H, Han B, Li W. Treatment of large impacted proximal ureteral stones: randomized comparison of percutaneous antegrade ureterolithotripsy versus retrograde ureterolithotripsy. J Endourol. 2008;22(5):913–7.
23. Bader MJ, Eisner B, Porpiglia F, Preminger GM, Tiselius HG. Contemporary management of ureteral stones. Eur Urol. 2012;61(4):764–72.
24. Maheshwari PN, Oswal AT, Andankar M, Nanjappa KM, Bansal M. Is antegrade ureteroscopy better than retrograde ureteroscopy for impacted large upper ureteral calculi? J Endourol. 1999;13(6):441–4.
25. Karami H, Arbab AH, Hosseini SJ, Razzaghi MR, Simaei NR. Impacted upper-ureteral calculi >1 cm: blind access and totally tubeless percutaneous antegrade removal or retrograde approach? J Endourol. 2006;20(9):616–9.
26. Basiri A, Simforoosh N, Ziaee A, Shayaninasab H, Moghaddam SM, Zare S. Retrograde, antegrade, and laparoscopic approaches for the management of large, proximal ureteral stones: a randomized clinical trial. J Endourol. 2008;22(12):2677–80.
27. Kumar A, Mohanty NK, Jain M, Prakash S, Arora RP. A prospective randomized comparison between early (<48 hours of onset of colicky pain) versus delayed shockwave lithotripsy for symptomatic upper ureteral calculi: a single center experience. J Endourol. 2010;24(12):2059–66.
28. Kreshover JE, Dickstein RJ, Rowe C, Babayan RK, Wang DS. Predictors for negative ureteroscopy in the management of upper urinary tract stone disease. Urology. 2011;78(4):748–52.

29. Knapp PM, Kulb TB, Lingeman JE, et al. Extracorporeal shock wave lithotripsy-induced perirenal hematomas. J Urol. 1988;139(4):700–3.
30. Dhar NB, Thornton J, Karafa MT, Streem SB. A multivariate analysis of risk factors associated with subcapsular hematoma formation following electromagnetic shock wave lithotripsy. J Urol. 2004;172(6 Pt 1):2271–4.
31. Soyupek S, Armağan A, Koşar A, et al. Risk factors for the formation of a steinstrasse after shock wave lithotripsy. Urol Int. 2005;74(4):323–5.
32. Padhye AS, Yadav PB, Mahajan PM, et al. Shock wave lithotripsy as a primary modality for treating upper ureteric stones: a 10-year experience. Indian J Urol. 2008;24(4):486–9.
33. Taie K, Jasemi M, Khazaeli D, Fatholahi A. Prevalence and management of complications of ureteroscopy: a seven-year experience with introduction of a new maneuver to prevent ureteral avulsion. Urol J. 2012;9(1):356–60.
34. Ramaswamy K, Shah O. Antibiotic prophylaxis after uncomplicated ureteroscopic stone treatment: is there a difference? J Endourol. 2012;26(2):122.
35. Joshi HB, Stainthorpe A, MacDonagh RP, Keeley Jr FX, Timoney AG, Barry MJ. Indwelling ureteral stents: evaluation of symptoms, quality of life and utility. J Urol. 2003;169(3):1065–9.
36. Michel MS, Trojan L, Rassweiler JJ. Complications in percutaneous nephrolithotomy. Eur Urol. 2007; 51(4):899–906.
37. de la Rosette J, Assimos D, Desai M, et al. The Clinical Research Office of the Endourological Society Percutaneous Nephrolithotomy Global Study: indications, complications, and outcomes in 5803 patients. J Endourol. 2011;25(1):11–7.
38. Soucy F, Ko R, Duvdevani M, Nott L, Denstedy JD, Razvi H. Percutaneous nephrolithotomy for staghorn calculi: a single center's experience over 15 years. J Endourol. 2009;23(10):1669–73.
39. Muslumanoglu AY, Tefekli A, Karadag MA, Tok A, Sari E, Berberogly Y. Impact of percutaneous access point number and location on complication and success rates in percutaneous nephrolithotomy. Urol Int. 2006;77(4):340–6.
40. Elsamra S, Pareek G. Complications of laparoscopic renal surgery. Int J Urol. 2010;17(3):206–14.
41. Liguori G, Antoniolli F, Trombetta C, et al. Comparative experimental evaluation of guidewire use in urology. Urology. 2008;72(2):286–9. discussion 289–90.
42. Clayman M, Uribe CA, Eichel L, Gordon Z, McDougall EM, Clayman RV. Comparison of guide wires in urology. Which, when and why? J Urol. 2004;171(6 Pt 1):2146–50.
43. Sarkissian C, Korman E, Hendlin K, Monga M. Systematic evaluation of hybrid guidewires: shaft stiffness, lubricity, and tip configuration. Urology. 2012;79(3):513–7.
44. Kourambas J, Byrne RR, Preminger GM. Does a ureteral access sheath facilitate ureteroscopy? J Urol. 2001;165(3):789–93.
45. Landman J, Venkatesh R, Ragab M, et al. Comparison of intrarenal pressure and irrigant flow during percutaneous nephroscopy with an indwelling ureteral catheter, ureteral occlusion balloon, and ureteral access sheath. Urology. 2002;60(4):584–7.
46. L'esperance JO, Ekeruo WO, Scales Jr CD, et al. Effect of ureteral access sheath on stone-free rates in patients undergoing ureteroscopic management of renal calculi. Urology. 2005;66(2):252–5.
47. Monga M, Bhayani S, Landman J, Conradie M, Sundaram CP, Clayman RV. Ureteral access for upper urinary tract disease: the access sheath. J Endourol. 2001;15(8):831–4.
48. Pietrow PK, Auge BK, Delvecchio FC, et al. Techniques to maximize flexible ureteroscope longevity. Urology. 2002;60(5):784–8.
49. De Sio M, Autorino R, Damiano R, Olivia A, Pane U, D'Armiento M. Expanding applications of the access sheath to ureterolithotripsy of distal ureteral stones. A frustrating experience. Urol Int. 2004;72 Suppl 1Suppl. 1:55–7.
50. Monga M, Gawlik A, Durfee W. Systematic evaluation of ureteral access sheaths. Urology. 2004;63(5): 834–6.
51. Pedro RN, Hendlin K, Durfee WK, Monga M. Physical characteristics of next-generation ureteral access sheaths: buckling and kinking. Urology. 2007;70(3):440–2.
52. Monga M, Best S, Venkatesh R, et al. Prospective randomized comparison of 2 ureteral access sheaths during flexible retrograde ureteroscopy. J Urol. 2004;172(2):572–3.
53. Hendlin K, Lund B, Dockendorf K, Ramani A, Monga M. Radial dilation of ureteral balloons: comparative in vitro analysis. J Endourol. 2005;19(5): 575–8.
54. Marguet CG, Sung JC, Springhart WP, et al. In vitro comparison of stone retropulsion and fragmentation of the frequency doubled, double pulse nd:yag laser and the holmium:yag laser. J Urol. 2005;173(5): 1797–800.
55. Teichman JM, Vassar GJ, Glickman RD. Holmium:yttrium-aluminum-garnet lithotripsy efficiency varies with stone composition. Urology. 1998;52(3):392–7.
56. Nazif OA, Teichman JM, Glickman RD, Welch AJ. Review of laser fibers: a practical guide for urologists. J Endourol. 2004;18(9):818–29.
57. Calvano CJ, Moran ME, White MD, Borhan-Manesh A, Mehlhaff BA. Experimental utilization of the holmium laser in a model of ureteroscopic lithotripsy: energy analysis. J Endourol. 1999;13(2):113–5.
58. Kuo RL, Aslan P, Zhong P, Preminger GM. Impact of holmium laser settings and fiber diameter on stone fragmentation and endoscope deflection. J Endourol. 1998;12(6):523–7.
59. Poon M, Beaghler M, Baldwin D. Flexible endoscope deflectability: changes using a variety of working instruments and laser fibers. J Endourol. 1997;11(4):247–9.

60. Maislos SD, Volpe M, Albert PS, Raboy A. Efficacy of the stone cone for treatment of proximal ureteral stones. J Endourol. 2004;18(9):862–4.
61. Wang CJ, Huang SW, Chang CH. Randomized trial of NTrap for proximal ureteral stones. Urology. 2011;77(3):553–7.
62. Vejdani K, Eisner BH, Pengune W, Stoller ML. Effect of laser insult on devices used to prevent stone retropulsion during ureteroscopic lithotripsy. J Endourol. 2009;23(4):705–7.
63. Ahmed M, Pedro RN, Kieley S, Akornor JW, Durfee WK, Monga M. Systematic evaluation of ureteral occlusion devices: insertion, deployment, stone migration, and extraction. Urology. 2009;73(5):976–80.
64. Farahat YA, Elbahnasy AW, Elashry OM. A randomized prospective controlled study for assessment of different ureteral occlusion devices in prevention of stone migration during pneumatic lithotripsy. Urology. 2011;77(1):30–5.
65. Salimi N, Mahajan A, Don J, Schwartz B. A novel stone retrieval basket for more efficient lithotripsy procedures. J Med Eng Technol. 2009;33(2):142–50.
66. Zeltser IS, Bagley DH. Basket design as a factor in retention and release of calculi in vitro. J Endourol. 2007;21(3):337–42.
67. Lukasewycz S, Hoffman N, Botnaru A, Deka PM, Monga M. Comparison of tipless and helical baskets in an in vitro ureteral model. Urology. 2004; 64(3):435–8. discussion 438.
68. Kesler SS, Pierre SA, Brison DI, Preminger GM, Munver R. Use of the Escape nitinol stone retrieval basket facilitates fragmentation and extraction of ureteral and renal calculi: a pilot study. J Endourol. 2008;22(6):1213–7.
69. Korman E, Hendlin K, Monga M. Small-diameter nitinol stone baskets: radial dilation force and dynamics of opening. J Endourol. 2011;25(9):1537–40.
70. Smith AD. Smith's textbook of endourology. 3rd ed. Oxford, UK: Wiley-Blackwell; 2011. p. 388–94.
71. Multescu DR, Mirciulescu V, Geavlete B, Geavlete P. C86 Digital semirigid ureteroscopy: a new standard in endoscopic imaging. Eur Urol. 2009;8:686.
72. Sung JC, Springhart WP, Marguet CG, et al. Location and etiology of flexible and semirigid ureteroscope damage. Urology. 2005;66(5):958–63.
73. Bagley DH. Removal of upper urinary tract calculi with flexible ureteropyeloscopy. Urology. 1990; 35(5):412–6.
74. Holden T, Pedro RN, Hendlin K, Durfee W, Monga M. Evidence-based instrumentation for flexible ureteroscopy: a review. J Endourol. 2008;22(7):1423–6.
75. Haberman K, Ortiz-Alvarado O, Chotikawanich E, Monga M. A dual-channel flexible ureteroscope: evaluation of deflection, flow, illumination, and optics. J Endourol. 2011;25(9):1411–4.
76. Semins MJ, George S, Allaf ME, Matlaga BR. Ureteroscope cleaning and sterilization by the urology operating room team: the effect on repair costs. J Endourol. 2009;23(6):903–5.
77. Monga M, Weiland D, Pedro RN, Lynch AC, Anderson K. Intrarenal manipulation of flexible ureteroscopes: a comparative study. BJU Int. 2007; 100(1):157–9.
78. Paffen ML, Keizer JG, de Winter GV, Arends AJ, Hendrikx AJ. A comparison of the physical properties of four new generation flexible ureteroscopes: (de)flection, flow properties, torsion stiffness, and optical characteristics. J Endourol. 2008;22(10): 2227–34.
79. Multescu R, Geavlete B, Georgescu D, Geavlete P. Conventional fiberoptic flexible ureteroscope versus fourth generation digital flexible ureteroscope: a critical comparison. J Endourol. 2010;24(1):17–21.
80. Zilberman DE, Lipkin ME, Ferrandino MN, et al. The digital flexible ureteroscope: in vitro assessment of optical characteristics. J Endourol. 2011;25(3):519–22.
81. Bach T, Geavlete B, Herrmann TR, Gross AJ. Working tools in flexible ureterorenoscopy—influence on flow and deflection: what does matter? J Endourol. 2008;22(8):1639–43.
82. Hendlin K, Weiland D, Monga M. Impact of irrigation systems on stone migration. J Endourol. 2008; 22(3):453–8.
83. Sprunger JK, Herrell III SD. Techniques of ureteroscopy. Urol Clin North Am. 2004;31(1):61–9.
84. Bhanot N, Sahud AG, Sepkowitz D. Best practice policy statement on urologic surgery antimicrobial prophylaxis. Urology. 2009;74(1):236–7.
85. Wolf Jr JS, Bennett CJ, Dmochowski RR, Hollenbeck BK, Pearle MS, Schaeffer AJ. Best practice policy statement on urologic surgery antimicrobial prophylaxis. J Urol. 2008;179(4):1379–90.
86. Knopf HJ, Graff HJ, Schulze H. Perioperative antibiotic prophylaxis in ureteroscopic stone removal. Eur Urol. 2003;44(1):115–8.
87. Christiano AP, Hollowell CM, Kim H, et al. Double-blind randomized comparison of single-dose ciprofloxacin versus intravenous cefazolin in patients undergoing outpatient endourologic surgery. Urology. 2000;55(2):182–5.
88. Meyer RS, White KK, Smith JM, Groppo ER, Mubarak SJ, Hargens AR. Intramuscular and blood pressures in legs positioned in the hemilithotomy position: clarification of risk factors for well-leg acute compartment syndrome. J Bone Joint Surg Am. 2002;84-A(10):1829–35.
89. Forrest JB, Clemens JQ, Finamore P, et al. AUA Best Practice Statement for the prevention of deep vein thrombosis in patients undergoing urologic surgery. J Urol. 2009;181(3):1170–7.
90. Elkoushy MA, Shahrour W, Andonian S. Pulsed fluoroscopy in ureteroscopy and percutaneous nephrolithotomy. Urology. 2012;79(6):1230–5.
91. Kipling M, Mohammed A, Medding RN. Guidewires in clinical practice: applications and troubleshooting. Expert Rev Med Devices. 2009;6(2):187–95.
92. Elashry OM, Elgamasy AK, Sabaa MA, et al. Ureteroscopic management of lower ureteric calculi:

a 15-year single-centre experience. BJU Int. 2008; 102(8):1010–7.

93. Borboroglu PG, Amling CL, Schenkman NS, et al. Ureteral stenting after ureteroscopy for distal ureteral calculi: a multi-institutional prospective randomized controlled study assessing pain, outcomes and complications. J Urol. 2001;166(5):1651–7.
94. Dickstein RJ, Kreshover JE, Babayan RK, Wang DS. Is a safety wire necessary during routine flexible ureteroscopy? J Endourol. 2010;24(10):1589–92.
95. Ordon M, Schuler TD, Honey RJ. Ureteral avulsion during contemporary ureteroscopic stone management: "the scabbard avulsion". J Endourol. 2011; 25(8):1259–62.
96. Kau EL, Ng CS, Fuchs GJ. Complications of ureteroscopic surgery. In: Taneja SS, editor. Complications of urologic surgery. 4th ed. Philadelphia, PA: Elsevier; 2010. p. 303–16.
97. Weedin JW, Coburn M, Link RE. The impact of proximal stone burden on the management of encrusted and retained ureteral stents. J Urol. 2011;185(2):542–7.
98. Krambeck AE, Walsh RS, Denstedt JD, et al. A novel drug eluting ureteral stent: a prospective, randomized, multicenter clinical trial to evaluate the safety and effectiveness of a ketorolac loaded ureteral stent. J Urol. 2010;183(3):1037–42.
99. Gupta M, Patel T, Xavier K, et al. Prospective randomized evaluation of periureteral botulinum toxin type A injection for ureteral stent pain reduction. J Urol. 2010;183(2):598–602.
100. Norris RD, Sur RL, Springhart WP, et al. A prospective, randomized, double-blinded placebo-controlled comparison of extended release oxybutynin versus phenazopyridine for the management of postoperative ureteral stent discomfort. Urology. 2008;71(5):792–5.
101. Adiyat KT, Meuleners R, Monga M. Selective postoperative imaging after ureteroscopy. Urology. 2009;73(3):490–3.
102. Weizer AZ, Auge BK, Silverstein AD, et al. Routine postoperative imaging is important after ureteroscopic stone manipulation. J Urol. 2002;168(1): 46–50.
103. Corcoran AT, Smaldone MC, Ricchiuti DD, Averch TD. Management of benign ureteral strictures in the endoscopic era. J Endourol. 2009;23(11): 1909–12.
104. Kozinn SI, Canes D, Sorcini A, Moinzadeh A. Robotic versus open distal ureteral reconstruction and reimplantation for benign stricture disease. J Endourol. 2012;26(2):147–51.
105. Lopes Neto AC, Korkes F, Silva II JL, et al. Prospective randomized study of treatment of large proximal ureteral stones: extracorporeal shock wave lithotripsy versus ureterolithotripsy versus laparoscopy. J Urol. 2011;187(1):164–8.

9 Ureteroscopy for Renal Stones with Case Discussion of Lower Pole Stones

Sri Sivalingam and Stephen Y. Nakada

Introduction

The management of renal calculi has evolved to the extent that percutaneous nephrolithotomy (PCNL), ureteroscopy (URS), and shock wave lithotripsy (SWL) are potential options depending on the stone type and anatomic characteristics. However, this presents new challenges in planning which modality is best suited for a given renal calculus. Established factors that influence management can be divided into stone factors (i.e. stone burden, stone composition, and stone location), anatomic factors (e.g. UPJO, hydronephrosis, calyceal diverticulum, lower pole) patient factors (e.g. infection, obesity, coagulopathy). Although these criteria are important in guiding treatment decisions, a comprehensive discussion of these is beyond the scope of this chapter. Presently, SWL is regarded as first-line therapy for renal calculi smaller than 20 mm; however, many studies have evaluated factors that predict SWL failure [1]. These include morbid obesity [2], stone volume [3], stone composition [4], or lower pole stone location [4, 5]. In such cases, URS and PCNL can achieve better success rates with fewer number of procedures per incident. It is therefore important to obtain accurate preoperative imaging for appropriate treatment planning and anticipate outcomes. Although plain films (KUB) are generally adequate to assess stone location and burden, we now know that more specific information such as skin-to-stone distance and stone density measurement using CT imaging can have significant impact on outcomes [2, 6, 7].

S. Sivalingam, M.D., F.R.C.S.C.
Department of Urology, University of Wisconsin Hospitals & Clinics, Madison, WI, USA

S.Y. Nakada, M.D., F.A.C.S. (✉)
Department of Urology, University of Wisconsin School of Medicine and Public Health, 1685 Highland Avenue, Madison, WI 53705, USA
e-mail: NAKADA@urology.wisc.edu

Indications for URS Management of Renal Calculi

The indications for URS treatment of renal calculi can be divided into anatomic characteristics, patient characteristics, and stone characteristics (Table 9.1). Renal calculi have traditionally been treated with ESWL or PCNL, but the improvement in ureteroscope technology permits the treatment of most renal calculi within 2 cm [8, 9]. The introduction of smaller diameter laser fibers, multistage deflecting, small caliber (5.3 F) flexible ureteroscopes, and improved displays has allowed for the treatment of all types and locations of renal calculi, with outcomes equal to, or better than SWL [10]. This is especially applicable for cases that are not suitable for SWL, in that URS is less invasive and potentially less morbid than PCNL. A diagrammatic algorithm as shown in Fig. 9.1 can be used to guide the decision-making process for SWL versus

S.Y. Nakada and M.S. Pearle (eds.), *Surgical Management of Urolithiasis: Percutaneous, Shockwave and Ureteroscopy*, DOI 10.1007/978-1-4614-6937-7_9, © Springer Science+Business Media New York 2013

Table 9.1 Indications for ureteroscopic management of renal calculi (adapted from Wignall et al. [10])

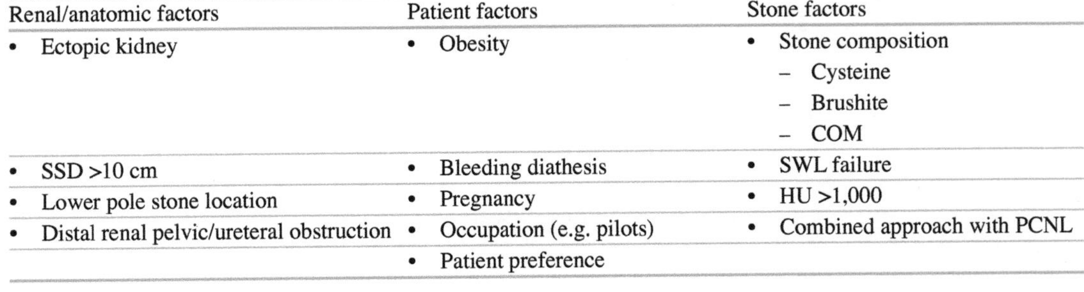

Renal/anatomic factors	Patient factors	Stone factors
• Ectopic kidney	• Obesity	• Stone composition – Cysteine – Brushite – COM
• SSD >10 cm	• Bleeding diathesis	• SWL failure
• Lower pole stone location	• Pregnancy	• HU >1,000
• Distal renal pelvic/ureteral obstruction	• Occupation (e.g. pilots)	• Combined approach with PCNL
	• Patient preference	

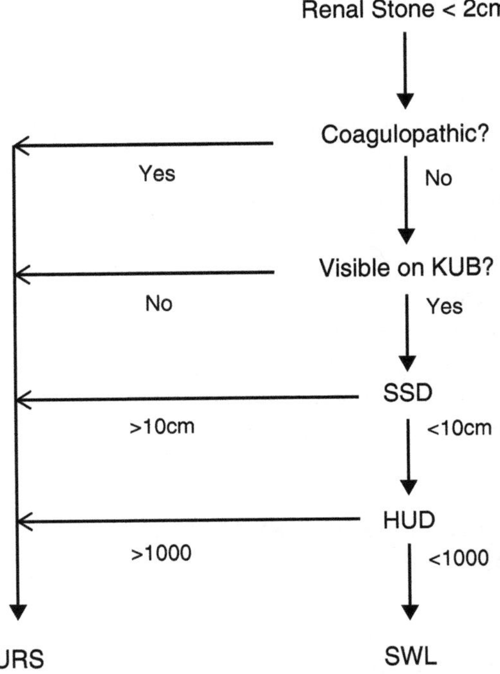

Fig. 9.1 Flow chart illustrating decision-making process in choosing SWL versus URS for the treatment of renal calculi

URS management of renal stones. Table 9.2 summarizes contemporary studies showing the outcomes of URS for renal calculi, and Table 9.3 highlights some key studies comparing URS versus SWL or PNL.

URS with Obesity and Other Comorbidities

Body habitus has an impact on planning the surgical approach for stone treatment, especially given the relatively high prevalence of obesity (36 %) in the USA [11]. Both SWL and, to a lesser extent, PCNL have some limitations and challenges in the obese/morbidly obese patient [12]. For example, the decreased efficacy of SWL in patients with large skin-to-stone distances, i.e. the obese, which is now an established predictor of SWL success [2, 6, 13], should be considered when attempting SWL in the obese. As far as PNL is concerned in the obese patient, cardiovascular compromise from the prone positioning can be an issue, and one must be equipped with extra-long instruments and accessories due to the longer access tract requirements. Some of the theoretical concerns regarding the safety and efficacy of PCNL in the obese have been refuted in more contemporary series [12, 14]. URS circumvents much of the challenges inherent to the obese patient, e.g. BMI >35, provided that the patient is a candidate for anesthesia. URS can be safely and effectively performed in the obese and morbidly obese patients, with similar SFRs and complication rates when matched for stone location and size [15–18]. The limits of URS has been pushed further for very large calculi, for example, as planned multisession URS for cases of staghorn calculi in instances where obesity and comorbidities preclude PCNL, achieving considerable reduction in stone burden [19, 20]. In experienced hands, the indications for URS can include large stones >2.0 cm or even 2.5 cm, pediatric patients, pregnant patients, patients on anticoagulation medications, and those with coagulopathy [21]. As reviewed by Preminger, some presentations may preclude the use of PNL or SWL, favoring URS as the more suitable approach. These include renal stones with the coexistence of ureteral calculi and/or ureteral

Table 9.2 Outcomes of URS for renal calculi

Study	Year	Energy	Number of patients	SFR	Comment
Breda et al. [46]	2008	Ho YAG	24	79 % after single URS; 100 % after 2nd URS	Stones <2 cm; 1.2 mean procedures/pt
			27	52 % with single URS; 85 % after 2nd URS	Stones >2 cm; 1.6 mean procedures/pt
Cocuzza et al. [54]	2008	Ho YAG	44	93 % after initial URS; 97.7 % after 2nd URS	Mean stone burden ~11.5 mm; 66 % had lower pole calculi
Mariani et al. [55]	2004	EHL+Ho YAG	15	92 % after initial URS procedure; 77 % of patients had single-stage procedure	Stones 2–4 cm
Bilgasem et al. [56]	2003	Ho-YAG	29	83 % after initial URS	Stones <1 cm (mean 5.7 mm; 89 % lower pole)
Riley et al. [20]	2009	Ho-YAG	22	90.9 % (average number of procedures = 1.85)	Stones >2.5 cm; mean stone size = 3.0 cm

Table 9.3 Outcomes of URS versus SWL or URS versus PCNL for lower pole calculi

Study	Year	*N*	SFR (SWL)	SFR (URS)	SFR (PCNL)	*p*	Comment
Bozkurt et al. [57]	2011	79	N/A	89.2 %	92.8 %		Longer OR time with URS; longer hospital stay with PCNL
Pearle et al. [51]	2005	67	35 %	50 %	N/A	0.92	Stones <1 cm
Koo et al. [58]	2011	89; 37 (URS); 51 (SWL)	45.1 %	59.4 %	N/A	NS	Reported SFRs after initial procedure, all stones <2 cm

strictures, bleeding diathesis, renal anomalies, solitary kidneys, and morbid obesity [22, 23].

Stone Composition and URS

The Holmium (Ho:YAG) laser can effectively fragment calculi of all compositions [24]. This is contrary to SWL, in which stone types such as cystine, brushite, and calcium oxalate monohydrate are relatively resistant to fragmentation. The Ho:YAG laser fragments stones through a photothermal mechanism [25]. The optimal settings to achieve maximal stone fragmentation and efficiency are not clearly defined and are based upon the fragmentation goals of the operator. Sea et al. tested a range of power settings and demonstrated Ho:YAG lithotripsy variation with pulse energy settings [26]. In their study, low pulse energy (0.2 J) resulted in less fragmentation and retropulsion, with smaller fragments. However, at high pulse energy (2.0 J), more fragmentation and retropulsion occurred, with larger fragments. Retropulsion increases with higher power settings, and the use of anti-retropulsion devices can help stabilize the stone and produce more efficient lithotripsy. Interestingly, retropulsion was not affected by changes in frequency when pulse energy was held constant. Laser fibers are available in varying core diameters (150–550 μm) as well as single-use and reusable variants. Kudsen et al., showed in a multicenter trial that reusable holmium:YAG optical laser fibers are a more cost-effective option for laser lithotripsy than single use variants [27]. Additionally, they demonstrated that laser fibers with larger core diameter (e.g. 365 μm) provide a greater number of uses compared to smaller fibers. We generally use a power setting of 0.8 J at a frequency of 8 Hz using a 270 μm laser fiber, and adjust if needed based on the principles of balancing fragmentation and retropulsion described above.

Case Discussion: Lower Pole Renal Calculi

Lower pole calculi have the unique disadvantages for stone clearance, caused by the inherent gravity effects, lengthier infundibula, and narrowed infundibulopelvic angles. While the three contemporary surgical techniques, i.e. shock wave lithotripsy (SWL), ureterorenoscopy, and percutaneous nephrolithotomy (PCNL) are all viable options, the success rates are different and should play a role in surgical decision-making.

Although SWL is generally the preferred form of treatment for symptomatic renal calculi smaller than 2 cm in diameter, the stone-free rates (SFR) are not as favorable for stones in the lower pole, or dependent portion of the kidney. PCNL was an alternative, albeit more invasive technique, that was reported to have higher SFRs with decreasing morbidity [28]. For this reason, the Lower Pole Study Group was created, to evaluate the unique challenges presented by lower pole calculi in 2001 [5].

Some of the challenges of lower pole calculi with respect to SFRs are attributed to the gravity-dependent position of the lower pole calyx, which prevents efficient stone clearance. However, the decreased SFRs in the lower pole owes to more than just the gravitation effect. Work by Sampaio and Aragao revealed that the spatial anatomy of the lower pole is a factor in stone passage [29]. In this study, three anatomic features that could possibly affect stone clearance were identified: the angle between the lower pole infundibulum and renal pelvis, diameter of the lower pole infundibulum, and third, the spatial distribution of the calices. Detailed studies on the infundibulo-pelvic angle (IPA) of the lower pole calices showed a significant correlation of these angles with SFRs. For example, at 9 months, 75 % of the patients presenting an angle of greater than 90° between the lower infundibulum where the stone was located and the renal pelvis became stone-free within 3 months. On the other hand, only 23 % of the patients presenting an angle smaller than 90° between the lower infundibulum where the stone was located and the renal pelvis became stone-free during the same follow-up [30]. Based on these and other similar findings, Elbahnasy et al. described a method to measure the IPA preoperatively using excretory urography (IVP) [31], which would be useful for surgical planning based on predicted stone clearance rates.

Currently available flexible ureteroscopes permit maximal deflections of up to 270°, or multi-staged deflection (i.e. primary and secondary deflection) which can gain access into the lower pole calyx. This is further facilitated by thin (200–270 μm) laser fibers and newer basket extraction devices, which minimize the effect on scope deflection [32, 33]. These developments allow for the treatment of lower pole stones in situ (Fig. 9.2a, b). In cases where the stone cannot be adequately targeted or accessed by the ureteroscope and laser, an appropriate next step is to reposition the stone into a more accessible upper pole calyx, which can be achieved with modern nitinol retrieval devices [33–35].

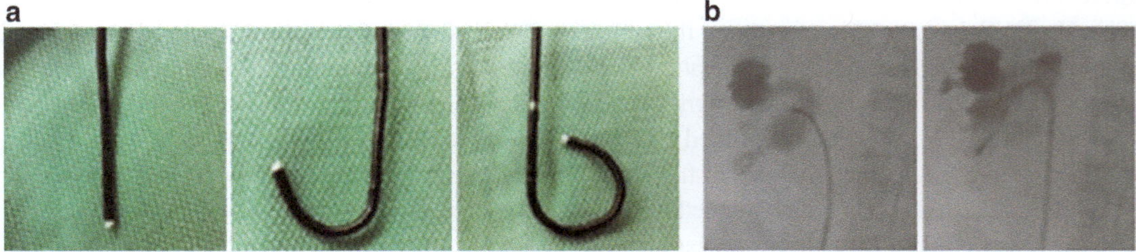

Fig. 9.2 (**a**) Active deflection shown in Olympus P-5 flexible ureteroscope. (**b**) Access to lower pole stone with Olympus P-5 Flexible ureteroscope with 270 μm laser fiber in place

Detailed Technical Approach

Instrument List

1. Flexible/rigid cystoscope
2. Open-ended 5 F ureteral catheter
3. Guide-wire (Sensor® PTFE-nitinol guidewire with hydrophilic tip (Boston Scientific), ± straight and angled Glidewire® nitinol hydrophilic guidewire (Boston Scientific) ± Amplatz super-stiff)
4. Flexible ureteroscope (Olympus P5 180-270)
5. Semirigid ureteroscope (ACMI Micro-6)
6. Light source and irrigation setup
7. Pathfinder™ endoscopic bulb irrigator (Utah medical products)
8. Sureseal adaptor (Applied medical)
9. Disposable laser fiber (270 μm) + Holmium laser set-up
10. Nitinol zero—tip basket
11. JJ ureteral stent (6 F)
12. Omnipaque Contrast—diluted 50 % in sterile water
13. C-arm Fluoroscopy
14. Optional: ureteral access sheath (12–14 F)
15. Optional: balloon dilator (15 F)
16. 60 cm^3 syringe

Current Ureteroscopes

Table 9.4 lists the currently available flexible ureteroscopes. Advancements in flexible ureteroscopy design and functionality have led to improved instrument longevity, and the ability to access more challenging stone locations such as the lower pole calyces. Newer, actively deflecting scopes offer increased lower pole access compared to the older passively deflecting scope by one of two mechanisms: either separate dual-lever primary and secondary deflection that offers increased unidirectional downward deflections of 270° (Gyrus-ACMI Dur8-E™ and Stryker Flexvision™) or increased bidirectional primary deflection that offers 270° of deflection in both directions (Gyrus-ACMI Dur-D™, Olympus URF-P5™, Karl Storz Flex-X2™, Wolf Viper™) [36]. Having variable deflection, such as 270/180, gives the surgeon even more options for access into multiple challenging calices.

Holden et al. [36], provide a detailed analysis of the various ureteroscopes listed above, and the pros and cons of each can be weighed to choose the ideal instrument for the urologist's needs. An important consideration is the durability of the flexible scope, which becomes even more critical when using it for advanced procedures such as lower pole calculi. Repair costs are expensive and it has been demonstrated that certain scope types, such as the Wolf Viper, Olympus URF-P5, and Stryker Flexvision U-500 have excellent and comparable durability, while the Gyrus-ACMI DUR-8 Elite suffered from early failure and major repair after the least use, in a recent prospective trial [37].

Patient Preparation

The patient should be counseled in the preoperative visit and informed consent is obtained, with appropriate discussion on potential complications, most commonly being that of urinary tract infections and stent-related symptoms. However, a more thorough discussion may include the risks of anesthesia, minor ureteral perforation, residual stones with the requirement of re-treatment or further treatment, long term complications of urethral/ureteral strictures, and rare complications such as major ureteral injury or hemorrhage. In complex cases involving ectopic kidneys, horseshoe kidney's etc., further discussion regarding obtaining access to the renal pelvis should be considered.

Preoperative investigations include a thorough history and physical examination, laboratory evaluation including complete blood count, serum creatinine, coagulation panel, urinalysis ± cultures, and imaging studies with either KUB, IVP, or CT KUB. The benefit of performing a CT study is that the Hounsfield density can be calculated, which provides key information on potential stone composition and fragility to shockwaves [7], as well as the SSD [2, 6]. URS is

Table 9.4 Specifications of current flexible ureteroscopes

	Olympus		Olympus ACMI-GYRUS					STORZ		WOLF		STRYKER
	URF-P5	URF-V	AUR-7	DUR-8 Elite	DUR-8	DUR-8 ULTRA	DUR-D	FLEX-X2	FLEX-X[c]	COBRA—Dual channel	VIPER	FlexVision U500
Tip diameter (F)	5.3F	8.5F	7.2F	6.75F	6.75F	8.6F	8.7F	7.5F	8.5F	6F	6F	6.9F
Maximal shaft diameter (F)	–	9.9F	11F	8.7F	8.7F	9.3F	9.3F	8.4F	8.5F	9.9F	8.8F	–
Inner channel diameter (F)	3.6F	3.6F	3.6F	3.6F	3.6F	3.6F	3.6F	3.6F	3.6F	3.3F×2	3.6F	3.6F
Active deflection in degrees (up/down)	180° up /275° down	180° up /275° down	120° up /160° down	170° up /180° down	175° up /185° down	270° up /270° down	250° up /250° down	270° up /270° down	270° up /270° down	270° up /270° down	270° up /270° down	250° up /250° down
Secondary deflection	No	No	No	Yes	No	No	No	No	No	No	No	Yes
View (°)	90	90	80	80	80	80	80	110	90	85	86	90
Lens	Analogue	Digital	Analogue	Analogue	Analogue	Analogue	Digital	Analogue	Digital	Analogue	Analogue	Analogue

particularly indicated in cases where the SSD is greater than 10 cm which has been shown to result in poor SWL outcomes.

Technique and Perioperative Setup

Routine preoperative antibiotics are given and anesthesia (sedation with local, regional, or general) is administered. The patient is positioned in dorsal lithotomy and prepped and draped appropriately with fluoroscopy using the C-arm positioned and draped over the ipsilateral kidney and ureter. The fluoroscopy and URS video monitors are positioned for easy viewing during the procedure. Cystoscopy is performed and the ureteral orifice is identified and canulated with the Sensor® PTFE-nitinol guidewire with hydrophilic tip (Boston Scientific) guidewire; if resistance is encountered, an open-ended ureteral catheter may be used to provide addition support for the guide wire to gain entry into the ureter. If further resistance is encountered, the open-ended catheter is advanced to the level of resistance under fluoroscopic guidance, and a retrograde ureterogram is performed to delineate the course and anatomy of the ureter. With a more detailed representation of the ureter and obstructing site, a hydrophilic wire can be used to negotiate entrance into the renal pelvis, followed by the open-ended catheter over it. It is prudent to exercise caution when manipulating a wire past an impacted or tortuous ureter to avoid perforation. Failing this, a semirigid or flexible ureteroscope must be used to advance a wire past the obstruction under direct vision. Once access is gained into the renal pelvis, the hydrophilic wire, if used, is replaced with the standard guide wire. This will serve as a safety wire, which can be secured to the drapes with a clamp.

The use of a safety wire is not routine in all renal stones, and select wireless approach cases, where the ureteroscope is the safety mechanism, have been demonstrated recently to be safe and efficacious [38, 39]. The wireless approach, along with the use of ureteral access sheaths and balloon dilatation of the ureteral orifice is discussed in detail in Chap. 7. Briefly, in the wireless technique, the flexible ureteroscope is initially advanced over a guide wire under fluoroscopic guidance. If resistance is encountered, an 8/10 F dilator may be used to calibrate the ureter with fluoroscopy. The ureteroscope can then be advanced over the wire. Once the ureteroscope is within the renal pelvis, the guide wire is withdrawn and ureterorenoscopy with laser lithotripsy is performed.

With the ureteroscope in place, laser lithotripsy can be initiated. Irrigation with NS should be maintained at a rate sufficient to obtain clear visibility, but not so high as to displace the stones being treated. A systematic approach should be used for proficiency and optimal outcomes. One such approach is to inspect the collecting system starting with the upper pole calyx and working systematically down to the lower pole calyx [10].

If the visualized stone is small enough to be extracted, a basket or grasper can be used to gently extract the stone, under direct vision. If this cannot be achieved with ease, the laser should be used to fragment/disintegrate the stone. Typically, a holmium:yttrium–aluminum–garnet (Ho:YAG) laser with a 200 μm laser fiber is used. The 200 μm fiber, being of smallest diameter, is ideal as it is the least restrictive on scope deflection, allowing better handling of the instrument during the procedure. It is critical to pass the laser fiber with the scope in a neutral position to avoid damaging the working channel. Additionally, it is important to leave adequate space between the tip of the laser fiber and the ureteroscope tip to avoid damage to the lens to prevent damage to lens. Of note, in cases where stone extraction is needed, we recommend using a sheath.

Lower Pole Stone Displacement

As described by Auge et al., lower pole calculi that are difficult to access due to reduced scope deflection with the laser fiber in place can be displaced into an upper pole calyx for easier fragmentation [35]. This technique utilizes a nitinol basket or grasper, which can be passed into the lower pole through the fully deflected ureteroscope without any loss of deflection (Fig. 9.3).

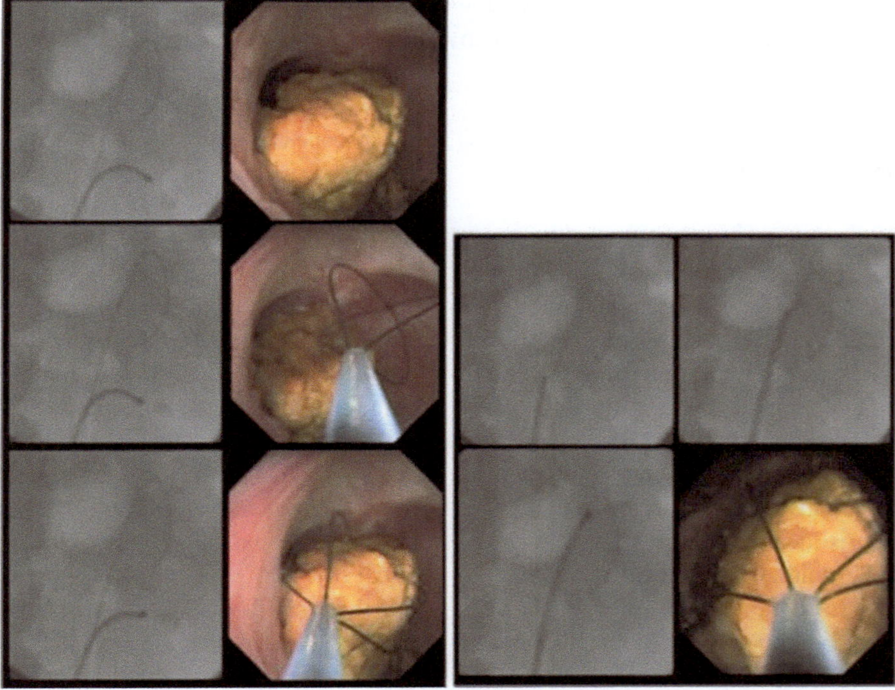

Fig. 9.3 Fluoroscopic and corresponding intraoperative images demonstrating the displacement of a lower pole calculus to an upper pole calyx prior to laser fragmentation

Although irrigant flow might be impeded with the basket in place, stone retrieval should not be affected. This technique allows the treatment of lower pole stones by displacing the stone to a less-dependent position, typically an upper pole calyx, which is easily accessed by the scope and laser fiber. Additionally, the upper pole location also facilitates spontaneous stone fragment clearance post procedure.

Stone Disintegration Technique

While a number of different endoscopic lithotrites have been used in endoscopy, such as ultrasonic, electrohydraulic, pneumatic and laser, the holmium laser has come to dominate intracorporeal lithotripsy [36]. Complete destruction of the calculus is the goal, so as to allow the tine fragments/dust to pass spontaneously. Although, the holmium laser is purported to fragment stones of any composition [24], this composition does affect the fragmentation pattern. As such, various approaches may be taken for stone destruction. The goal of completely disintegrating the stone may be met by "brushing" or "painting" the stone with the tip of the laser fiber by moving the fiber back and forth across the surface of the stone. This is particularly useful for soft stones, and the resulting dust will easily be washed out with urine flow. Another approach is to break the stone into fragments with a "drilling" technique, which is more appropriate for harder stones, and the resulting fragments can be extracted by basket or grasping devices. Once several fragments are formed, the "popcorning" technique, in which the laser is placed within a mound of fragments to created random shattering, can be helpful to gradually reduce the fragments' size [40]. This technique is generally better if the fragments are contained within a calyx. A targeted application of the laser onto distinct fragments by "pinning" them onto the mucosa is more efficacious, albeit more laborious.

Basket Extraction of Stone Fragments

The aim of laser lithotripsy is to disintegrate the stone into gravel that will easily be passed by the patient. The Ho-YAG laser causes a pitting or drilling effect on calculi [41] which can produce stone dust and tiny fragments rather than larger fragments as in SWL. This enables spontaneous passage of the remnant stone fragments, and potentially obviates basket extraction of individual fragments. A recent study by Schatloff et al. evaluated basket extraction of all fragments versus allowing for spontaneous passage [42]. The spontaneous passage group had a higher rate of unplanned visits (3 % versus 30 %, $p=0.01$), with trends toward higher rates of rehospitalization (0 % versus 10 %, $p=0.24$), need for ancillary treatment (0 % versus 7 %, $p=0.49$), and a lower stone-free rate (100 % versus 87 %, $p=0.1$).

Patients with a large stone burden (e.g. stones >15 mm) may benefit from placement of a ureteral access sheath to aid in basket extraction of residual fragments and minimize morbidity from repeat passage the instruments. Patients with smaller stones (mean <11 m) do not necessarily need an access sheath, nor do they need meticulous extraction of fragments after URS as complete destruction of the calculi is the goal, and the resulting gravel will often clear spontaneously. Stone basketing itself is not without complications, and over-zealous basketing can potentially lead to iatrogenic injury to the ureter. As reviewed by de la Rosette et al., such complications include ureteral avulsion, major perforation necessitating surgical repair, minor ureteral perforation, mucosal abrasion, and ureteral stricture [43].

At the end of lithotripsy, contrast is used via the scope to opacify the collecting system, and if it is felt that a stent is needed, the guide wire can be placed in exchange for the ureteroscope.

Flexible Versus Rigid URS

With currently available endoscopic instruments, flexible ureteroscopy is the instrument of choice for the treatment of intrarenal calculi, as it allows for access into individual calyces with excellent maneuvering capabilities and potential to maintain lower intrapelvic pressures through the use of ureteral access sheaths. However, the semirigid ureteroscope has some advantages, such as a larger working channel, and increased durability. There is a paucity of literature on the use of semirigid ureteroscopes for the treatment of renal calculi; however, some recent series have shown the operating time to be lower, with similar SFRs, complication rates, and length of hospital stay when compared to flexible ureteroscopy [9].

Results

Ureteroscopic management of renal calculi has gained popularity and higher success rates owing to the improvement in flexible ureteroscopes. Overall SFR for ureteroscopy are very high, with most patients rendered stone-free after a single procedure [44, 45]. SFRs following ureteroscopy is comparable to that of PCNL, even for large stones >2 cm in contemporary series [46]. The overall success rates of retrograde intrarenal surgery have been reported as 75–95 % for intrarenal stones greater than 2 cm after the first or second treatment, whereas the major and minor complication rates vary from 1.5 to 12 %, which are less frequent than rates in PCNL procedures. For multiple intrarenal stones <2 cm, the ureteroscopic SFRs are as high as 92 % after one or two procedures [8], which is comparable to the rates reported after PCNL or SWL [44, 47]. Complication rates for ureteroscopic management of renal calculi are lower than that encountered after PCNL, with overall rates of 13 % [8] with minimal major complications [48] in contemporary studies. URS is also an excellent salvage procedure for SWL-refractory stones and should be considered in symptomatic patients as opposed to repeat SWL procedures [49, 50]. However, in such situations, it is important to note that the success rates of the salvage URS may be influenced by the same negative factors that reduced the effectiveness of SWL, and SFRs are lower when compared to primary URS series [50].

SFRs for lower pole calculi are generally lower than the overall SFRs for renal calculi. Although many studies have shown relatively modest SFRs of 50 % [51], more recent data suggest that the gap between lower pole calculi and upper and middle calyces is narrowing, owing to the more advanced flexible ureteroscopes today. For example, Perlmutter et al. showed in their series that the SFRs were 100 %, 96 % and 91 % for the upper, middle, and lower pole calyces, respectively [52]. The use of current scopes with deflection angles of 270° has allowed for SFRs as high as 100 % in the lower pole [53].

There has been a shift in the way the stone is treated over the years, for example, a shift away from basket extraction toward mechanical pulverization of the stone [48]. Krambeck et al. reported a decrease from 69.4 % of stones being basket-extracted in 1988 to 47.7 % in their 2006 series. On the same token, the number of procedures with laser mechanical pulverization had substantially increased to 48.7 % in their 2006, up from 6.5 % in 1997, speaking to the popularity of the laser as the lithotripter of choice. Interestingly, in this 2006 report, electrohydraulic lithotripsy was second to laser in popularity, at 42.4 %.

Another interesting trend in the ureteroscopic management of upper tract calculi is that there has been a shift from rigid to flexible instruments. The use of flexible ureteroscopes in the Mayo series increased from 12 % in 1992 to 37 % in 2006. The development of the flexible ureteroscope has continued to evolve, and this usage trend will likely continue to increase with ongoing refinements in flexible instrument technology.

Key Points

1. URS has improved optics and mechanics and has gained widespread popularity for its indications for the treatment of renal calculi.
2. URS has higher overall SFRs for renal calculi when compared to SWL.
3. SFRs for URS may be better than SWL for lower pole calculi, but the difference was not shown to be statistically significant.
4. URS is a good salvage option for failed SWL.
5. URS is an option even for very large (>2 cm) or staghorn calculi, with acceptable SFRs when PCNL is not an option.

References

1. Argyropoulos AN, Tolley DA. Optimizing shock wave lithotripsy in the 21st century. Eur Urol. 2007;52(2):344–52.
2. Pareek G, Hedican SP, Lee FT, Nakada SY. Shock wave lithotripsy success determined by skin-to-stone distance on computed tomography. Urology. 2005; 66(5):941–4.
3. Bandi G, Meiners RJ, Pickhardt PJ, Nakada SY. Stone measurement by volumetric three-dimensional computed tomography for predicting the outcome after extracorporeal shock wave lithotripsy. BJU Int. 2009;103(4):524–8.
4. Grasso M, Loisides P, Beaghler M, Bagley D. The case for primary endoscopic management of upper urinary tract calculi: I. A critical review of 121 extracorporeal shock-wave lithotripsy failures. Urology. 1995;45(3):363–71.
5. Albala DM, Assimos DG, Clayman RV, Denstedt JD, Grasso M, Gutierrez-Aceves J, et al. Lower pole I: a prospective randomized trial of extracorporeal shock wave lithotripsy and percutaneous nephrostolithotomy for lower pole nephrolithiasis-initial results. J Urol. 2001;166(6):2072–80.
6. Patel T, Kozakowski K, Hruby G, Gupta M. Skin to stone distance is an independent predictor of stone-free status following shockwave lithotripsy. J Endourol. 2009;23(9):1383–5.
7. Nakada SY, Hoff DG, Attai S, Heisey D, Blankenbaker D, Pozniak M. Determination of stone composition by noncontrast spiral computed tomography in the clinical setting. Urology. 2000;55(6):816–9.
8. Breda A, Ogunyemi O, Leppert JT, Schulam PG. Flexible ureteroscopy and laser lithotripsy for multiple unilateral intrarenal stones. Eur Urol. 2009;55(5):1190–6.
9. Atis G, Gurbuz C, Arikan O, Canat L, Kilic M, Caskurlu T. Ureteroscopic management with laser lithotripsy of renal pelvic stones. J Endourol. 2012; 26(8):983–7.
10. Wignall GR, Canales BK, Denstedt JD, Monga M. Minimally invasive approaches to upper urinary tract urolithiasis. Urol Clin North Am. 2008;35(3):441–54. viii.
11. Flegal KM, Carroll MD, Kit BK, Ogden CL. Prevalence of obesity and trends in the distribution of body mass index among US adults, 1999–2010. JAMA. 2012;307(5):491–7.
12. Calvert RC, Burgess NA. Urolithiasis and obesity: metabolic and technical considerations. Curr Opin Urol. 2005;15(2):113–7.
13. Wiesenthal JD, Ghiculete D, D'A Honey RJ, Pace KT. Evaluating the importance of mean stone density and

skin-to-stone distance in predicting successful shock wave lithotripsy of renal and ureteric calculi. Urol Res. 2010;38(4):307–13.
14. Pearle MS, Nakada SY, Womack JS, Kryger JV. Outcomes of contemporary percutaneous nephrostolithotomy in morbidly obese patients. J Urol. 1998; 160(3 Pt 1):669–73.
15. Best SL, Nakada SY. Flexible ureteroscopy is effective for proximal ureteral stones in both obese and nonobese patients: a two-year, single-surgeon experience. Urology. 2011;77(1):36–9.
16. Aboumarzouk OM, Somani B, Monga M. Safety and efficacy of ureteroscopic lithotripsy for stone disease in obese patients: a systematic review of the literature. BJU Int. 2012;110(8 Pt B):E374–80.
17. Dash A, Schuster TG, Hollenbeck BK, Faerber GJ, Wolf Jr JS. Ureteroscopic treatment of renal calculi in morbidly obese patients: a stone-matched comparison. Urology. 2002;60(3):393–7. discussion 397.
18. Delorme G, Huu YN, Lillaz J, Bernardini S, Chabannes E, Guichard G, et al. Ureterorenoscopy with holmium-yttrium-aluminum-garnet fragmentation is a safe and efficient technique for stone treatment in patients with a body mass index superior to 30 kg/m^2. J Endourol. 2012;26(3):239–43.
19. Wheat JC, Roberts WW, Wolf Jr JS. Multi-session retrograde endoscopic lithotripsy of large renal calculi in obese patients. Can J Urol. 2009;16(6):4915–20.
20. Riley JM, Stearman L, Troxel S. Retrograde ureteroscopy for renal stones larger than 2.5 cm. J Endourol. 2009;23(9):1395–8.
21. Eisner BH, Kurtz MP, Dretler SP. Ureteroscopy for the management of stone disease. Nat Rev Urol. 2010;7(1):40–5.
22. Preminger GM. Management of lower pole renal calculi: shock wave lithotripsy versus percutaneous nephrolithotomy versus flexible ureteroscopy. Urol Res. 2006;34(2):108–11.
23. Weizer AZ, Springhart WP, Ekeruo WO, Matlaga BR, Tan YH, Assimos DG, et al. Ureteroscopic management of renal calculi in anomalous kidneys. Urology. 2005;65(2):265–9.
24. Bagley D, Erhard M. Use of the holmium laser in the upper urinary tract. Tech Urol. 1995;1(1):25–30.
25. Vassar GJ, Chan KF, Teichman JM, Glickman RD, Weintraub ST, Pfefer TJ, et al. Holmium:YAG lithotripsy: photothermal mechanism. J Endourol. 1999;13(3):181–90.
26. Sea J, Jonat LM, Chew BH, Qiu J, Wang B, Hoopman J, et al. Optimal power settings for holmium:YAG lithotripsy. J Urol. 2012;187(3):914–9.
27. Knudsen BE, Pedro R, Hinck B, Monga M. Durability of reusable holmium:YAG laser fibers: a multicenter study. J Urol. 2011;185(1):160–3.
28. Lingeman JE, Siegel YI, Steele B, Nyhuis AW, Woods JR. Management of lower pole nephrolithiasis: a critical analysis. J Urol. 1994;151(3):663–7.
29. Sampaio FJ, Aragao AH. Limitations of extracorporeal shockwave lithotripsy for lower caliceal stones: anatomic insight. J Endourol. 1994;8(4):241–7.
30. Sampaio FJ, D'Anunciação AL, Silva EC. Comparative follow-up of patients with acute and obtuse infundibulum-pelvic angle submitted to extracorporeal shockwave lithotripsy for lower caliceal stones: preliminary report and proposed study design. J Endourol. 1997;11(3):157–61.
31. Elbahnasy AM, Shalhav AL, Hoenig DM, Elashry OM, Smith DS, McDougall EM, et al. Lower caliceal stone clearance after shock wave lithotripsy or ureteroscopy: the impact of lower pole radiographic anatomy. J Urol. 1998;159(3):676–82.
32. Pasqui F, Dubosq F, Tchala K, Tligui M, Gattegno B, Thibault P, et al. Impact on active scope deflection and irrigation flow of all endoscopic working tools during flexible ureteroscopy. Eur Urol. 2004;45(1):58–64.
33. Landman J, Monga M, El-Gabry EA, Rehman J, Lee DI, Bhayani S, et al. Bare naked baskets: ureteroscope deflection and flow characteristics with intact and disassembled ureteroscopic nitinol stone baskets. J Urol. 2002;167(6):2377–9.
34. Kourambas J, Delvecchio FC, Munver R, Preminger GM. Nitinol stone retrieval-assisted ureteroscopic management of lower pole renal calculi. Urology. 2000;56(6):935–9.
35. Auge BK, Dahm P, Wu NZ, Preminger GM. Ureteroscopic management of lower-pole renal calculi: technique of calculus displacement. J Endourol. 2001;15(8):835–8.
36. Holden T, Pedro RN, Hendlin K, Durfee W, Monga M. Evidence-based instrumentation for flexible ureteroscopy: a review. J Endourol. 2008; 22(7):1423–6.
37. Knudsen B, Miyaoka R, Shah K, Holden T, Turk TM, Pedro RN, et al. Durability of the next-generation flexible fiberoptic ureteroscopes: a randomized prospective multi-institutional clinical trial. Urology. 2010;75(3):534–8.
38. Patel SR, McLaren I, Nakada SY. The ureteroscope as a safety wire for ureteronephroscopy. J Endourol. 2012;26(4):351–4.
39. Johnson GB, Portela D, Grasso M. Advanced ureteroscopy: wireless and sheathless. J Endourol. 2006; 20(8):552–5.
40. Desai MR, Ganpule A. Flexible ureterorenoscopy. BJU Int. 2011;108(3):462–74.
41. Erhard MJ, Bagley DH. Urologic applications of the holmium laser: preliminary experience. J Endourol. 1995;9(5):383–6.
42. Schatloff O, Lindner U, Ramon J, Winkler HZ. Randomized trial of stone fragment active retrieval versus spontaneous passage during holmium laser lithotripsy for ureteral stones. J Urol. 2010;183(3): 1031–5.
43. de la Rosette JJ, Skrekas T, Segura JW. Handling and prevention of complications in stone basketing. Eur Urol. 2006;50(5):991–8. discussion 998–9.
44. Preminger GM, Tiselius HG, Assimos DG, Alken P, Buck C, Gallucci M, et al. 2007 guideline for the management of ureteral calculi. J Urol. 2007;178(6): 2418–34.

45. Smith RD, Patel A. Impact of flexible ureterorenoscopy in current management of nephrolithiasis. Curr Opin Urol. 2007;17(2):114–9.
46. Breda A, Ogunyemi O, Leppert JT, Lam JS, Schulam PG. Flexible ureteroscopy and laser lithotripsy for single intrarenal stones 2 cm or greater—is this the new frontier? J Urol. 2008;179(3):981–4.
47. Tiselius HG, Ackermann D, Alken P, Buck C, Conort P, Gallucci M, et al. Guidelines on urolithiasis. Eur Urol. 2001;40(4):362–71.
48. Krambeck AE, Murat FJ, Gettman MT, Chow GK, Patterson DE, Segura JW. The evolution of ureteroscopy: a modern single-institution series. Mayo Clin Proc. 2006;81(4):468–73.
49. Jung H, Nørby B, Osther PJ. Retrograde intrarenal stone surgery for extracorporeal shock-wave lithotripsy-resistant kidney stones. Scand J Urol Nephrol. 2006;40(5):380–4.
50. Holland R, Margel D, Livne PM, Lask DM, Lifshitz DA. Retrograde intrarenal surgery as second-line therapy yields a lower success rate. J Endourol. 2006; 20(8):556–9.
51. Pearle MS, Lingeman JE, Leveillee R, Kuo R, Preminger GM, Nadler RB, et al. Prospective, randomized trial comparing shock wave lithotripsy and ureteroscopy for lower pole caliceal calculi 1 cm or less. J Urol. 2005;173(6):2005–9.
52. Perlmutter AE, Talug C, Tarry WF, Zaslau S, Mohseni H, Kandzari SJ. Impact of stone location on success rates of endoscopic lithotripsy for nephrolithiasis. Urology. 2008;71(2):214–7.
53. Wendt-Nordahl G, Trojan L, Alken P, Michel MS, Knoll T. Ureteroscopy for stone treatment using new 270 degrees semiflexible endoscope: in vitro, ex vivo, and clinical application. J Endourol. 2007;21(12):1439–44.
54. Cocuzza M, Colombo JR, Cocuzza AL, Mascarenhas F, Vicentini F, Mazzucchi E, et al. Outcomes of flexible ureteroscopic lithotripsy with holmium laser for upper urinary tract calculi. Int Braz J Urol. 2008;34(2):143–9. discussion 149–50.
55. Mariani AJ. Combined electrohydraulic and holmium:YAG laser ureteroscopic nephrolithotripsy for 20 to 40 mm renal calculi. J Urol. 2004;172(1): 170–4.
56. Bilgasem S, Pace KT, Dyer S, Honey RJ. Removal of asymptomatic ipsilateral renal stones following rigid ureteroscopy for ureteral stones. J Endourol. 2003; 17(6):397–400.
57. Bozkurt OF, Resorlu B, Yildiz Y, Can CE, Unsal A. Retrograde intrarenal surgery versus percutaneous nephrolithotomy in the management of lower-pole renal stones with a diameter of 15 to 20 mm. J Endourol. 2011;25(7):1131–5.
58. Koo V, Young M, Thompson T, Duggan B. Cost-effectiveness and efficiency of shockwave lithotripsy vs. flexible ureteroscopic holmium:yttrium-aluminium-garnet laser lithotripsy in the treatment of lower pole renal calculi. BJU Int. 2011;108(11):1913–6.

10 Ureteroscopy: Stents and Other Adjuncts

Patrick Lowry

Introduction

The action of ureteral instrumentation with a ureteroscope for the purpose of lithotripsy or stone extraction causes some degree of trauma to the ureter. Traditionally, ureteral stents were placed routinely to prevent renal colic from either ureteral edema or passage of small clots, and in some cases to prevent ureteral stricture [1]. These benefits of stenting can be accompanied, however, by symptoms such as bladder irritation, flank pain, dysuria, or hematuria.

In the early years of ureteroscopy, the use of larger caliber rigid scopes always required dilation and subsequent stenting. At that time, only externalized ureteral catheters were available. These were uncomfortable, and the symptoms required hospitalization. Over time, indwelling double J-type stents of more tolerable materials were developed, which allowed for internal stenting, decreased levels of patient symptoms, and outpatient surgery [2]. As advances in technology have given us scopes with decreasing diameter, surgery became less traumatic for the ureteral tissues, prompting Urologists to question the need for routine stenting. Clearly, properly selected ureteroscopic procedures may be routinely performed without the need for postoperative stents.

Stent Evolution

The initial utilization of ureteral stents occurred during open surgery to repair or realign the ureter. Gustav Simon was credited with the first ureteral stent placement back in the nineteenth century when he placed a tube in the ureter during a cystostomy. Joaquin Albarrano created the first stent designed for use in the ureter in the early 1900s [3].

In 1967, the first cystoscopically placed indwelling ureteral stent was described, which was made of silicone [4]. These had no curl at either end, and were susceptible to migration. Various alterations in design attempted to minimize the chance of migration, yet no major breakthrough occurred for over a decade. In 1978, the double J stent design was described, which prevented both proximal and distal migration while allowing for adequate urine flow [2, 5]. The double J stent has progressed from a J-shaped half curl to a full curl "pigtail" shape, which decreases stent migration (Fig. 10.1). Currently, the double pigtail design is overwhelmingly the most utilized stent design. Since the advent of the pigtail shape, stent progress has primarily been through advancements in stent composition.

P. Lowry, M.D. (✉)
Section of Laparoscopy and Endourology, Texas A&M College of Medicine, Scott & White Memorial Hospital, Temple, TX, USA
e-mail: PLOWRY@swmail.sw.org

S.Y. Nakada and M.S. Pearle (eds.), *Surgical Management of Urolithiasis: Percutaneous, Shockwave and Ureteroscopy*, DOI 10.1007/978-1-4614-6937-7_10, © Springer Science+Business Media New York 2013

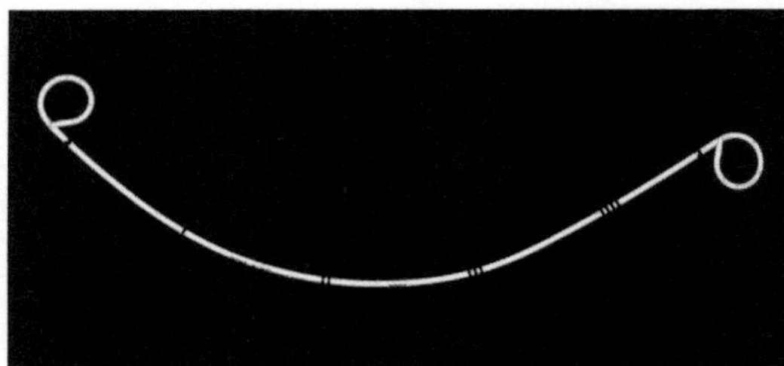

Fig. 10.1 Double Pigtail Ureteral Stent (Cook Urological)

Stent Composition

Polymers

A perfect stent would have rigidity to allow ease of placement, pliability to provide patient comfort, and radial strength to prevent blockage from external compression. In an ideal situation, the stent would have intrinsic resistance to encrustation as well as the ability to limit bacterial adherence to decrease infection. Currently, no single polymer has the strength and rigidity needed for function combined with the pliability to maximize patient comfort.

Polyethylene was the first polymer used for stent composition. Although successfully used at the time for orthopedic and soft tissue applications, exposure of polyethylene to urine resulted in depolymerization by hydrolytic degradation. Long-term usage would result in spontaneous breakage as the stents became more fragile over time [6, 7].

The most flexible and elastic of the stent biomaterials is silicone. These properties may lead to less patient discomfort; however, by itself, silicone lacks radial strength and compresses easily. Additionally, pure silicone does not have adequate rigidity to allow ease of placement.

Almost all stents today are composed of some type of polyurethane. Polyurethane is a class of condensation polymers made from polyisocyanate and polylol. Various polyurethanes have differing properties, allowing for creation of differing types for different purposes. Polyurethanes used for ureteral stents are generally blended with silicone and other polyurethanes to develop an advantageous combination of strength, patient comfort, and biocompatibility. The addition of elastomers provides the "memory" of the double J coils so they return to their coils after being straightened over a guidewire during placement [6]. Manufacturers currently produce various stents made with different polyurethane combinations and other additives to offer stent products with unique properties to meet the varying needs of the clinical situation.

As an example, Cook Medical currently produces stent product lines in all lengths and diameters of their proprietary materials C-Flex®, Universa®, and Sof-flex®. Each of these has a different composition with differing clinical advantages. By comparison, Boston Scientific also has several product lines made from their proprietary material Percuflex®, in either a firm or soft variety, as well a line of stents composed of Flexima®. Each stent product, depending on the composition, will be approved for different maximum indwelling time varying from 90 days to up to a year although clinical scenarios may require more frequent replacement.

Reinforced/Metal Stents

Ureteral strictures and extrinsic obstruction from pathology such as cancer or retroperitoneal fibrosis often requires long-term stenting, and requires radial strength to avoid failure due to compressive forces. The Applied Medical Silhouette series offers two to three times the radial strength of comparable polyurethane stents due to radial coil reinforcement built into the stent [8].

Metal stents provide additional radial strength. The Resonance stent (Cook Medical) is made of a nickel-cobalt-chromium-molybdenum alloy and compared to typical polyurethane stents, increases radial strength by a factor of seven or eight, although at a significantly increased cost [8]. The design employs a tightly wound metallic coil that is not dependent on a central lumen, but allows urine to flow in an extraluminal manner (Fig. 10.2). Under proper conditions, patients with this stent can safely undergo MRI examinations (see product guide for specifics). Despite the proven superiority of the radial strength, failure rate in malignant obstruction may be similar to polymer stents [9].

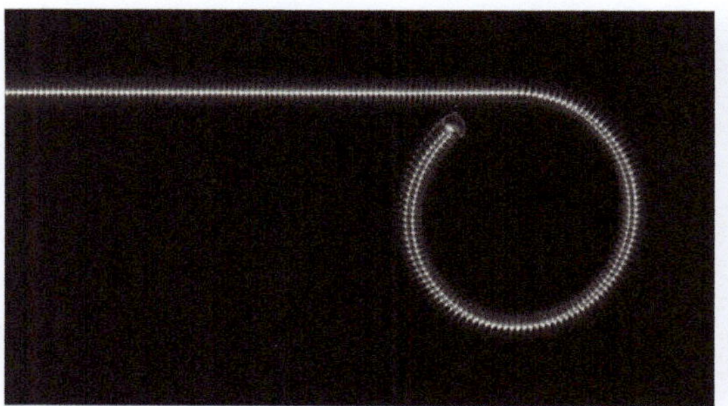

Fig. 10.2 Magnified view of coiled tip of Resonance Stent, which is made from nickel-cobalt-chromium-molybdenum alloy (Cook International)

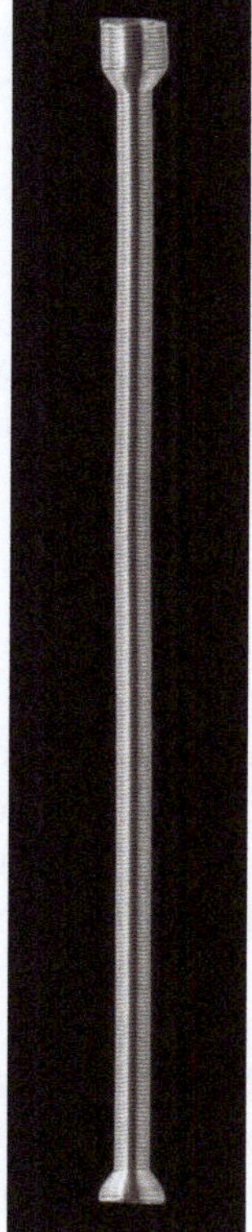

Fig. 10.3 Memokath Stent, dual cone design (PNN Medical)

A retrospective study in patient with malignant obstruction showed a 35 % failure rate, especially in patient with malignant bladder invasion.

Although unavailable in the USA, the Memokath metallic stent (PNN Medical, Denmark) offers another option (Fig. 10.3). Unlike the previously described stents, the Memokath is not a double pigtail-type design, but instead offers a dual cone design with one cone above and one cone below the focal area to be stented. The Memokath does not extend into the bladder, and consequently neither causes flank pain from reflux nor does it cause as significant bladder symptomatology (Fig. 10.4). The Memokath has a nickel-titanium alloy coiled wire composition with a shape memory based on temperature, which aids in deployment. One simply places the stent into the proper position across the strictured ureteral segment, after which hot water (60 °C) is injected across the stent. The stent expands to fit the stricture in the hot water, and retains the expanded shape. For stent removal, ice cold water is injected in a retrograde manner to cool the stent below 10 °C. As the stent shrinks to original diameter, the lower edge may be grasped and the stent is carefully removed while keeping the temperature cold [10, 11]. A study reported only a 4.5 % failure rate for the Memokath, both instances due to infiltration by transitional cell carcinoma [12].

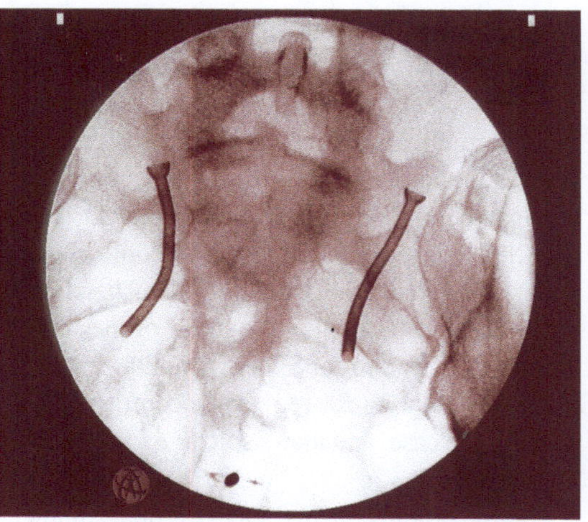

Fig. 10.4 Memokath Stent, deployed bilaterally in the distal ureters. The stent does not extend into the bladder (PNN Medical)

Speciality Stents for Specific Situations

Retrograde injection stents allow injection of contrast media into the renal collecting system for the illumination of the collecting system to confirm proper placement prior to stent deployment. Alternatively, these stents may facilitate stone localization during shock wave lithotripsy prior to their deployment. After the proximal tip arrives in the renal pelvis, the wire is removed to deploy the proximal curl. X-ray contrast is then instilled in a retrograde manner to confirm placement, after which the distal end is localized under fluoroscopy, and deployed with a proper curl in the bladder. If used for Shockwave lithotripsy, the stent may be used for retrograde contrast instillation for the case, and then deployed when the case is complete.

Endopylotomy stents have a dual diameter design with a larger diameter at the proximal end to hypothetically allow for healing of a larger diameter lumen at the ureteropelvic junction than a standard stent with the same diameter from proximal to distal end would allow. Distal stent diameter remains the same size as the usual stent (6–7 French, depending on manufacturer), with a proximal end larger, ranging from 9.5 to 14 French. No consensus exists in the literature as to whether or not endopyelotomy stents convey an advantage in long-term patency rates [13, 14].

Variable length stents are designed to accommodate the need for varying stent lengths with one stent set. This stent type has a single coil on the proximal (kidney) end to prevent distal migration. The distal (bladder) end has several coils that either maintain the tight multicoil shape for shorter ureters or can unwind to accommodate longer ureters.

Stent Designs

Tail Stent

The vast majority of stents in use today are of the Double Pigtail design. Since stent discomfort remains a challenging morbidity to manage, different stent designs have been put forth as having potential for decreasing stent discomfort. The Tail stent (Boston Scientific) did not have a distal curl in the bladder but instead had a smaller diameter, 3f, soft lumenless distal end. The premise was that a smaller, softer stent tip would be less irritating to the bladder, thereby decreasing bothersome effects. Although an early study supported this hypothesis by showing significantly fewer irritative bladder symptoms [15], the tail stent is no longer available.

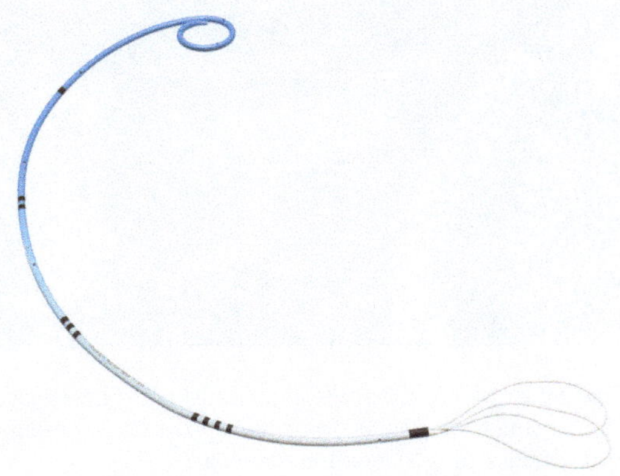

Fig. 10.5 Polaris Loop Stent (Images Courtesy of Boston Scientific Corporation. Opinions expressed are those of the author alone and not of Boston Scientific)

Loop Tail

Another attempt at making the distal stent tip less irritating to the bladder involved decreasing the mass and material inside the bladder by replacing the existing 6f pigtail with 2 loops that measure <3f. Although a prospective randomized study using the validated Ureteric Stent Symptoms Questionnaire showed somewhat lower pain scores for the loop stent cohort, no significant difference was noted when compared to controls [16]. A version of this design is currently manufactured by Boston Scientific (Fig. 10.5).

Dual Durometer Stents

This concept in stent design does not alter the shape of the distal portion, but instead changes the composition. The proximal portion of this double pigtail stent is comprised of a firm polymer to prevent distal migration, and the distal portion

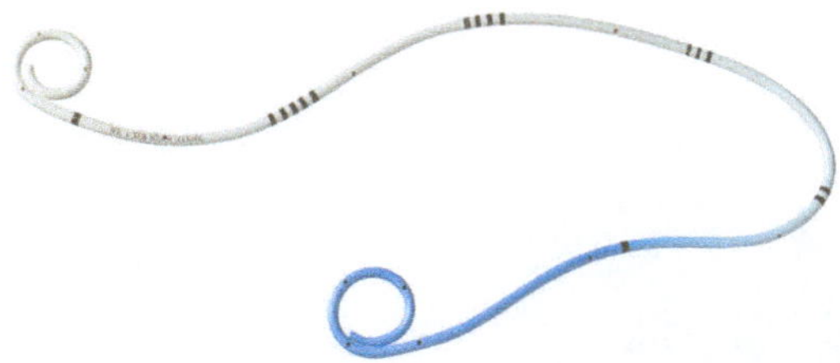

Fig. 10.6 Polaris Dual Durometer stent (Images Courtesy of Boston Scientific Corporation. Opinions expressed are those of the author alone and not of Boston Scientific)

is made from a much softer material, designed to put less pressure on the bladder, thereby decreasing irritative voiding symptoms. The Boston Scientific Polaris stent product line utilizes this design (Fig. 10.6).

Are Stents Always Necessary?

With the development of rigid ureteroscopy, routine postoperative stenting was the standard of care. This was first questioned in 1999 [17], and further studies have clearly shown that not all procedures need stent placement [18, 19]. One must remember that in the early 1980s, ureteroscopy was a more morbid procedure. At that time, the ureteroscope was 11.5 French (Fr) in diameter, and the technology available for lithotripsy was primarily electrohydraulic. This combination was certainly more traumatic to the collecting system, and postoperative stenting was performed routinely. Although this was done solely on the premise that stenting was necessary, not on evidence-based medicine, the large caliber scope and more traumatic lithotripsy likely warranted stenting the vast majority of the time.

Over time, scopes have decreased to 6 Fr, and additionally, lithotripsy is now overwhelmingly performed with Holmium laser, a much less morbid combination. Despite advances in technology and the knowledge that stentless ureteroscopy was a safe practice, routine stenting persisted. Primarily, this was due to the inability to foresee which patients could be safely treated without stents. Accurate predictors are imperative to avoid having a patient return with flank pain requiring delayed stenting (likely more difficult), a second anesthesia, or potentially even a nephrostomy if stent placement was not possible or if ureteral injury occurred.

Almost 10 years ago, Hollenbeck et al. helped to determine operative and patient-specific risk factors associated postoperative morbidity [19]. Various stone and postoperative variables were evaluated; patients who had bilateral stentless procedures, lithotripsy performed, or operative time greater than 45 min with lithotripsy performed were significantly more likely to experience postoperative complications. Additionally, patients with recurrent or recent infections, history of stones, prior stone treatment, and no preoperative stent were more likely to experience symptoms secondary to obstruction. Stone location was not a predictor of morbidity if the patient was stented preoperatively; however, location in the renal pelvis was a risk for postoperative morbidity for patients without preoperative stents. Additional studies are needed to further clarify criteria that would help determine which patients would best treated without postoperative stent placement. If intraoperative concern regarding ureteral damage or edema exists, patient safety supports ureteral stent placement.

How Long Should Stents Remain?

If the urothelium remains intact, but the surgeon has concern about ureteral edema causing renal colic, 2–3 days of ureteral stenting should be adequate to allow the edema to resolve. No adequate data exists to dictate the duration of stenting after various types of potential injury to the ureter (wire perforation, laser injury, mucosal split, full thickness tear, etc.) In case of more serious, full thickness, injury, 4–6 weeks of stenting is required to allow the ureter to properly heal. This is based on the Davis intubated ureterotomy, which described a 6-week period of ureteral stenting to allow for proper healing [20]. For injuries that are not full thickness and perhaps perceived as minor, such as a linear split during balloon dilation, the length of time required for stenting is not well studied. If question exists as to the severity of injury, or for

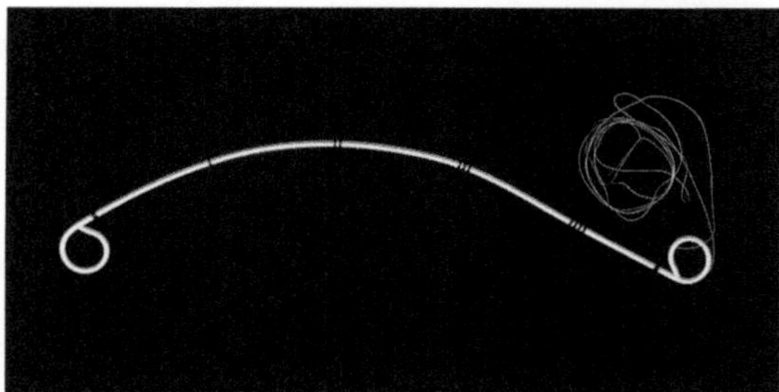

Fig. 10.7 Double Pigtail Stent with tether attached (Cook Urological)

thermal (laser) injury, patient safety would dictate leaving a stent in long enough for the most potential serious injury to heal. After stents are removed, and injuries have presumably healed, follow-up imaging must be performed to rule out stricture formation.

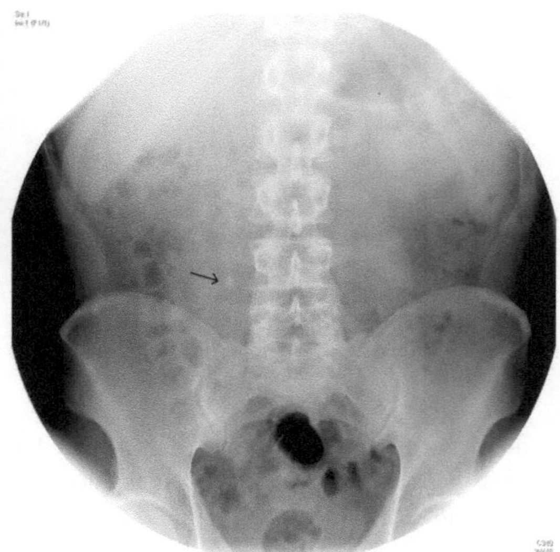

Fig. 10.8 Right Ureteral Calculus seen at the level of L1 (see *arrow*)

Tether

The stitch attached to the distal curl of polyurethane stents (Fig. 10.7) may facilitate stent removal in several ways. For stents left in situ for just a few days, the tether may be taped to the thigh of female patients at the time of stent placement. If taped to the thigh in male patients, nocturnal erections cause the tether to pull on the stent, causing bladder discomfort and disrupting sleep. Consequently, in the case of male patients, the tether should be taped to the shaft of the phallus. After a few days, the patient may then remove the stent at home without the need for cystoscopic instrumentation. Premedication with anticholinergics help to decrease uncomfortable bladder spasms that may result from stent removal. Patients should be warned that urine may wick along the tether through the sphincter, leaking small amounts of urine through the urethra.

Some urologists shorten the tether to a few inches. This floating tether in the bladder is easier to grasp cystoscopically, with less lateral maneuvering of the scope, and a resultant decrease in patient discomfort. Alternatively, in men, a shortened tether may be positioned in the bulbar urethra, which allows for cystoscopic removal without having to traverse the urethral sphincter or bladder neck, again decreasing the morbidity of the procedure. As with an externalized tether attached to the leg or phallus, this may result in small amounts of incontinence.

Stent Placement

Placement of a stent through a rigid cystoscope should begin by advancing a guidewire up through the ureter to the level of the kidney under fluoroscopic guidance. If there is question about the anatomy, a retrograde pyelogram may be performed to delineate the collecting system. At this point, the stent is advanced over the wire, and the pusher is utilized to advance the stent into the renal pelvis. Under fluoroscopic guidance, the wire is slowly backed up to allow the proximal end of the stent to curl in the renal pelvis. Using the pusher to hold the distal tip of the stent just inside the bladder neck, the wire is then removed, allowing the distal stent to curl in the bladder.

Alternatively, stents may be placed fluoroscopically, without need for the cystoscope.

Step 1: An obstructing right ureteral calculus can be seen at the level of L1 (Fig. 10.8). Using a flexible cystoscope, a guidewire is advanced past the stone to the level of the kidney under

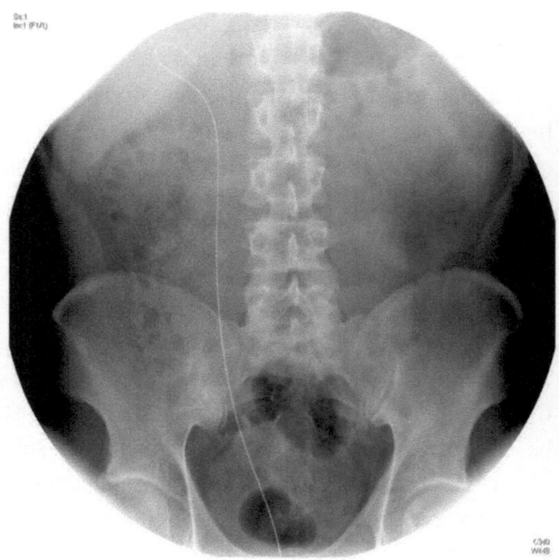

Fig. 10.9 A guidewire is advanced past the stone to the level of the kidney

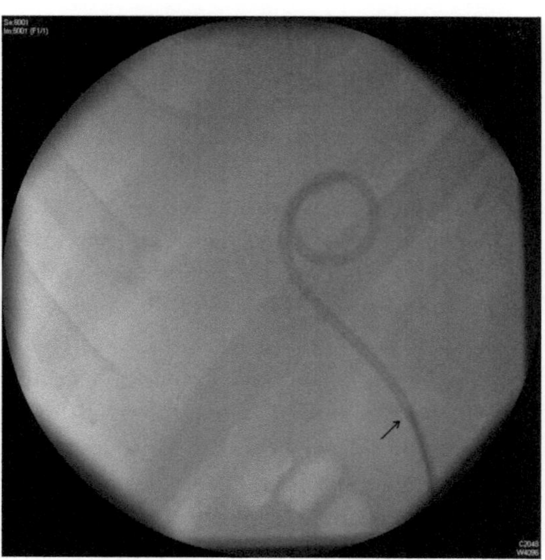

Fig. 10.11 Without moving the metal tip pusher, under fluoroscopic guidance the wire is retracted just enough to allow the proximal curl of the stent to deploy. Note the guidewire just below the curl (see *arrow*)

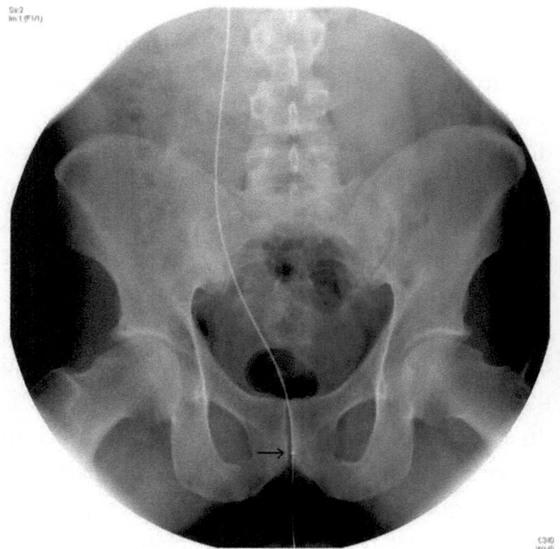

Fig. 10.10 Keeping the pubic symphysis in fluoroscopic view, a stent is advanced over the guidewire until the radiopaque metal tip pusher reaches the lower edge of the pubic symphysis (see *arrow*)

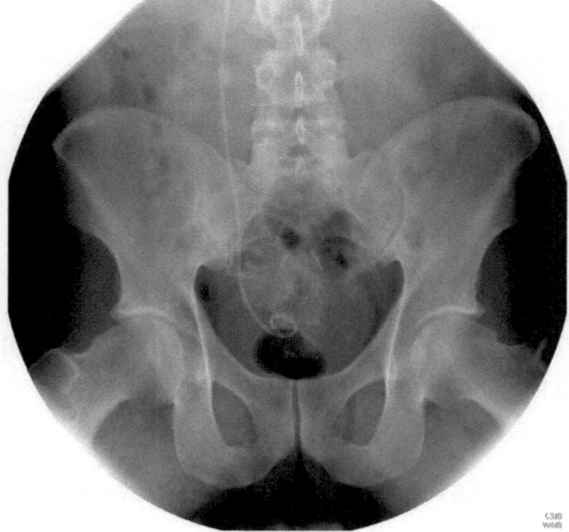

Fig. 10.12 Keeping the metal tip pusher at the same location on the lower aspect of the pubic symphysis, the wire is removed to allow the distal tip to deploy

fluoroscopic guidance (Fig. 10.9). After ureteroscopic procedures, the stent may be placed over the existing safety guidewire, alleviating the need for step 1.

Step 2: Over the wire, a stent is advanced up the ureter until the metal radiopaque tip of the pusher reaches the lower edge of the pubic symphysis (Fig. 10.10).

Step 3: Using fluoroscopy to insure that the position of the pusher does not change, the wire is pulled back just enough to allow the proximal curl of the stent to deploy (Fig. 10.11).

Step 4: Keeping the metal tip of the pusher at the lower edge of the pubic symphysis, the wire is then completely removed, deploying the distal curl in the bladder (Fig. 10.12).

Stent Discomfort

Clearly, stents cause significant morbidity. Although some patients are minimally affected by the presence of a stent, symptoms are significant for others, and even debilitating for some. The problem for Urologists remains the inability to effectively treat the stent symptoms for those who are symptomatic. The mechanism by which stents cause discomfort is not well characterized. The flank pain that may accompany stenting likely comes from reflux along the stent. Lower tract symptoms (dysuria, urgency, frequency, suprapubic pain) probably result from direct irritation of the distal stent portion on the bladder.

Multiple variables were evaluated in an effort to define predictors of stent discomfort. Using a validated questionnaire, univariable and multivariable analysis assessed patient age, sex, body mass index, stent length, stent caliber, stent side, and distal loop location for association with morbidity at day 7 and 28. Of the variables studied, visualization of the distal loop of the stent crossing the midline had the strongest association with morbidity than the other variables [21]. Additionally, stents with incomplete loop deployment in the bladder have been associated with increased severity of stent-related symptoms [22].

Further study is necessary to better elucidate which patient and stent characteristics lead to stent-related morbidity. Careful placement with attention to the curl and placement of the distal portion will help to minimize discomfort.

Stent Discomfort: Medical Treatment

Attempts to alleviate stent-related irritative bladder symptoms have been tried with several classes of oral medication. The various medication options may be taken individually or in combination decrease symptoms.

Alpha adrenergic receptors are present in the smooth muscle cells of the bladder trigone and distal ureter. Since the distal stent tip is located in this area, alpha adrenergic blocking agents have been used reduce smooth muscle activity for the treatment of stent-related symptoms. Two meta-analyses have concluded that randomized, controlled studies show that alpha blockers provide an improvement in the symptoms caused by ureteral stents [23, 24]. Patients must be warned about the potential for orthostatic hypotension, especially with the first dose. Patients with cataracts who have not undergone surgical correction should discuss alpha blockers with their ophthalmologist prior to usage to avoid the surgical implications of floppy iris syndrome.

Oral anticholinergics are generally quite effective for stent-related bladder symptoms, but must be used with caution. The most common side effect is dry mouth, and patients may also experience dry eyes, headache, constipation, dizziness, somnolence, arrhythmia, or nausea. Use may be inappropriate in the elderly as this population may suffer memory loss, confusion, delirium, cardiac effects, or constipation. Anticholinergics are contraindicated in patients with narrow angle glaucoma, gastric retention, and urinary retention.

Phenazopyridine is primarily excreted through the urine, and acts as a local analgesic on the bladder mucosa. For many patients, phenazopyridine effectively minimizes stent morbidity. One must be cautious, as its use is contraindicated in renal insufficiency. Additionally, use in patients with glucose-6-dehydrogenase deficiency must be avoided to prevent hemolytic anemia.

An interesting prospective, randomized, double-blinded, placebo-controlled study evaluated the benefit of oxybutynin versus phenazopyridine versus placebo. There was no difference in bother scores for flank pain, suprapubic pain, urinary frequency, urinary urgency, or dysuria [25]. We know that oxybutynin and phenazopyridine are effective, yet their failure to show improvement over placebo underscores the challenge in treating patients who endure the morbidity of ureteral stents.

Future Directions

The next advancement in stent technology appears to be improvements using stent coatings. These coatings have primarily been used to decrease biofilm formation, bacterial adhesion, encrustation, and stent discomfort. Certain coated stents currently exist, although not currently available in the United States.

Glycosaminoglycans naturally inhibit crystal formation by binding to stone forming elements in the urine [26, 27]. Heparin, a glycosaminoglycan, was shown to inhibit stent encrustation in vitro compared to placebo over a 7-day period of continuous exposure to artificial urine [28]. A small clinical study subsequently followed five patients with bilateral ureteral obstruction. Each patient had both a heparin-coated stent and a traditional stent (control) placed and then evaluated with electron microscopy, energy dispersive spectroscopy, and micro infrared spectrophotometry. The heparin-coated stents had a significant decrease in the amount of encrustation. Even after 10 and 12 months, no changes were noted in the heparin layer, suggesting that the ability to prevent encrustation is not reduced over time [29]. A novel stent coated with a diamond like carbon coating was evaluated in a population of 10 patients notorious for significant encrustation problems resulting in stent change intervals of less than 6 weeks. A total of 26 stents were trialed over an experience period of 2,467 days, and no encrustation was seen [30].

A commercially available heparin-coated stent (Radiance®, Cook Medical) and a commercially available Triclosan-coated stent (Triumph®, Boston Scientific) and controls were evaluated for their resistance to bacterial adherence [31]. No significant difference between the heparin-coated stents and controls were noted with regard to the amount of bacterial adhesion. Of the bacteria in the study, the Triclosan-coated stent was resistant to *S. aureus*, *Klebsiella*, and *E. coli*, but not *Enterococcus* or *Pseudomonas*. Additionally, an in vitro study showed that Triclosan eluting stents have shown a decrease in pro-inflammatory cytokine release when compared to control stents [32]. This early study has been supported with a prospective randomized trial in which 20 patients were given either a Triumph stent or a traditional stent. Those with the Triclosan-coated stent had significant reductions in flank pain scores during activity, flank pain during urination, abdominal pain during activity, and urethral pain during urination. Although a small series, the results are promising, and further study with larger groups are needed to confirm the effectiveness of this stent [33].

Drug eluting stents have also been evaluated in an effort to decease stent discomfort. In an animal study, a paclitaxel eluting stent has been shown to decrease inflammation and hyperplasia compared to controls [34]. Further study will reveal if these findings translate to clinical benefits. Ketorolac is particularly effective for the treatment of renal colic, and has been shown to relieve stent-related symptoms when used intravesically [35]. Presumably, the bladder symptoms result from direct irritation of the stent, so a drug eluting stent may help treat the symptoms where they originate at the location of the distal stent. A ketorolac eluting stent (Lexington™, Boston Scientific) was studied in a prospective, randomized, double-blinded trial; although no significant difference was shown between drug eluting stents and controls, young men trended towards a lower requirement for pain medication [36]. Perhaps if certain patient groups are studied, a more significant difference may be seen.

Biodegradable Stents

Biodegradable stents have the potential to provide post-ureteroscopy ureteral drainage, yet by dissolving, alleviate the need for a cystoscopic removal. Previously, dissolvable stents were studied, but the concern was that retained fragments, although uncommon, resulted in additional surgical procedures [37]. A newer type of biodegradable stent is an absorbable, elastic matrix made from components similar to those in absorbable sutures, and reinforced with a radial coil to give enough rigidity for placement (Uriprine, Poly Med Inc). Porcine studies show second- and third-generation stents completely degrade by 10 and 4 weeks, respectively [38, 39]. This very promising technology requires further human trials to determine whether or not this technology will allow degradation of the stents without retained fragments resulting in morbidity from obstruction or the need for surgical removal.

Conclusion

Currently, from a drainage standpoint, stents function without problem. They unfortunately cause morbidity, which is bothersome for many patients and outright severe for others. Our advancements and current areas of study are driven by these symptoms. If stent morbidity were absent or easily controlled, we would likely have never seen the significant effort made towards improving stent design and composition, or the studies that show ureteroscopy can be safely done without stenting. Future study must elucidate the mechanism that causes morbidity, which will in turn allow for better-guided development in stent design and medical management of symptoms.

Disclosure

The author discloses that he has no financial or other interest from any stent manufacturer. The author has little input on the stents used at his institution, as administrators negotiate for the lowest possible prices. Currently, his institution uses Cook stents. The author's bias is that the stent type makes little difference for the vast majority of endourologic uses.

References

1. Harmon WJ, Sershon PD, Blute ML, Patterson DE, Segura JW. Ureteroscopy: current practice and long-term complications. J Urol. 1997;157(1):28–32.
2. Finney RP. Experience with new double-J ureteral stent. J Urol. 1978;120(6):678–81.
3. Saltzman B. Ureteral stents: indications, variations, and complications. Urol Clin North Am. 1988;15(3):481–91.
4. Zimskind PD, Fetter TR, Wilkerson JL. Clinical use of long-term indwelling silicone rubber ureteral splints injected cystoscopically. J Urol. 1967;97(5):840–4.
5. Hepperlen TW, Mardis HK, Kammandel H. Self-retained internal ureteral stents: a new approach. J Urol. 1978;119(6):731–4.
6. Mardis HK, Kroeger RM. Ureteral stents: materials. Urol Clin North Am. 1988;15(3):471–9.
7. Hepperlen TW, Mardis HK, Malashock E. Spontaneous breakage of polyethylene double pigtail ureteral stents (abstract). Proceedings of the American Urological Association. 1982: 198.
8. Christman MS, L'esperance JO, Choe CH, Stroup SP, Auge BK. Analysis of ureteral stent compression force and its role in malignant obstruction. J Urol. 2009;181(1):392–6.
9. Goldsmith ZG, Wang AJ, Bañez LL, Lipkin ME, Ferrandino MN, Preminger GM, et al. Outcomes of metallic stents for malignant ureteral obstruction. J Urol. 2012;188(3):851–5.
10. Kulkarni RP, Bellamy EA. A new thermo-expandable shape-memory nickel-titanium alloy stent for the management of ureteric strictures. BJU Int. 1999; 83(7):755–9.
11. Kulkarni R, Bellamy E. Nickel-titanium shape memory alloy Memokath 051 ureteral stent for managing long-term ureteral obstruction: 4-year experience. J Urol. 2001;166(5):1750–4.
12. Zaman F, Poullis C, Bach C, Moraitis K, Junaid I, Buchholz N, et al. Use of a segmental thermoexpandable metal alloy stent in the management of malignant ureteric obstruction: a single centre experience in the UK. Urol Int. 2011;87(4):405–10.
13. Moon YT, Kerbl K, Pearle MS, Gardner SM, McDougall EM, Humphrey P, et al. Evaluation of optimal stent size after endourologic incision of ureteral strictures. J Endourol. 1995;9(1):15–22.
14. Danuser H, Hochreiter WW. Influence of stent size on the success of antegrade endopyelotomy for primary ureteropelvic junction obstruction: results of 2 consecutive series. J Urol. 2001;166(3):902–9.
15. Dunn MD, Portis AJ, Kahn SA, Yan Y, Shalhav AL, Elbahnasy AM, et al. Clinical effectiveness of new stent design: randomized single-blind comparison of tail and double-pigtail stents. J Endourol. 2000;14(2): 195–202.
16. Lingeman JE, Preminger GM, Goldfischer ER, Krambeck AE. Comfort study team. Assessing the impact of ureteral stent design on patient comfort. J Urol. 2009;181(6):2581–7.
17. Hosking DH, McColm SE, Smith WE. Is stenting following ureteroscopy for removal of distal ureteral calculi necessary? J Urol. 1999;161(1):48–50.
18. Hollenbeck BK, Schuster TG, Faerber GJ, Wolf Jr JS. Routine placement of ureteral stents is unnecessary after ureteroscopy for urinary calculi. Urology. 2001; 57(4):639–43.
19. Hollenbeck BK, Schuster TG, Seifman BD, Faerber GJ, Wolf Jr JS. Identifying patients who are suitable for stentless ureteroscopy following treatment of urolithiasis. J Urol. 2003;170(1):103–6.
20. Davis DM. Intubated uroterostomy: a new operation for ureteral and ureteropelvic strictures. Surg Gynecol Obstet. 1943;76:513–23.
21. Giannarini G, Keeley Jr FX, Valent F, et al. Predictors of morbidity in patients with indwelling ureteric stents: results of a prospective study using the validated Ureteric Stent Symptoms Questionnaire. BJU Int. 2011;107(4):648–54.

22. Rane A, Saleemi A, Cahill D, Sriprasad S, Shrotri N, Tiptaft R. Have stent-related symptoms anything to do with placement technique? J Endourol. 2001;15(7): 741–5.
23. Lamb AD, Vowler SL, Johnston R, Dunn N, Wisemann OJ. Meta-analysis showing the beneficial effect of a-blockers on ureteric stent discomfort. BJU Int. 2011;108(11):1894–902.
24. Yakoubi R, Lemdani M, Monga M, Villers A, Koenig P. Is there a role for a-blockers in ureteral stent related symptoms? A systematic review and meta-analysis. J Urol. 2011;186(3):928–34.
25. Norris RD, Sur RL, Springhart WP, Marguet CG, Mathias BJ, Pietrow PK, et al. A prospective, randomized, double-blinded placebo-controlled comparison of extended release oxybutynin versus phenazopyridine for the management of postoperative ureteral stent discomfort. Urology. 2008;71(5):792–5.
26. Yoshimura K, Yoshioka T, Miyake O, Honda M, Yamaguchi S, Koide T, et al. Glycosaminoglycans in crystal-surface binding substances and their role in calcium oxalate crystal growth. Br J Urol. 997;80(1):64–8.
27. Angell AH, Resnick MI. Surface interaction between glycosaminoglycans and calcium oxalate. J Urol. 1989;141:1255–8.
28. Hildebrandt P, Sayyad M, Rzany A, Schaldach M, Seiter H. Prevention of surface encrustation of urological implants by coating with inhibitors. Biomaterials. 2001;22(5):503–7.
29. Cauda F, Cauda V, Fiori C, Onida B, Garrone E. Heparin coating on ureteral Double J stents prevents encrustations: an in vivo case study. J Endourol. 2008;22(3):465–72.
30. Laube N, Kleinen L, Bradenahl J, Meissner A. Diamond-like carbon coatings on ureteral stents–a new strategy for decreasing the formation of crystalline bacterial biofilms? J Urol. 2007;177(5):1923–7.
31. Lange D, Elwood CN, Choi K, Hendlin K, Monga M, Chew BH. Uropathogen interaction with the surface of urological stents using different surface properties. J Urol. 2009;182(3):1194–200.
32. Elwood CN, Chew BH, Seney S, Jass J, Denstedt JD, Cadieux PA. Triclosan inhibits uropathogenic Escherichia coli-stimulated tumor necrosis factor-alpha secretion in T24 bladder cells in vitro. J Endourol. 2007;21(10):1717–22.
33. Mendez-Probst CE, Goneau LW, Macdonald KW, Nott L, Seney S, Elwood CN, et al. The use of triclosan eluting stents effectively reduces ureteral stent symptoms: a prospective randomized trial. BJU Int. 2012;110(5):749–54.
34. Liatsikos EN, Karnabatidis D, Kagadis GC, Rokkas K, Constantinides C, Christeas N, et al. Application of paclitaxel-eluting metal mesh stents within the pig ureter: an experimental study. Eur Urol. 2007; 51(1):217–23.
35. Beiko DT, Watterson JD, Knudsen BE, Nott L, Pautler SE, Brock GB, et al. Doubleblind randomized controlled trial assessing the safety and efficacy of intravesical agents for ureteral stent symptoms after extracorporeal shockwave lithotripsy. J Endourol. 2004;18(8):723–30.
36. Krambeck AE, Walsh RS, Denstedt JD, Preminger GM, Li J, Evans JC, et al. A novel drug eluting ureteral stent: a prospective, randomized, multicenter clinical trial to evaluate the safety and effectiveness of a ketorolac loaded ureteral stent. J Urol. 2010; 183(3):1037–42.
37. Lingeman JE, Preminger GM, Berger Y, Denstedt JD, Goldstone L, Segura JW, et al. Use of a temporary ureteral drainage stent after uncomplicated ureteroscopy: results from a phase II clinical trial. J Urol. 2003;169(5):1682–8.
38. Chew BH, Lange D, Paterson RF, Hendlin K, Monga M, Clinkscales KW, et al. Next generation biodegradable ureteral stent in a yucatan pig model. J Urol. 2010;183(2):765–71.
39. Chew BH, Paterson RF, Clinkscales KW, Levine BS, Shalaby SW, Lange D. The in vivo evaluation of the third generation biodegradable uriprene™ stent—a novel approach to avoiding the forgotten stent syndrome. J Urol. 2013;189(2):719–25.

11 Complications of Ureteroscopy

Ryan B. Pickens and Nicole L. Miller

Introduction

Rigid and flexible ureteroscopy (URS) is a well-established and widely used modality for both the therapeutic and diagnostic treatment of urologic conditions affecting the ureter and kidney. The continued improvements in technology and instruments have expanded the applications of URS within the scope of urologic surgery, and greatly improved its safety. Originally used to treat mainly ureterolithasis, ureteroscopy has extended its use to include: nephrolithiasis, malignancies, congenital anomalies, and iatrogenic injuries within these organs. However, unexpected events or poor technique can still lead to complications of ureteroscopy. This chapter will explore complications associated with URS and discuss their recognition, prevention, and appropriate management.

R.B. Pickens, M.D. (✉)
Department of Urologic Surgery, Vanderbilt University Medical Center, Nashville, TN, USA
e-mail: ryan.pickens@vanderbilt.edu

N.L. Miller, M.D.
Department of Urologic Surgery, Vanderbilt University School of Medicine, Nashville, TN, USA

Safety Techniques in Modern Ureteroscopy

Over the past few decades, there have been significant technologic advancement breakthroughs within the field of Endourology. Compared to earlier decades when urologists were using blind basketing techniques, URS under direct vision has decreased the complication rate associated with this procedure [1, 2]. Furthermore, high definition technology provides image clarity that can help identify iatrogenic complications such as small perforations in the urothelium; or small urothelial tumors previously missed.

Another important advancement in the safety of URS has been the widespread use of safety wires. These wires provide a protected access from the kidney to the urethral meatus. They can help straighten out a ureter that may be tortuous due to obstruction, and can also help guide the ureteroscope up the ureter in the event of decreased vision due to bleeding or a narrow lumen. The wires can identify strictures within the ureter and aid in treating these by providing access for the use of a balloon dilator. When lasering stones in the ureter, the wire can be used as a reference point to judge when the stones are small enough to pass on their own or be safely retrieved with a basket. Perhaps the most important use of a safety wire is to provide an immediate tool to guide placement of a ureteral stent should a complication occur during URS.

S.Y. Nakada and M.S. Pearle (eds.), *Surgical Management of Urolithiasis: Percutaneous, Shockwave and Ureteroscopy*, DOI 10.1007/978-1-4614-6937-7_11,

The ability to use contrast medium has also helped the urologist map out the collecting system during URS. With intraoperative fluoroscopy, this allows the surgeon to visualize the diameter of the ureter as well as the level of obstruction within the ureter due to a stone, mass, or stricture. Contrast can identify complications such as extravasation due to perforation or avulsion, and provide important information about the length of a stricture. Contrast medium and fluoroscopy can also aid the surgeon during flexible panrenoscopy to ensure that all calices have been visualized, and to determine if a calyceal diverticulum is accessible through endoscopic means by visualizing contrast entering the diverticulum. Contrast should be injected at a low pressure to prevent extravasation of contrast or pyelovenous backflow. In the case of an infected system, increased intraluminal pressure during contrast injection can lead to bacteremia and sepsis.

Ureteral access sheaths used in flexible ureteroscopy have made treatment of large proximal ureteral and renal stones more feasible due to the ability of the surgeon to make multiple passes up the ureter. A safety wire can be left through or alongside the access sheath or "naked" ureteroscopy without a wire can be performed through these sheaths with reasonable safety [3]. The access sheath allows the surgeon to basket multiple stones safely, especially within the proximal ureter where the muscularis layer is thinner and the ureter is more prone to injury [4]. These sheaths also keep renal intrapelvic pressures low, potentially being a significant benefit in patients with an infected stone [5].

Even with smaller instruments and safety wires, some stones still remain difficult to access or can be impacted with severe inflammation preventing one stage treatment. Should this situation be encountered, it is recommended the surgeon place a ureteral stent for 10–14 days to allow the ureter to passively dilate which will provide easier access to the ureter for definitive treatment of the stone during the second procedure.

The holmium:YAG laser is a multimodality tool that has greatly aided the field of Endourology. Its current uses include: stone fragmentation, endoscopic treatment of short ureteral strictures, and ureteral and renal pelvic tumors. It has added to the safety of URS by its pinpoint end firing capability and the fact that is highly absorbed in water, which makes treatment of ureteral and renal stones much safer than electrohydraulic lithotrite (EHL).

Classification

For convenience of discussion, URS complications can be divided into minor or major complications and by the timeline that they occur with relation to the surgery, intraoperative or postoperative. Although most complications occur during the procedure, some become apparent only in the postoperative period, and the surgeon must be able to recognize these issues.

Fortunately, most complications of URS are minor but major complications still occur at a rate of 1 % or less [6]. The major complications can result in significant morbidity or even mortality, including prolonged hospital stays and even multiple procedures such as open or laparoscopic surgeries to correct these complications.

Intraoperative Complications

Bleeding

Bleeding during URS can lead to decreased visualization and is the most common reason for reoperation. It occurs in 0.3 % of all URS cases [7]. Bleeding can occur during placement of safety wires, fragmentation of a stone or tumor, laser treatment of a stricture or aggressive basket extraction of a stone. Bleeding occurring during URS is usually minor and most times removal of the ureteroscope and placement of a ureteral stent is all that is needed. Bleeding can occur in the prostate due to instrumentation in patients with a high bladder neck, enlarged prostate, or median lobe, and may require foley catheter placement postoperatively. Continuous bladder irrigation postoperatively is rarely required. In a series of 290 patients, bleeding severe enough to halt a procedure occurred at a rate of 2.1 % but the transfusion rate was 0 % [8].

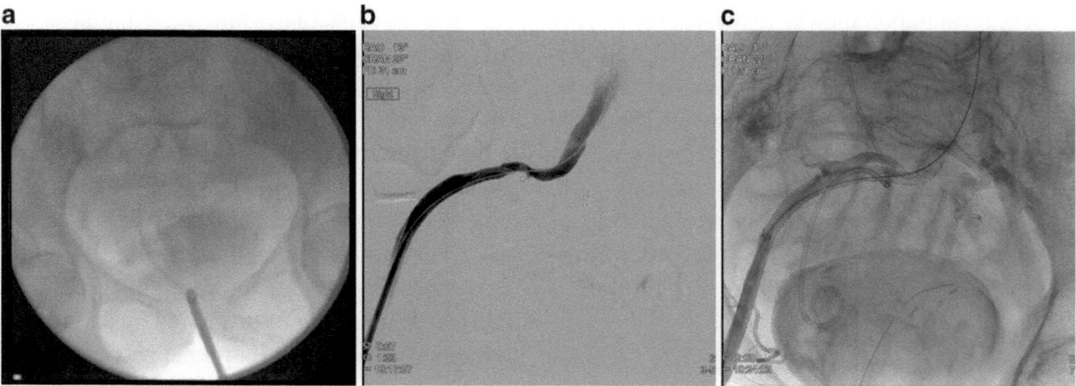

Fig. 11.1 (**a**) Fluoroscopic image of ureteral stent placement after pulsatile blood seen coming from ureteral orifice. (**b**) Arteriogram picture of connection between right common iliac artery and right ureter. (**c**) Successful endovascular graft placement to close stricture

Severe bleeding is rare but can cause significant morbidity or even mortality. This is usually due to a nearby or crossing vessel at places such as the ureteropelvic junction (UPJ), intrarenal artery at an infundibulum or the common iliac artery [9]. Knowing the arterial anatomy and its relation to the ureter or renal pelvis can obviate these injuries especially when attempting endoscopic treatment of ureteral stricture near these vascular structures. The ureter during these procedures should be incised at the side opposite the nearby vessel. At the UPJ, the ureter should be cut on the lateral posterior side of the lumen to avoid an anterior crossing vessel. In the rare instance that a crossing vessel is identified posterior, then the UPJ should be cut on the anterior side. A preoperative CT of the abdomen and pelvis with IV contrast and 3D reconstructions can help delineate the vascular anatomy. In the distal ureter, the stricture should be cut on the medial side to avoid pelvic sidewall vessels. At the iliac vessels, the ureteral stricture should be cut on the anterior side. If severe bleeding does occur, a balloon can be used to tamponade the bleeding until it stops. If the bleeding does not halt, further treatments may be required such as embolization using interventional radiology or vascular surgery. A rare, but often devastating cause of severe bleeding is an ureteroiliac fistula. If encountered, immediate placement of a ureteral stent and foley catheter placement is advised. If the patient is stable, an endovascular stent can be placed by interventional radiology or vascular surgery as seen in Fig. 11.1a–c; however if the patient is hemodynamically unstable, emergent open exploration to get proximal control of the iliac artery should be attempted.

Holding anticoagulation 5–7 days preoperatively may help decrease the risk of intraoperative or postoperative bleeding. This may not be possible for some patients due to the increased use of drug-eluting cardiac stents or recent pulmonary embolus or deep vein thrombus. Fortunately, the safety of URS in patients on anticoagulation has been established in the literature. A recent study of 37 patients undergoing URS on anticoagulation showed no increase in the risk of bleeding or reduction in stone-free rates [10].

Mucosal Injury

Mucosal injury of the ureter or renal pelvis is reported to occur between 2.5 and 24 % [6, 11]. These injuries can happen during placement of the guide wire, balloon dilation of the ureter, placement of a ureteral access sheath, laser lithotripsy, or stone basket extraction. The recent advances in smaller instruments have decreased the incidence from 24 to 6 % when compared to larger caliber instruments [12]. These injuries can usually be managed conservatively and most do not require termination of the case. However, recognition is helpful in guiding the decision to place a ureteral stent at the end of the operation.

The most important way to prevent these types of injuries is appropriate technique during URS. If there is a need for multiple passes of the ureteroscope, then a ureteral access sheath should be used or the scope should be passed over a wire to help prevent contact with the ureteral wall. Whenever the ureteroscope is advanced up or down the ureter, it should be done under direct vision to avoid collision with the ureteral wall.

False Passage

False passage during placement of a guide wire can create a mucosal flap or submucosal tunnel with or without total ureteral perforation. This is most likely to occur when the surgeon is attempting to place a wire adjacent to an obstructing or impacted stone, and should be suspected when the wire does not advance easily. Even if recognized during the procedure, a false passage is associated with a postoperative ureteral stricture rate of 0.4–0.9 % [6].

Extravasation of contrast particularly in a periadventitial pattern can identify a false passage and aid in placing a wire into the correct position. If a false passage occurs, the wire should not be used for further dilation or placement of catheters as this will cause a more severe injury. A wire should be placed under direct vision sometimes with the help of a ureteroscope into the ureteral lumen and renal pelvis followed by placement of a ureteral stent to allow healing [6].

Thermal Injuries

Thermal injuries of the ureter were much more common with the use of the EHL. These injuries can be superficial or deep abrasions that can lead to necrosis of the ureter. The EHL can cause a significant rise in intraluminal temperature and was associated with a 1 % perforation rate in a study of 207 patients [13].

The widespread use of the holmium:YAG laser has decreased the risk of thermal injury mainly due to its pinpoint end firing application and penetration depth of 0.4 mm. However, improper visualization while using the laser can still cause thermal injury leading to stricture formation of 1 % as was reported in one study of 598 patients [14]. The Nd:YAG laser has a penetration depth five times that of the holmium laser so care should be taken when ablating urothelial tumors within the ureter or renal pelvis with this laser. This penetration ability can lead to bowel or vascular injuries if not carefully used [15]. Thermal injuries can be prevented by careful use of lasers near the ureteral or renal pelvic mucosa, and placing the EHL probe parallel to the mucosa edge. Furthermore, adequate visualization is the key to preventing thermal injury.

If a thermal injury is apparent or suspected during URS at the time of the procedure, ureteral stenting alone should be adequate treatment. However, imaging should be performed after removal of the stent to ensure there is no late sequela of this injury such as a ureteral stricture.

Ureteral Perforation

The overall incidence of ureteral perforation has decreased over the years due to smaller instruments and flexible scopes with a range as low as 0 % [16] in a recent study to 17 % [17] in earlier studies. Francesca et al. reported a ureteral perforation rate of 11 % with conventional ureteroscopes (9.5–11.5 F) when compared to a 2 % rate with smaller caliber (6.5–7.5 F) ureteroscopes [12]. A large study of over 5,000 URS procedures showed an overall incidence of ureteral perforation to be 6.1 % [18] In a series of over 1,500 URS procedures, there were 29 reported ureteral perforations, 20 were minor mucosal injuries, five required prolonged stenting, and four required open surgery to fix a severe injury [19].

Ureteral perforation can be minor or major depending on the instrument that causes the perforation. Identifying defects within the ureteral mucosa or even periureteral fat can help the surgeon diagnose these injuries. Perforation can be caused by advancement of a guide wire past an obstructing or impacted stone as discussed earlier in this chapter, overly forceful passage of ureteral dilators, or in the case of a fixed ureter due to

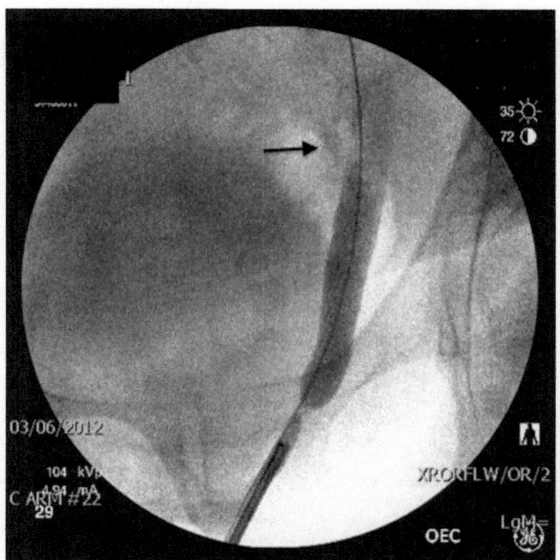

Fig. 11.2 Distal ureteral perforation (*arrow*) during ureteroscopic treatment of impacted distal ureteral stone

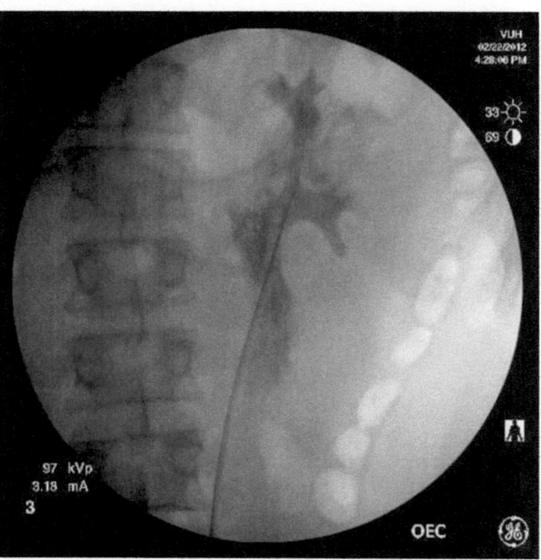

Fig. 11.3 Large amount of extravasation at the proximal ureter during ureteroscopic laser lithotripsy due to large perforation

retroperitoneal pathology. Placing contrast into the collecting system before advancement of the wire can help identify or prevent wire perforation as seen in Fig. 11.2. Stiffer wires are more likely to cause perforation so a wire with a hydrophilic tip such as a Glide wire or Sensor™ should be placed first and confirmed to be in the correct position. If a stiff wire is needed for instance to place an access sheath then an open-ended ureteral catheter should be placed over the hydrophilic wire first up to the renal pelvis under fluoroscopic guidance. Once the open-ended catheter is in the renal pelvis, the hydrophilic wire may be removed and the stiff wire can be placed through the catheter into the correct position.

One important thing to remember during URS is to keep the irrigation pressure only as high as needed to have good visualization. We use 150 Hg of pressure during a rigid or flexible URS without an access sheath and 200 Hg of pressure with an access sheath in place. Hand irrigation through the scope needs to be done slowly to prevent large increases in intraluminal pressure. Irrigation pressures too high can cause ureteral perforation or forniceal rupture. In the event of an infected stone and/or urine, this can lead to bacteremia or even sepsis.

Laser fibers can cause perforation due to direct contact with the ureteral wall causing small or even large defects within the mucosa. Knowing the depth of penetration of the laser once again can prevent these complications. Basket extraction of stones can cause accidental perforation if a piece of mucosa is grasped along with the stone fragment or too large a stone fragment is attempted to be pulled through a narrow ureter. The attempted basket extraction of a ureteral or renal pelvis tumor can lead to perforation if the biopsy taken is too deep.

The ureteroscope itself can cause a large perforation in the ureteral wall if aggressive force is applied to it while trying to advance the scope through a tight ureteral lumen, or the ureteroscope is not kept in the middle of the lumen during advancement of the scope as seen in Fig. 11.3. Careful advancement and removal of the ureteroscope under direct vision can prevent these types of injuries. If the patient suddenly moves during the procedure, this can cause perforation so general anesthesia is preferred while doing URS, especially if working in the upper ureter or renal pelvis. Spinal anesthesia for middle or distal ureteral stones is acceptable. It is also important to remember that longer operative times have been

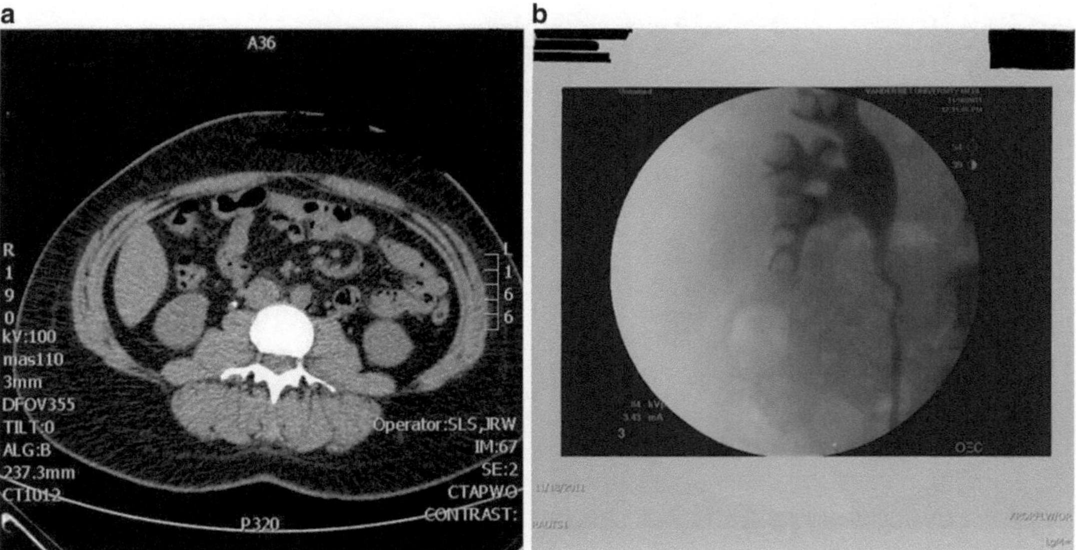

Fig. 11.4 (**a**) Submucosal stone seen in patient's right proximal ureter. (**b**) Intraoperative retrograde pyelogram showing stone outside the collecting system

associated with an increased incidence of ureteral perforation [20].

Using good technique during URS can help prevent most of these injuries, yet when they occur, the most important thing is prompt recognition. Treatment of a ureteral perforation includes termination of the procedure and placement of a ureteral stent. Typically, the stent should be left in place for 4–6 weeks before removal or second procedure is undertaken. If a ureteral stent is unable to be placed, we recommend placement of a percutaneous nephrostomy tube for proximal drainage of the collecting system to prevent further extravasation or urinoma/abscess formation [6, 21]. Following stent removal, an imaging study should be performed approximately 4 weeks later to ensure a stricture or urinoma has not formed. If a stent or percutaneous nephrostomy tube is unable to be placed then open or laparoscopic surgery is warranted.

Submucosal or Lost Stone

The submucosal or lost stone is a problematic issue for the treating surgeon as it is difficult to treat. The incidence of extrusion of stones is up to 2 % of URS cases [6, 11, 21]. A stone that migrates into the submucosa can lead to formation of a stone granuloma and/or ureteral stenosis. Grasso et al. showed that submucosal stones less than 4 mm imbedded in the submucosa have a high rate of long-term stricture formation and should be extracted [22].

Removal of a submucosal stone requires laser fragmentation of the stone to release it from the ureter for extraction followed by prolonged ureteral stenting. This can lead to perforation of the ureter or retroperitoneal urinoma if care is not taken during laser extraction of the stone. If the stone is pushed out of the lumen of the ureter into the retroperitoneal space, the surgeon should not attempt to remove the stone as this may exacerbate the injury [23]. An example of a CT scan and retrograde pyelogram of a submucosal stone can be seen in Fig. 11.4. Submucosal stones that are unable to be removed through endoscopic means, often result in stone granuloma formation and eventual stricture of the ureter which usually requires laparoscopic or even open reconstruction [24, 25].

Imaging postoperatively is imperative in both situations. With the submucosal stone, the risk of ureteral stenosis or stricture formation is prevalent so imaging 4–6 weeks later and perhaps in addition 3–6 months postoperatively should be done to ensure this did not occur or to diagnose a "silent stricture" that can lead to decreased renal function or atrophy of the renal parenchyma. If the patient has a stone that is completely outside the ureter, imaging postoperatively will show the surgeon where the stone is located so in the future this stone will not be mistaken for an intraluminal stone causing obstruction or pain as seen in Fig. 11.4a, b. The patient should be aware of this as well to help inform other physicians who may care for the patient.

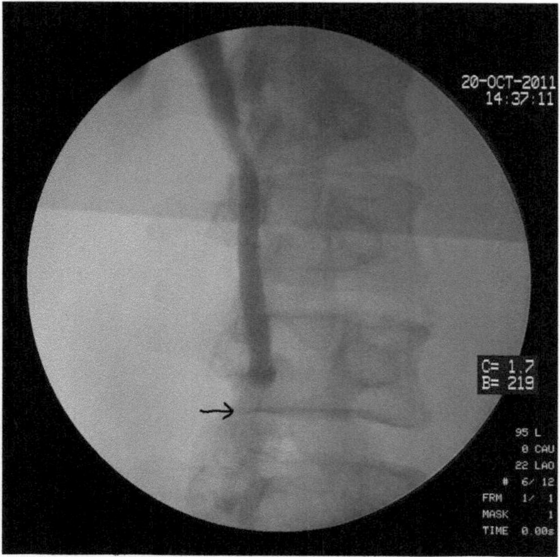

Fig. 11.5 Antegrade nephrostogram picture of contrast extravasation at proximal ureter after ureteral avulsion (*arrow*). Picture courtesy of Jared Moss, M.D.

Ureteral Avulsion

Ureteral avulsion is a rare but devastating complication of URS usually occurring in the proximal third of the ureter where it has the least amount of muscle within its wall [4]. It is caused by elongation of the ureter itself followed by rupture in the area of minimal resistance. This complication generally arises during aggressive manipulation of a large or impacted ureteral stone with an endourologic basket [6, 26]. The overall incidence is less than 1 % of all cases [2, 7], and a recent study of 1,000 cases showed no incidence of ureteral avulsion [2, 6, 11, 16].

The decreased risk of a ureteral avulsion has mainly been impacted by the abolishment of blind basketing maneuvers under fluoroscopy. The use of lasers to fragment stones into very small pieces has also lead to a decrease in the incidence of ureteral avulsion. Basket extraction should be reserved for small stones [27]. When a stone is engaged by the basket, it should be kept in direct vision during the entire extraction from the ureter. If the stone will not come down with the scope, the basket should be disengaged and the stone fragmented into smaller pieces for removal or passage. If the basket cannot be disengaged, it should be disassembled at the handle so the ureteroscope can be removed over the basket. The ureteroscope can then be placed alongside the basket up to the level of the stone and laser lithotripsy performed on the stone until the basket is freed. The basket can then be removed under direct vision and then the stone fragments can either be allowed to pass or a new basket used to remove the fragments. A safety wire should be in place during this time so that a ureteral stent can be placed if the stone cannot be removed or integrity of the ureter is compromised.

Ureteral avulsion is usually diagnosed at the time of the procedure when part of the ureter is found attached to the basket upon removal, or on retrograde pyelography. In the latter case, there will be complete extravasation at the level of the avulsion with no contrast in the collecting system above this as seen in Fig. 11.5. If this injury is not diagnosed at the time of the procedure, the patient will usually present in the immediate postoperative period with fever, flank pain, and a retroperitoneal urinoma or possible abscess. Diagnosis can be confirmed with: CT Urogram, intravenous pyelogram (IVP) or in the operating room with a retrograde pyelogram. Immediate placement of a percutaneous nephrostomy tube for proximal drainage of the collecting system is recommended when the injury is diagnosed.

Management of this injury depends on the timing of diagnosis, length of injury, and the patient's age and renal function. If the avulsion is diagnosed at the time of the operation and a wire

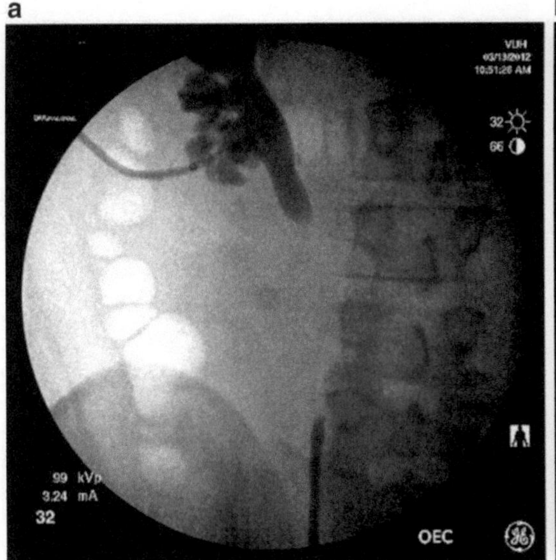

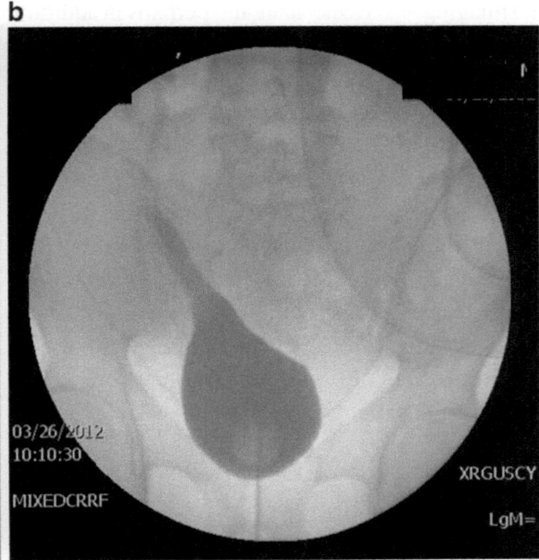

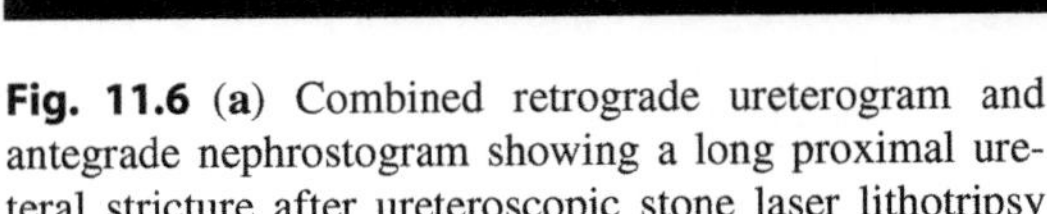

Fig. 11.6 (**a**) Combined retrograde ureterogram and antegrade nephrostogram showing a long proximal ureteral stricture after ureteroscopic stone laser lithotripsy for impacted stone. (**b**) Postoperative image of cystogram showing a Boari Flap up to the renal pelvis

can be placed across the injury, then a ureteral stent for a few months may allow secondary healing. The stent may save the patient from a major operation; however, they must be followed closely due to the high risk of stricture formation. The ability to place a ureteral stent usually occurs during partial ureteral avulsion not complete avulsion.

If a wire or continuity of the ureter cannot be accomplished, the procedure should be stopped and the patient should undergo percutaneous nephrostomy tube placement as a staged repair is recommended more than an immediate repair to fully prepare and inform the patient [26, 28]. Repair of these injuries requires an open or complex laparoscopic/robotic-assisted ureteral reconstruction depending on the level and length at which the injury occurred. Distal ureteral avulsion can be repaired with reimplantation of the ureter into the bladder and often a psoas hitch procedure. Middle ureteral injuries may be repaired with either a ureteroureterostomy if the defect is short or a psoas hitch and/or Boari flap if the defect is long. Proximal ureteral injuries may require a Boari flap or ileal ureter especially if the defect is long. A long proximal ureteral stricture can be seen on antegrade and retrograde pyelogram in Fig. 11.6 along with the postoperative cystogram showing the Boari flap. Auto-transplantation of the kidney to the common iliacs may be used if only a short amount of ureter remains with good results if the patient is young [29]. An ileal ureter can lead to significant metabolic abnormalities and should be refrained from use in a young patient if possible [30]. Transureteroureterostomy while feasible is contraindicated in stone formers.

Technology Failures

URS is highly dependent on technology, and failure of equipment or instruments can compromise patient safety. A retrospective study by Geavlete et al. of over 2,500 hundred cases showed an overall incidence of equipment failure to be 1.4 % [11]. These equipment failures range from loss of optics on the ureteroscope, locked deflection of a flexible ureteroscope while in the kidney, broken laser fibers or guidewires, or baskets that will not disengage. As always, the use of a safety wire will allow the surgeon to place a ureteral stent and come back another time if any significant technology failure occurs.

The most important way to prevent these failures is to have routine maintenance of the lasers and ureteroscopes. All equipment should be checked before every case. Checking the flexible ureteroscope to make sure it deflects properly and can return to a straightforward position is also important. The basket should be opened and closed before engaging a stone. The laser fiber should be examined to ensure the fiber is not fractured or stripped along the entire length of the fiber to prevent injury to the patient or operating room staff. All surfaces should be wet where any potential contact of the laser may occur with the patient, and all operating room personnel credentialed in laser safety.

Postoperative Complications

Infection/Sepsis

Infection is the most common postoperative complication associated with URS. The overall incidence of urinary tract infection (UTI) after URS is 6.9 % even with administration of appropriate preoperative antibiotics and negative preoperative urine culture [4, 11, 21]. The most common manifestation is postoperative fever, but, while rare, pyelonephritis and sepsis can occur [1, 6]. The incidence of post-URS sepsis is low with an incidence of only 0.3 % while UTI incidence is only 1.2 % [31]. With the rise in fluoroquinolone and trimethoprim-sulfamethoxazole resistant bacteria, the rate of infectious complications may increase as a fluoroquinolone is still the preoperative antibiotic of choice by the AUA Best Practice Policy for endoscopic cases [32]. Cephalosporins were shown to be just as effective in preventing infectious complications as a fluoroquinolone but were not as cost-effective [33–36]

Preoperative antibiotics have been shown to reduce the risk of postoperative infection and sepsis [4, 11, 21]. One study showed a 22 % incidence of fever in a patient cohort not given any antibiotics except if considered a complicated case, and a UTI was only diagnosed with a positive urine culture in 3.7 % of these patients [19].

Patients with a history of infection stones may be at an increased risk for postoperative infection. These stones are usually struvite stones and are made from urea-splitting bacteria such as Proteus. If the surgeon suspects that the stone is infected, a sample of the stone should be ground up in saline and sent off for Gram stain and stone culture at the time of the procedure.

One of the most important things the surgeon can do is to prevent infection and sepsis is to make sure the patient is optimized for surgery. A preoperative urine culture should be performed and be negative before taking the patient to the operating room. If the urine culture is positive, then the patient should be treated with culture-specific antibiotics for the recommended time and a reculture should show no growth before proceeding. Patients colonized with bacteria (indwelling catheter, urinary diversion, neurogenic bladder) should receive culture-specific antibiotics pre-op even in the absence of symptomatic infection as instrumentation may increase the risk of a postoperative infectious complication. The urine should be dipped the day of the procedure to ensure the patient has nitrite negative urine. If the infection cannot be eradicated due to the infected stone, we recommend the patient be adequately drained for 1–2 weeks with a percutaneous nephrostomy tube or stent and given appropriate culture sensitive antibiotics during this time to decrease the chance of postoperative sepsis or fever. If these patients become febrile or hypotensive during the case due to possible infection/sepsis, the surgeon should stop and place either a stent or percutaneous nephrostomy tube immediately and come back 48–72 h later if the patient is stable. If purulent urine is discovered at the time of a case, we recommend the case be terminated and the patient adequately drained with a stent or percutaneous nephrostomy tube.

Another way to reduce the risk of bacteremia or sepsis during URS when dealing with an infected stone is to use the least amount of irrigation pressure to allow the surgeon to have adequate vision during the case. It may also help to periodically depressurize the system by removing fluid through the ureteroscope. Furthermore, we recommend the use of a ureteral access sheath if an infectious stone is suspected, as it provides an excellent drainage tool to lower the intraluminal pressure while providing adequate visualization [5].

Vesicoureteral Reflux

Vesicoureteral reflux (VUR) after URS is usually transient in nature and occurs with an incidence of up to 5–10 % of cases [4, 6, 37]. The VUR is usually due to active dilation of the ureteral orifice either with ureteral dilators, access sheaths, or balloon dilators [37]. The predominant symptom is flank pain with voiding, and can usually be treated with oral pain medication. Persistent VUR is rare but may need treatment with endoscopic measures or open/laparoscopic measures if the patient is symptomatic with recurrent pyelonephritis. The diagnosis of persistent VUR is made with a voiding cystourethrogram.

Ureteral Stricture

Ureteral strictures are a late complication of ureteroscopy that can lead to significant morbidity including pain, infection, or even loss of renal function. The overall incidence of ureteral stricture has improved over the past two decades from nearly 10 % down to 0.5–4 % in recent studies [2, 21, 38, 39]. This decline is most likely due to improvements in technology such as smaller diameter ureteroscopes, flexible instruments, lasers, and baskets. Another factor in this decline may be the increase in routine imaging among patients and widespread use of CT scans which allows diagnosis of stones earlier on in their clinical course before they can become impacted stones.

The cause of ureteral strictures is multifactorial. Stones themselves can become impacted into the wall of the ureter causing severe inflammation and vascular compromise that may lead to stricture formation. Robert et al. showed a 24 % stricture rate for stones impacted for an average of 11 months [31]. Ureteral perforation is another cause of stricture formation due to injury to the ureter and subsequent stenosis of the lumen. In one study of 156 rigid ureteroscopies, ureteral perforation was recognized in 24 patients leading to a postoperative ureteral stricture rate of 5.9 vs. a 3.5 % of patients without a recognized ureteral perforation [38]. Ureteral stenting can help decrease the risk of ureteral stricture if the perforation is noticed at the time of the procedure but there is no consensus in the literature on how long to leave the stent in place. Most urologist leave a stent for 6 weeks based on the endopyleotomy literature [40]. A history of pelvic radiation or prior surgery on the ureter can lead to vascular compromise, which increases the risk of stricture formation following URS. The use of a ureteral access sheath was hypothesized to be a cause of ureteral stricture, but Delvecchio et al. saw only 1 of 71 patients in whom an access sheath was used who formed a stricture along the path of the sheath [39]. The use of lasers and baskets within the ureter can lead to stricture formation due to mucosal injuries, perforations, or thermal injuries which were discussed earlier. Trauma or perforation from the ureteroscope itself can lead to stricture formation and constant care and diligence should be used during URS to prevent complications as in Figs. 11.7 and 11.8.

With the decrease in the incidence of ureteral strictures over the last several years, there has been a debate on whether or not asymptomatic patients after uncomplicated URS need postoperative imaging. Weizer et al. showed a 3.7 % stricture rate of asymptomatic patients after routine URS within 3 months of their procedure and currently recommend routine imaging evaluation in the first 3 months postoperatively to diagnose asymptomatic "silent" ureteral obstruction [41]. The authors routinely perform a renal ultrasound 6 weeks postoperatively to check for hydroureteronephrosis in all URS patients.

The current management of ureteral strictures entirely depends on the length and location of the stricture. Short, nonischemic strictures (<2 cm)

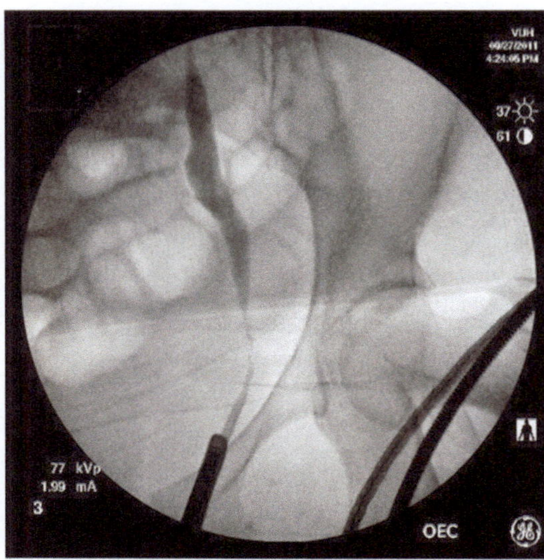

Fig. 11.7 Retrograde pyelogram photo showing a long distal ureteral stricture after ureteroscopic stone extraction with proximal ureteral dilation

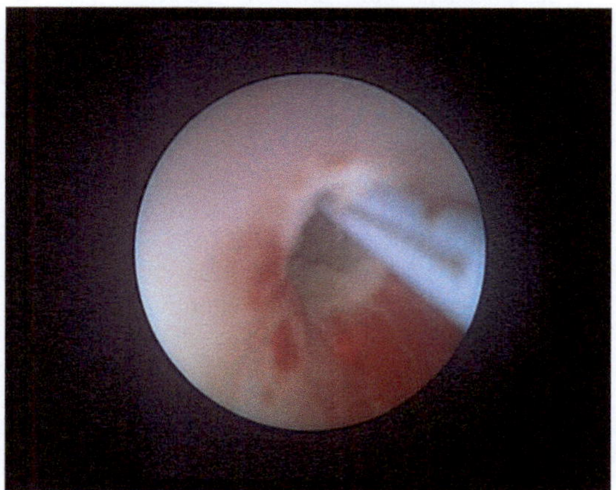

Fig. 11.8 Endoscopic view of a ureteral stricture

can either be treated endoscopically with holmium laser incision or with open/laparoscopic repair, usually ureteroureterostomy. Short ischemic appearing strictures should be treated with open/laparoscopic/robotic-assisted excision and repair. Strictures longer than 2 cm should all be treated with open/laparoscopic/robotic-assisted repair unless contraindicated. These types of repairs are the same as the discussion for the repair of ureteral avulsion including the following: ureteroureterostomy, Boari flap, psoas hitch, ileal ureter, and auto transplantation as seen in Fig. 11.8a, b.

Table 11.1 Intraoperative complications of ureteroscopy

Ureteroscopic complication	Incidence
Bleeding	0.3–2.1 % [7, 8]
Mucosal injury	2.5–24 % [6, 11]
False passage	0.4–0.9 % [6]
Thermal injury	1 % [13]
Perforation	0–17 % [16, 17]
Submucosal or lost stone	2 % [6, 11, 21]
Avulsion	0–1 % [6, 7, 11, 16]
Technology failures	1.4 % [11]

Table 11.2 Postoperative complications of ureteroscopy

Ureteroscopic complication	Incidence
Infection (UTI)	1.2–6.9 % [4, 31]
Urosepsis	0.3 % [31]
Ureteral stricture	0.5–10 % [38, 39]
Vesicoureteral reflux	5–10 % [4, 6, 37]

Summary

Ureteroscopy is a safe and efficacious tool for treatment of ureteral and renal stones along with diagnosis and treatment of urothelial cancers of the upper urinary tract. Complications of ureteroscopy are fortunately low, but major complications, while rare, often require additional surgical intervention. Prompt recognition of ureteral perforation, avulsion, or impending sepsis is critically important in reducing the morbidity or mortality of these complications. Furthermore, application of safety techniques such as the use of guidewires, glide wires, preoperative urine cultures, smaller, flexible ureteroscopes, safer lasers and baskets, and better image quality have lowered the incidence of these complications. A list of these complications can be seen in Tables 11.1 and 11.2.

References

1. Schuster TG, Hollenbeck BK, Gaeber GJ, Wolf Jr JS. Complications of ureteroscopy: analysis of predictor factors. J Urol. 2001;166(2):538–40.
2. Harmon WJ, Sershon PD, Blute ML, Patterson DE, Segura JW. Ureteroscopy: current practice and long-term complications. J Urol. 1997;157(1):28–32.

3. Patel SR, McLaren ID, Nakada SY. The ureteroscope as a safety wire for ureteronephroscopy. J Endourol. 2012;26(4):351–4.
4. Zattoni F. Ureteroscopy: complications. In: Smith AD, editor. Smith's textbook of endourology. 2nd ed. Hamilton, ON: BC Decker; 2007.
5. Rehman J, Monga M, Landman J. Characterization of intrapelvic pressure during ureteropyeloscopy with ureteral access sheaths. Urology. 2003;61(4): 713–8.
6. Johnson DB, Pearle MS. Complications of ureteroscopy. Urol Clin North Am. 2004;31(1):157–71.
7. Blute ML, Sergura JW, Patterson DE. Ureteroscopy. J Urol. 1988;139(3):510–2.
8. Abdel-Razzak OM, Bagley DH. Clinical experience with flexible ureteropyeloscopy. J Urol. 1992;148: 1788–92.
9. Meretyk I, Meretyk S, Clayman RV. Endopyelotomy: comparison of ureteroscopic retrograde and antegrade percutaneous techniques. J Urol. 1992;148(3):775–82. discussion 782–3.
10. Turna B, Stein RJ, Smaldone MC, et al. Safety and efficacy of flexible ureterorenoscopy and holmium:YAG lithotripsy for intrarenal stones in anticoagulated cases. J Urol. 2008;179(4):1415–9.
11. Geavlete P, Georgescu D, Ni G, Mirciulescu V, Cauni V. Complications of 2735 retrograde semirigid ureteroscopy procedures: a single center experience. J Endourol. 2006;20(3):179–85.
12. Francesca F, Scattoni V, Nava L, Pompa P, Grasso M, Rigatti P. Failures and complications of transurethral ureteroscopy in 297 cases: conventional rigid instruments vs. small caliber semirigid ureteroscopes. Eur Urol. 1995;28(2):112–5.
13. Ba ar H, Ohta N, Kageyama S, Suzuki K, Kawabe K. Treatment of ureteral and renal stone by electrohydraulic lithotripsy. Int Urol Nephrol. 1997;29(3):275–80.
14. Sofer M, Watterson JD, Wollin TA, Nott L, Razvi H, Denstedt JD. Holmium:YAG laser lithotripsy for upper urinary tract calculi in 598 patients. J Urol. 2002;167(1):31–4.
15. Chen GL, Bagley DH. Ureteroscopic surgery for upper tract transitional-cell carcinoma: complications and management. J Endourol. 2001;15(4):399–404. discussion 409.
16. Grasso M. Ureteropyeloscopic treatment of ureteral and intrarenal calculi. Urol Clin North Am. 2000;27(4):623–31.
17. Leveillee RJ, Hulbert JC. Complications. In: Smith AD, editor. Smith's Textbook of endourology. St. Louis: Quality Medical Publishing; 1996. p. 513–25.
18. Stoller ML, Wolf JS. Endoscopic ureteral injuries. In: McAnnich JW, editor. Traumatic and reconstructive uology. Philadelphia, PA: WB Saunders; 1996. p. 199–211.
19. Jeromin L, Sosnowski M. Ureteroscopy in the treatment of ureteral stones: over ten years' experience. Eur Urol. 1998;34(4):344–9.
20. Schuster TG, Hollenbeck BK, Faerber GJ, Wolf Jr JS. Complications of ureteroscopy: analysis of predictive factors. J Urol. 2001;166(2):538–40.
21. Siddiq FM, Leveillee RJ. Complications of ureteroscopic approaches, including incisions. In: Nakada SY, Pearle MS, editors. Advanced endourology: the complete clinical guide. Totowa, NJ: Humana Press Inc; 2005. p. 299–320.
22. Grasso M, Lui JB, Goldberg B, Bagley DH. Submucosal calculi: endoscopic and intramural sonographic diagnosis and treatment options. J Urol. 1995;153(5):1384–9.
23. Kriegmair MN. Paraureteral calculi caused by ureteroscopic perforation. Urology. 1995;45(4): 578–80.
24. Doddamani D, Kumar R, Hemal AK. Stone granuloma–not to be forgotten as a delayed complication of ureteroscopy. Urol Int. 2002;68(2):129–31.
25. Dretler SP, Young RH. Stone granuloma: a cause of ureteral stricture. J Urol. 1993;150(6):1800–2.
26. de la Rosetter JJ, Skrekas T, Segura JW. Handling and prevention complications in stone basketing. Eur Urol. 2006;50(5):991–8.
27. Grasso M. Complications of ureteropyeloscopy. In: Taneja SS, Smith RB, Ehrlich RM, editors. Complications of urologic surgery. 3rd ed. Philadelphia, PA: Saunders; 2001. p. 268–76.
28. Abdelrahim AF, Abdelmaguid A, Abuzeid H, Amin M, Mousa el S, Abdelrahim F. Rigid ureteroscopy for ureteral stones: factors associated with intraoperative adverse events. J Endourol. 2008;22(2):277–80.
29. Martin X, Ndoye A, Knoan PG, et al. Hazards of lumber ureteroscopy: apropos of 4 cases of avulsion of the ureter. Prog Urol. 1998;8(3):358–62.
30. Shokeir AA. Interposition of ileum in the ureter: a clinical study of long-term follow up. Br J Urol. 1997;79(3):324–7.
31. Roberts WW, Cadeddu JA, Micali S, Kavoussi LR, Moore RG. Ureteral stricture formation after removal of impacted calculi. J Urol. 1998;159(3):723–6.
32. American Urologic Association [homepage on the Internet]. Baltimore: Best Practice Policy Statement on Urologic Surgery Antimicrobial Prophylaxis; 2008. (Reviewed and validity confirmed 2011, updated February 2012). AUA Guidelines for Antibiotic Prophylaxis. Available from: www.auanet.org/content/media/antimicroprop08.pdf.
33. Cox CE. Comparison of intravenous ciprofloxacin and intravenous cefotaxime for Antimicrobial prophylaxis in transurethral surgery. Am J Med. 1989; 87(5A):252S–4.
34. Gombert ME, duBouchet L, Aulicino TM, Berkowitz LB, Macchia RJ. Intravenous ciprofloxacin versus cefotaxime prophylaxis during transurethral surgery. Am J Med. 1989;87(5A):250S–1.
35. Lukkarinen O, Hellström P, Leppilahti M, Kontturi M, Tammela T. Antimicrobial prophylaxis in patients with urinary retention undergoing transurethral

prostatectomy. Ann Chir Gynaecol. 1997;86(3): 239–42.
36. Christiano AP, Hollowell CM, Kim H, et al. Double-blind randomized comparison of single-dose ciprofloxacin versus intravenous cefazolin in patients undergoing outpatient endourologic surgery. Urology. 2000;55(2):182–5.
37. Richter S, Shalev M, Lobik L, Buchumensky V, Nissenkorn I. Early postureteroscopy vesicoureteral reflux–a temporary and infrequent complication: prospective study. J Endourol. 1999;13(5):365–6.
38. Stoller ML, Wolf JS, Hofmann R, Marc B. Ureteroscopy without routine balloon dilation: an outcome assessment. J Urol. 1992;147(5):1238–42.
39. Delvecchio FC, Auge BK, Brizuela RM, et al. Assessment of stricture formation with the ureteral access sheath. Urology. 2003;61(3):518–22.
40. Davis DM. Intubated ureterostomy: a new operation for ureteral and ureteropelvic strictures. Surg Gynecol Obstet. 1943;76:513.
41. Weizer AZ, Auge BK, Silverstein AD, et al. Routine postoperative imaging is important after ureteroscopic stone manipulation. J Urol. 2002;168(1): 46–50.
42. Alapont JM, Broseta E, Oliver F, Pontones JL, Boronat F, Jiménez-Cruz JF. Ureteral avulsion as a complication of ureteroscopy. Int Braz J Urol. 2003; 29:18–22.

ESWL Principles

12

James Lingeman and Naeem Bhojani

Introduction

The treatment of stone disease has changed dramatically over the past 30 years. This is due in large part to the arrival of extracorporeal shock wave lithotripsy (ESWL). Before the arrival of ESWL in the early 1980s, the vast majority of urinary stones were treated with open surgery. Many stone patients are recurrent stone formers and would have to undergo multiple highly complicated surgeries in order to treat their stones. The virtual extinction of open surgical treatment of urinary stones is due in large part to ESWL. The first successful ESWL treatment was accomplished in 1980, in Germany by Dr. Christian Chaussy using a Dornier HM1 lithotriptor. Due to the effectiveness of ESWL and its minimal side effects, the FDA quickly approved ESWL. Dr. James Lingeman at the Methodist Hospital in Indianapolis using the unmodified Dornier HM3 lithotriptor performed the first ESWL procedure in North America. Since this time, ESWL has been used on millions of stone patients with great success and minimal detrimental effects.

ESWL uses high-intensity acoustic pulses to break up urinary tract stones. This technique offers an entirely noninvasive approach with minimal complications. When ESWL was first used to treat urinary stone disease, ESWL was seen as a technique that would be able to treat all urinary stones. This was quickly found to be inaccurate as limitations began to emerge.

Studies quickly discovered that some urinary stones (calcium oxalate monohydrate, cystine, and brushite) were resistant to ESWL and their fragmentation could not be accomplished using this technique [1–3]. Furthermore, some stones that could be fragmented would not fragment completely, and secondary treatments were necessary. As well, renal anatomy (calyceal diverticulum or acute infundibulopelvic angles) and location (lower pole calix) of the stone were crucial to stone-free outcomes [4]. Finally, many have reported on the frequent minor complications and the rare major complications [5, 6].

In response to the above mentioned issues concerning ESWL, much research has gone into understanding how ESWL fragments urinary stone. The objective of this chapter is to discuss the principles of ESWL including the mechanism of action, the different generators used to produce acoustic pulses, the different variables that impact the effectiveness of ESWL and the imaging techniques used during ESWL to target stones.

Mechanism of Action

All shock waves (acoustic pulses) have both a positive and a negative portion (Fig. 12.1). The positive portion of the wave, also known as the compressive phase causes pressure gradients

J. Lingeman • N. Bhojani (✉)
Department of Urology, Indiana University School of Medicine, Indianapolis, IA, USA
e-mail: naeem.bhojani@gmail.com

S.Y. Nakada and M.S. Pearle (eds.), *Surgical Management of Urolithiasis: Percutaneous, Shockwave and Ureteroscopy*, DOI 10.1007/978-1-4614-6937-7_12, © Springer Science+Business Media New York 2013

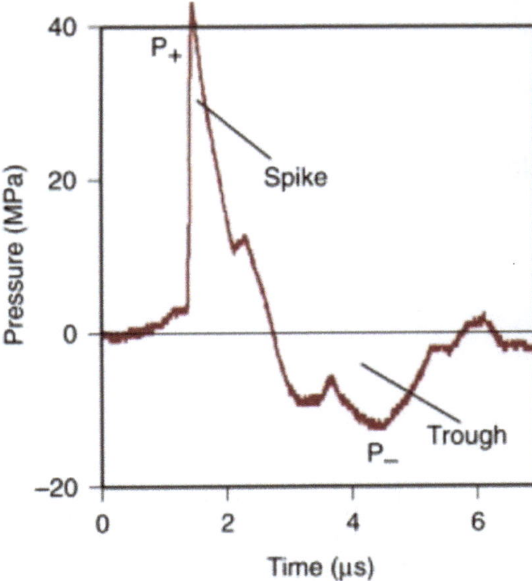

Fig. 12.1 Acoustic pulse

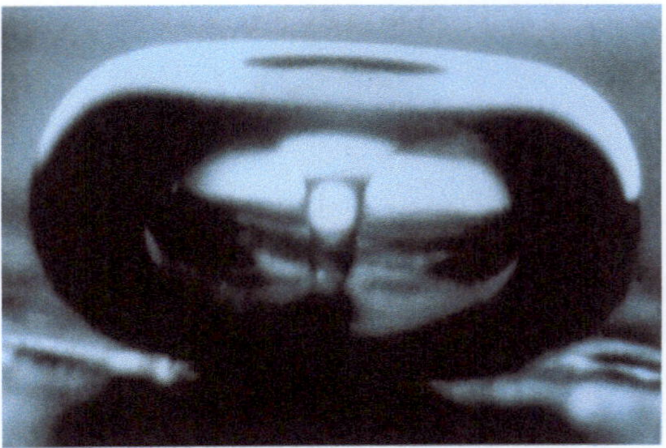

Fig. 12.2 Cavitation bubble

within stones leading to shear and tensile stress. This compressive phase produces pressures of about 20–100 MPa depending on the lithotripter. The negative portion of the wave, which has a lower amplitude causes mainly tensile stress (−5 to −15 MPa) but also causes cavitation in the fluid surrounding the stone. Both these forces are believed to contribute to stone fragmentation.

In general, fragmentation of stones occurs due to cracks that occur secondary to stresses that are caused by applied shock waves. With repetitive stresses these cracks grow and lead to fragmentation. The initial cracking of stones occurs secondary to different theorized shock-wave mechanisms including tear/shear forces, spallation, quasi-static squeezing, cavitation, and dynamic squeezing.

Tear/Shear Forces

Shear stresses are generated by a combination of both shear waves and compressive waves. These waves develop as the shock wave travels through the kidney stone. As a result, the shear and compressive waves cause large shear stresses at the crystal interfaces, which contribute to the fracture of the kidney stones. Shock waves move at different speeds in solid versus liquid mediums. This mismatch of the compressive waves results in shear stress.

Spallation

This theory hypothesizes that once the acoustic pulse has traversed the stone, it is inverted and reflected back from the distal surface of the stone. This creates a tensile (negative wave) force that can fragment the stone.

Quasi-Static Squeezing

Quasi-static squeezing occurs when the focal zone is greater than the diameter of the stone itself. Fragmentation occurs due to the difference in sound speed between the stone and the surrounding fluid. The acoustic pulse traveling through the stone is faster than the pulse that is traveling in the fluid outside the stone. This pulse produces a circumferential force on the stone, which results in a tensile stress on the stone. The force is maximal at the proximal and distal ends of the stone.

Cavitation

Cavitation bubbles (Fig. 12.2) are generated from the negative pressure phase of shock waves that occurs in both the fluid surrounding the stone and within micro-cracks of the stone. As the cavitation bubble collapses near a solid surface (kidney stone) a microjet of fluid is formed that pierces the bubble and impacts the surface of the stone. The collapse of the cavitation bubble also results in the formation of secondary shock waves. These secondary shock waves have amplitudes comparable to the focused shock wave.

Dynamic Squeezing

Dynamic squeezing hypothesizes that the damage caused by ESWL accumulates during the treatment session, which leads to the eventual fragmentation of the stone. All of the previously discussed mechanisms have the ability to generate progressive damage to the stone.

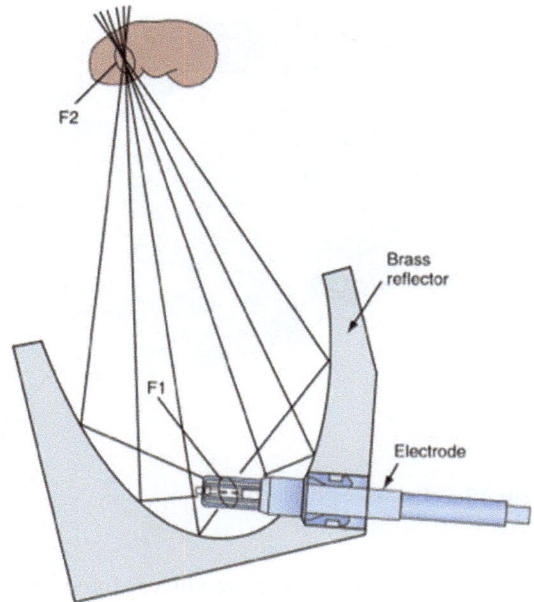

Fig. 12.3 Electrohydraulic lithotripter

Generators

There are three main generators that are used to produce shock waves. These include electrohydraulic (EHL), electromagnetic (EML), and piezoelectric (PZL).

Electrohydraulic

The EHL generator (Fig. 12.3) uses an underwater spark discharge between two electrodes to generate an spherically expanding shock wave. High voltage is applied to two electrodes that are separated by 1 mm. The spark discharge results in the vaporization of water at the electrode tips. The generated shock wave is focused by an ellipsoidal reflector. The focusing of the shock wave is dependent on the placement of the spark at the first focus of the ellipse (F1). Misalignment of the spark, even by just a few millimeters can lead to a significant loss in focusing of the shock wave.

Advantages

– Effectiveness in breaking kidney stones

Disadvantages

– Substantial pressure fluctuations from shock to shock
– Short electrode life

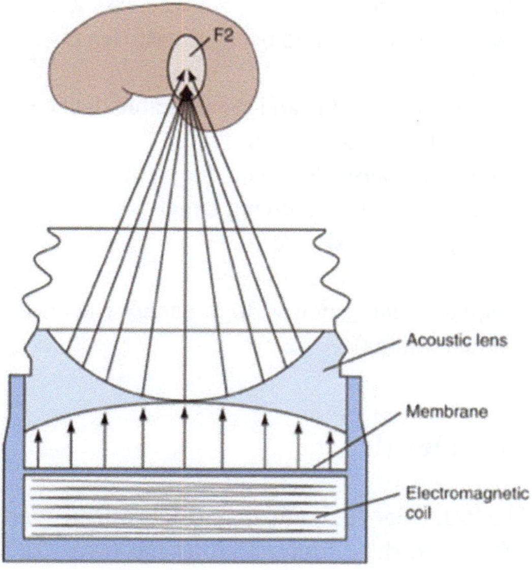

Fig. 12.4 Electromagnetic lithotripter

Electromagnetic

The EML generates shockwaves through a magnetic field, which is created between electromagnetic coil conductors (like the vibration of a base speaker) (Fig. 12.4). When the coil is excited by an electrical pulse, a metal plate placed in close

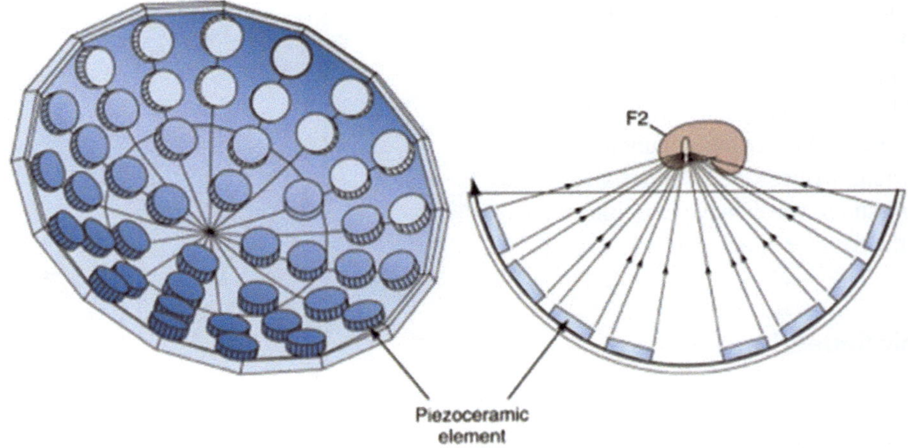

Fig. 12.5 Piezoelectric lithotripter

proximity experiences a repulsive force and this is used to generate an acoustic pulse. This lithotriptor can produce either cylindrical or plane shockwaves. The cylindrical shockwaves are reflected by a parabolic reflector whereas the plane shockwaves are focused by an acoustic lens.

Advantages

- More controllable and reproducible than electrohydraulic generators
- Possibly causes less pain due to the large surface area of the receiving target
- Longer electrode life

Disadvantages

- Small focal region of high energy (increased renal trauma)
- Decreased stone fragmentation effectiveness
- Small focal zone

Piezoelectric

The PZL (Fig. 12.5) utilizes crystals oriented in a spherical dish to form an ultrasonic wave. This lithotriptor produces plane shockwaves generated by rapid expansion of ceramic elements after application of a high-voltage pulse. The acoustic wave form with this lithotriptor starts as an acoustic pulse, and a shock wave is created by nonlinear propagation distortion.

Advantages

- Longer service-free life

Disadvantages

- Inadequate power

Variables Affecting ESWL Efficacy

Different variables can be manipulated in order to improve or modify the effectiveness of ESWL. These variables include the focal zone, coupling, monitoring, and rate.

Focal Zone

Acoustic energy is focused to a relatively small zone surrounding the focal point of the lithotriptor. The focal point is a geometric point and is usually the location of the kidney stone of interest. This zone can be small or large and the amount of energy or peak pressure that is applied can be manipulated (Fig. 12.6). In vitro studies have shown that larger focal zones can improve stone breakage [7]. Similarly, it was hypothesized that higher peak pressures can be used to break harder stones. However, higher peak pressures have been shown to cause greater damage to renal tissue [8–10]. The smaller, tighter focal zone, found in EML and PZL would appear at first glance to be advantageous as it would limit damage to the surrounding tissue. However, in vitro studies have demonstrated that the EML and the

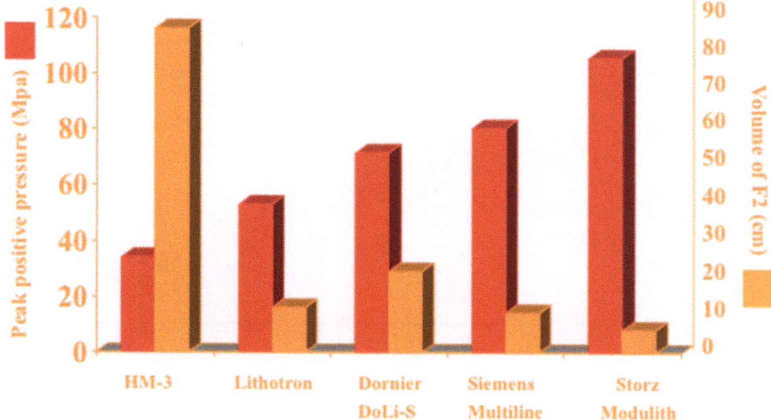

Fig. 12.6 Lithotriptors: Volume of focal zone versus peak pressure

PZL, with their high peak positive pressures, are no better at breaking stones and are often less effective [11]. The decreased effectiveness can be attributed to the lack of compressive waves associated with small focal zones. Recently it has been found that lower peak pressures are adequate to break stone, which also reduces the associated complications [12]. Due to respiratory movement, urinary stones are in continual motion. The hypothesis is that the stone will have a greater chance of staying within the target focal zone if it is larger. Pishchalnikov et al. have tested this hypothesis in an in vitro study [13]. Additionally, due to the tighter focal zones of the EML and PZL fewer shock waves actually hit the stone and more shock wave energy is deposited directly into tissue [14]. This excess shock wave energy can explain why EML and PZL have and increased incidence of subcapsular hematomas [15, 16].

Coupling

One of the most important factors affecting the effectiveness of ESWL to break stone is coupling. With good coupling, stone breakage is optimized. The HM-3 uses water as a medium for coupling which has been found to be ideal. The reason for this is that body tissue has an acoustical impedance very close to that of water, and therefore, a shock wave generated in water will pass into the body with minimal reflection or absorption of energy at the water/skin interface. Alternatively, other lithotriptors, also known as dry-head lithotriptors must be coupled to patients using other mediums such as gel or oil. In these dry-head lithotriptors, air pockets can get caught in the gel medium, which reduces the transmission of the shock wave energy. Pishchalnikov et al. demonstrated in an in vitro study a negative relationship between increasing air pockets and ESWL efficiency [17]. Jain et al. found that optimal fragmentation was obtained using bubble-free ultrasound gel [18]. Additionally, Bergsdorf et al. demonstrated clinically that gel with lower viscosity and better quality provided significantly better fragmentation [19]. Finally, it has been demonstrated that a defect in the gel medium of only 8 % by air pockets, reduced the breakage of stones by 60 % [20, 21] (Fig. 12.7). The implications of poor coupling include poor stone breakage, poor stone clearance, and possibly an increased number of shock waves applied to the kidney.

Monitoring

Once a stone has been localized, its movement in and out of the focal zone is crucial to its fragmentation. The longer the stone remains within

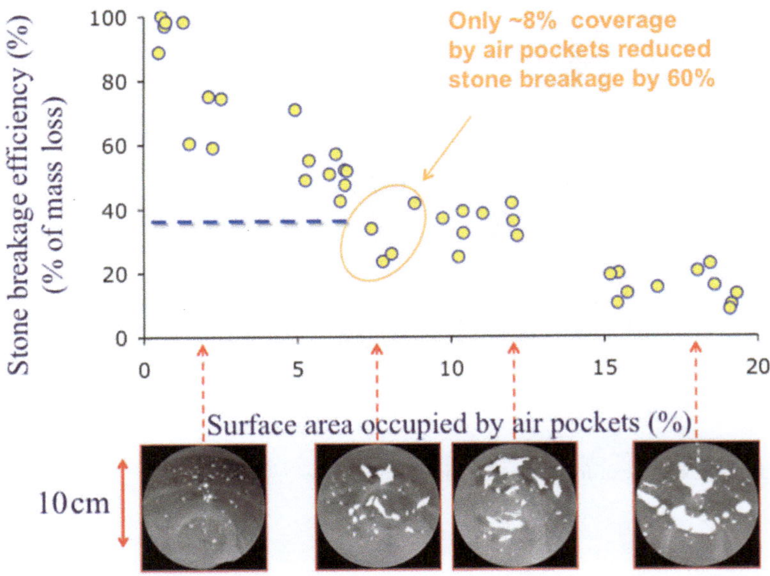

Fig. 12.7 Graph demonstrating reduced stone breakage with increasing air pocket coverage of coupling interface

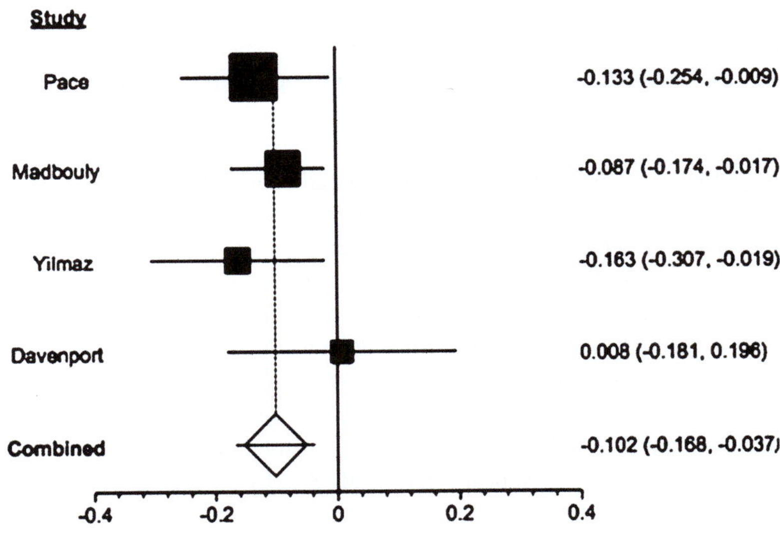

Fig. 12.8 Successful lithotripsy procedures using fast versus slow rate

the focal zone, the more likely it is to fragment. Respiratory motion can move the stone in and out of the focal zone. Previous attempts at high-frequency ventilation was effective but was found to be too invasive. Other systems used respiratory belts and shock wave triggering but these were found to increase treatment times considerably. The ideal strategy incorporates reduced respiratory movements with larger focal zones [22].

Rate

The rate at which shock waves are delivered has been discovered to have a significant impact on the fragmentation of urinary stones. Multiple randomized controlled trials have demonstrated that better fragmentation outcome can be achieved when shock waves are delivered at 60–80 shock waves per minute compared to the typical 120 shock waves per minute [23–28]. A meta-analysis by Semins et al. demonstrated that a treatment rate of 60 shocks per minute is associated with a higher rate of treatment success than treatment performed at a rate of 120 shocks per minute (Fig. 12.8) [28]. Additionally, a lower rate has also been associated with less renal tissue damage [8–10]. One drawback of this treatment method is the increased timed required to break urinary stones, which may extend the time that the patient is subjected to sedation. The reason behind the decreased stone fragmentation with increasing shock wave rate was hypothesized to be caused by an increase in the formation of cavitation bubbles, which would create an acoustic barrier to the transmission of positive-pressure phase of shock waves. However, Pishchalnikov et al. proposed an alternative explanation suggesting that the main reason was actually due to the loss of the negative pressure portion of the shock wave and not the interference with the positive pressure portion of the shock wave [29].

ESWL Imaging

Stone fragmentation using ESWL is only possible if the stone can be localized. The two ways to localize urinary stones for ESWL are with fluoroscopy or ultrasound. Both techniques have advantages and disadvantages. Fluoroscopy is the easier of the two methods as it requires only a C-arm and most urologists are familiar with this technology and its clinical application. As well, the majority of stones can be identified using fluoroscopy including ureteral stones. However, uric acid stones cannot be identified with fluoroscopy and this is one main advantage of ultrasound. Ultrasound requires more technical expertise and identifying kidney stones in obese patients and ureteral stones in the general population can be challenging at times. The main advantage of ultrasound is that there is no ionizing radiation, it can be done continuously and it is cheaper.

Conclusion

The ideal lithotriptor produces a very high stone-free rate with minimal complications. Through much research it is evident that this can be accomplished only using different strategies. Most important is the large focal zone of the lithotriptor in order to decrease complications and increase stone breakage. Additionally, slower pulse rates and meticulous coupling are paramount to realizing the ideal lithotriptor (please refer to Chap. 13).

References

1. Dretler SP. Stone fragility–a new therapeutic distinction. J Urol. 1988;139(5):1124–7.
2. Klee LW, Brito CG, Lingeman JE. The clinical implications of brushite calculi. J Urol. 1991;145(4):715–8.
3. Kim SC, Burns EK, Lingeman JE, Paterson RF, McAteer JA, Williams Jr JC. Cystine calculi: correlation of CT-visible structure, CT number, and stone morphology with fragmentation by shock wave lithotripsy. Urol Res. 2007;35(6):319–24.
4. Lingeman J, Matlaga BR, Evan AP. Surgical management of upper urinary tract calculi. In: Wein AJ, Kavoussi LR, Novick AC, Partin AW, Peters CA, editors. Campbell-walsh urology. Philadelphia, PA: Saunders; 2007. p. 1431–507.
5. Kaude JV, Williams CM, Millner MR, Scott KN, Finlayson B. Renal morphology and function immediately after extracorporeal shock-wave lithotripsy. AJR Am J Roentgenol. 1985;145(2):305–13.
6. McAteer JA, Evan AP. The acute and long-term adverse effects of shock wave lithotripsy. Semin Nephrol. 2008;28(2):200–13.
7. Neucks JS, Pishchalnikov YA, Zancanaro AJ, VonDerHaar JN, Williams Jr JC, McAteer JA. Improved acoustic coupling for shock wave lithotripsy. Urol Res. 2008;36(1):61–6.
8. Willis LR, Evan AP, Connors BA, et al. Shockwave lithotripsy: dose-related effects on renal structure, hemodynamics, and tubular function. J Endourol. 2005;19(1):90–101.
9. Connors BA, Evan AP, Blomgren PM, et al. Reducing shock number dramatically decreases lesion size in a juvenile kidney model. J Endourol. 2006;20(9):607–11.

10. Connors BA, Evan AP, Willis LR, Blomgren PM, Lingeman JE, Fineberg NS. The effect of discharge voltage on renal injury and impairment caused by lithotripsy in the pig. J Am Soc Nephrol. 2000; 11(2):310–8.
11. Kerbl K, Rehman J, Landman J, Lee D, Sundaram C, Clayman RV. Current management of urolithiasis: progress or regress? J Endourol. 2002;16(5):281–8.
12. Evan AP, McAteer JA, Connors BA, et al. Independent assessment of a wide-focus, low-pressure electromagnetic lithotripter: absence of renal bioeffects in the pig. BJU Int. 2008;101(3):382–8.
13. Cleveland RO, McAteer JA. The physics of shock wave lithotripsy. In: Smith AD, Badlani GH, Bagley DH, Clayman RV, Docimo SG, Jordan GH, Kavoussi LR, Lee BR, Lingeman JE, Preminger GM, Segura JW, editors. Smith's Textbook on endourology. Hamilton, ON: BC Decker, Inc; 2007. p. 317–32.
14. Cleveland RO, Anglade R, Babayan RK. Effect of stone motion on in vitro comminution efficiency of Storz Modulith SLX. J Endourol. 2004;18(7):629–33.
15. Köhrmann KU, Rassweiler JJ, Manning M, et al. The clinical introduction of a third generation lithotriptor: Modulith SL 20. J Urol. 1995;153(5):1379–83.
16. Ueda S, Matsuoka K, Yamashita T, Kunimi H, Noda S, Eto K. Perirenal hematomas caused by SWL with EDAP LT-01 lithotripter. J Endourol. 1993;7(1):11–5.
17. Pishchalnikov YA, Neucks JS, VonDerHaar RJ, Pishchalnikova IV, Williams Jr JC, McAteer JA. Air pockets trapped during routine coupling in dry head lithotripsy can significantly decrease the delivery of shock wave energy. J Urol. 2006;176(6 Pt 1):2706–10.
18. Jain A, Shah TK. Effect of air bubbles in the coupling medium on efficacy of extracorporeal shock wave lithotripsy. Eur Urol. 2007;51(6):1680–7. discussion 1686–7.
19. Bergsdorf T, Chaussy C, Türoff S. Energy coupling in extracorporeal shock wave lithotripsy-the impact of coupling quality on disintegration efficacy. J Endourol. 2008;22(Suppl):A161.
20. Bierkens AF, Hendrikx AJ, de Kort VJ, et al. Efficacy of second generation lithotriptors: a multicenter comparative study of 2,206 extracorporeal shock wave lithotripsy treatments with the Siemens Lithostar, Dornier HM4, Wolf Piezolith 2300, Direx Tripter X-1 and Breakstone lithotriptors. J Urol. 1992;148(3 Pt 2):1052–6. discussion 1056–7.
21. Lingeman JE. Extracorporeal shock wave lithotripsy. Development, instrumentation, and current status. Urol Clin North Am. 1997;24(1):185–211.
22. Rassweiler JJ, Knoll T, Köhrmann KU, et al. Shock wave technology and application: an update. Eur Urol. 2011;59(5):784–96.
23. Pace KT, Ghiculete D, Harju M, Honey RJ. University of Toronto Lithotripsy Associates. Shock wave lithotripsy at 60 or 120 shocks per minute: a randomized, double-blind trial. J Urol. 2005;174(2):595–9.
24. Madbouly K, El-Tiraifi AM, Seida M, El-Faqih SR, Atassi R, Talic RF. Slow versus fast shock wave lithotripsy rate for urolithiasis: a prospective randomized study. J Urol. 2005;173(1):127–30.
25. Yilmaz E, Batislam E, Basar M, Tuglu D, Mert C, Basar H. Optimal frequency in extracorporeal shock wave lithotripsy: prospective randomized study. Urology. 2005;66(6):1160–4.
26. Chacko J, Moore M, Sankey N, Chandhoke PS. Does a slower treatment rate impact the efficacy of extracorporeal shock wave lithotripsy for solitary kidney or ureteral stones? J Urol. 2006;175(4):1370–3. discussion 1373–4.
27. Eisenmenger W, Du XX, Tang C, et al. The first clinical results of "wide-focus and low-pressure" ESWL. Ultrasound Med Biol. 2002;28(6):769–74.
28. Semins MJ, Trock BJ, Matlaga BR. The effect of shock wave rate on the outcome of shock wave lithotripsy: a meta-analysis. J Urol. 2008;179(1):194–7. discussion 197.
29. Pishchalnikov YA, McAteer JA, Williams Jr JC. Effect of firing rate on the performance of shock wave lithotriptors. BJU Int. 2008;102(11):1681–6.

Improving Shockwave Lithotripsy Outcomes

13

Margaret S. Pearle, Jodi Antonelli, and Paurush Babbar

Introduction

Shock wave lithotripsy (SWL) has consistently constituted the most commonly utilized procedure for the treatment of upper urinary tract stones. In both the Medicare population and among commercially insured individuals, SWL has comprised approximately 50–55 % of surgical procedures performed for upper tract stones, followed by ureteroscopy (URS) as a close second [1]. The reasons for the popularity of SWL among patients and physicians are readily apparent. SWL is the only noninvasive treatment for urinary tract stones, has low morbidity, is well tolerated by patients, requires relatively little training on the part of the physician and reimburses well [2]. Accordingly, SWL was initially applied widely to upper tract stones until the limitations of the technology became apparent with time and analyses of SWL failures. As the indications for SWL have narrowed, there has been disappointingly little technologic progress in lithotripters to maintain its widespread applicability. On the other hand, there has been a trend towards increased use of URS and reduced use of SWL in contemporary practice that may not be reflected yet in national datasets [3].

Over the last decade, however, a number of advances have been introduced that have improved SWL outcomes without the use of new or improved lithotripters. These advances include refining patient selection to increase the chance of successful treatment, optimizing SWL treatment parameters to enhance stone fragmentation and potentially reduce SWL-induced renal injury, initiation of pharmacologic and mechanical measures to improve stone clearance and medical therapy to reduce post-SWL recurrences. This chapter will review these nontechnologic measures that have been introduced to enhance SWL outcomes.

Refining Patient Selection

The effect of stone size, location, and composition on SWL outcomes have long been recognized. SWL stone-free rates have been shown in many published series with stratified SWL data to vary inversely with stone size: 85 % for <1 cm stones, 71 % for 1–2 cm stones and 59 % for >2 cm stones [4]. Likewise, retreatment and auxiliary procedure rates increase with stone size. Indeed, a meta-analysis by the American Urologic Association Nephrolithiasis Clinical Guideline

M.S. Pearle, M.D., Ph.D. (✉)
Department of Urology, University of Texas Southwestern Medical Center, 5323 Harry Hines Blvd., J8.106, Dallas, TX 75390-9110, USA
e-mail: Margaret.Pearle@UTsouthwestern.edu

J. Antonelli, M.D.
Department of Urology, University of Texas Southwestern Medical Center, 5323 Harry Hines Blvd., J8.106, Dallas, TX 75390-9110, USA

P. Babbar
Department of Urology, Wake Forest School of Medicine, Winston Salem, NC, USA

S.Y. Nakada and M.S. Pearle (eds.), *Surgical Management of Urolithiasis: Percutaneous, Shockwave and Ureteroscopy*, DOI 10.1007/978-1-4614-6937-7_13, © Springer Science+Business Media New York 2013

Panel for Staghorn Calculi found a stone-free rate of only 54 % after a mean of 2.8 primary procedures/patient and a 19 % rate of significant complications, leading the panel to discourage the use of SWL for most patients with staghorn calculi [5].

Stone size also predictably affects stone-free rates for ureteral stones. The EAU/AUA Ureteral Stones Clinical Guidelines Panel performed a meta-analysis of published series for which outcomes for surgical management of ureteral stones were available [6]. For each location in the ureter—proximal, middle and distal—stone-free rates were superior for stones <10 mm in size compared to stones ≥10 mm: 90 % versus 68 % for proximal ureteral stones, 84 % versus 76 % for middle ureteral stones and 86 % versus 74 % for distal ureteral stones, respectively.

Stone location also influences stone-free rates, with lower pole location typically associated with the poorest stone-free rates, likely reflecting the limited clearance of fragments from the dependent lower pole calices. In a meta-analysis of SWL and percutaneous nephrolithotomy (PCNL) series with stone-free rates stratified according to stone location, lower pole stones were associated with a success rate of only 60 % for SWL compared with 90 % for PCNL [7]. Based on these findings, Lingeman led a multicenter randomized trial comparing SWL and PCNL for the management of symptomatic lower pole renal calculi and found an even greater discrepancy in stone-free rates between the two treatment modalities: 37 % for SWL and 95 % for PCNL. When stone-free rates were stratified by stone size, the disparity was magnified for larger stone sizes: 63 % versus 100 % for stones <1 cm, 23 % versus 93 % for 1–2 cm stones and 14 % versus 86 % for >2 cm stones, respectively. A second phase of the Lower Pole Stone Study compared SWL with URS for the management of stones ≤1 cm in size, but used more rigorous criteria for stone-free status by using computed tomography (CT) instead of nephrotomography as was used in the first Lower Pole Stone Study to identify residual stones [8]. Stone-free rates were disappointingly low for both treatment modalities, and despite a 15 % higher stone-free rate for URS (50 %) over SWL (35 %), the differences were not statistically significantly different.

These randomized clinical trials (RCTs) underscore the limitation of SWL in the treatment of lower pole renal calculi and suggest that this modality may be reasonably utilized only for lower pole stones <1 cm in size. As such, although the 2012 European Association of Urology Guidelines on Urolithiasis recommends SWL as first line therapy for <2 cm nonlower pole renal calculi, SWL was included as first line therapy only for lower pole renal calculi <15 mm in size or with favorable anatomic factors [9].

A number of anatomic factors have been suggested to impact the clearance of fragments from the lower pole calices after SWL. Infundibular length, infundibular width, infundibulopelvic angle, spacial anatomy of the lower pole calices, caliceal pelvic height, and infundibular length-to-width ratio have all been investigated for their effect on the clearance of fragments after SWL with conflicting results [10–16]. Although it is likely that some anatomic factors influence SWL stone-free rates, the specific parameters and their critical cut-points remain elusive. Furthermore, the widespread use of CT and limited use of intravenous urography and other contrast studies in the diagnosis of renal calculi make these factors unobtainable and therefore less relevant in current practice.

Stone location also impacts SWL success in the ureter, although the relationship between location and stone-free rate is less consistent. According to a meta-analysis for the EAU/AUA Ureteral Stones Clinical Guidelines, SWL stone-free rates for proximal, middle, and distal ureteral stones were 82 %, 73 % and 74 %, respectively [6]. Despite the shorter distance for fragments to travel from the middle and distal ureter to the bladder, stone-free rates for stones in these locations were lower than for proximal ureteral stones, perhaps because of the greater difficulty localizing the stone and positioning the patient when the stone resides in the middle or distal ureter.

Fragility describes the ease with which a stone fragments with SWL, and fragility varies according to stone composition [17]. Brushite and cysteine stones are the most shockwave-resistant stone compositions, with calcium oxalate monohydrate, struvite, calcium oxalate dihydrate, and uric acid following in descending order [18]. Unfortunately, stone composition is frequently unknown prior to treatment. Consequently, investigators have attempted to predict stone composition based on standard CT characteristics (Hounsfield units), but their efforts have met with limited success because of overlapping values for stones of different composition [19–21]. However, a number of parameters that can be readily measured on standard CT images have recently been investigated for their ability to predict SWL success. Stone density, as measured by CT attenuation coefficient, is thought to act as a surrogate for stone composition and reflects stone fragility. Joseph and coworkers reviewed a group of 30 patients undergoing SWL for 5–20 mm renal calculi and found a strong inverse correlation between CT Hounsfield units (HU) and shock wave number ($r=0.779$) [22]. Additionally, CT HU correlated inversely with SWL success: 100 % success for stones with HU < 500 but only 54.5 % for stones with HU > 1,000. On the other hand, Shah and associates found no difference in stone-free rates for 42 patients with stones of HU < 1,200 and 57 patients with stones of HU > 1,200 (88.1 % vs. 82.5 %, respectively, $p=\text{NS}$) [23]. However patients in the higher HU group had a higher retreatment rate than those in the lower HU group (14 % vs. 0 %, respectively, $p<0.0001$). Gupta and colleagues reviewed a series of 112 patients with 5–20 mm renal calculi treated with SWL and found a linear relationship between HU and number of SWL sessions [24]. Using a cut-point of 750 HU, they showed that stone-free rate was superior for stones with HU ≤ 750 compared with stones with HU > 750 (88 % vs. 65 %, respectively). Although the precise HU cut-point distinguishing success from failure has not been firmly established, there is relative consensus that stones with higher CT attenuation coefficient are less successfully treated with SWL than stones with lower attenuation coefficient.

Although standard single source CT has shown limited success in predicting stone composition, dual energy CT (DECT) holds greater promise in distinguishing among stones of different composition. In a group of 40 patients undergoing (DECT) prior to definitive surgical management of their stones, Manglaviti and colleagues found concordance between DECT and X-ray crystallography in 45 of 49 stones [25]. The stones for which composition was not accurately predicted by DECT were all of mixed composition. Others have used DECT to reliably distinguish uric acid from non-uric acid stones [26]. With further modification of CT parameters including the use of a tin filter and varying the combination of tube voltages, the ability of DECT to distinguish among stones of different compositions will likely be strengthened [27].

Pareek and coworkers introduced another parameter, skin-to-stone distance (SSD), that is easily gleaned from standard CT by averaging the distance from the skin to the stone at 0, 45, and 90° [28]. They reviewed 64 patients with 5–15 mm lower pole stones and divided them into those rendered stone free ($n=30$) and those left with residual fragments ($n=34$). They found a significant difference in mean SSD between the two groups (8.1 cm vs. 11.5 cm, respectively, $p<0.01$) and determined through logistic regression analysis that a SSD of 10 cm distinguished success from failure. Wiesenthal and colleagues also used logistic regression analysis, based on 422 patients who underwent SWL for renal or ureteral calculi, to determine that HU, mean stone density, and SSD were independent predictors of outcome, and the cut-points identified in their analysis revealed that HU>900 (OR 0.49, 95 % CI 0.32–0.75, $p>0.01$) and SSD > 11 cm (OR 0.49, 95 % CI 0.31–0.78, $p<0.01$) best predicted SWL failure. Although some authors have corroborated the importance of SSD in predicting SWL success [29], the validity of this parameter has not been uniformly embraced [30–32].

To facilitate treatment selection for a patient with a renal or ureteral calculus, several investigators have incorporated a variety of clinical parameters to construct nomograms that predict SWL success in a given clinical scenario. Using logistic regression analysis, Ng and coworkers determined that stone volume and mean stone density were independent predictors of SWL outcomes while SSD showed only a marginal effect [33]. After constructing ROC curves, they determined that the optimum cut-points for each parameter were stone volume 0.2 cm^3, mean stone density 593 HU and SSD 9.2 cm. Incorporating these three factors with equal weighting they developed a scoring system by which 1 point was assigned for each positive factor (stone volume $\leq$0.2 cm^3, mean stone density $\leq$593 HU, SSD$\leq$9.2 cm). A score of 2 or more was associated with an SWL success rate of 77 %.

Kanao and coworkers were the first to develop a nomogram that incorporated stone length, location, and number—parameters that were shown on multivariate analysis to be independent predictors of stone-free status—to predict stone-free rate 3 months after SWL for both single and multiple stones [34]. According to their nomogram for solitary calculi, the poorest stone-free rate is obtained with caliceal stones $\geq$21 mm in diameter (23 %) while the highest stone-free rate is achieved with proximal ureteral stones $\leq$5 mm in diameter (94 %).

Kacker and associates utilized the Kanao nomogram and incorporated average stone attenuation into the calculation as they determined that is the best independent predictor of SWL success [35]. They then created a table that reported the average HU cut-points required to reach levels of success (stone-free status) from 60 to 80 % for stones <6, 6–10, and 11–15 mm using the stone-free probabilities derived from Kanao et al. [34]. According to their nomogram, for example, in order for a 6–10 mm proximal ureteral stone to be treated with an 80 % success rate, the average HU density must be less than 480; in order for the same stone to achieve a 60 % success rate, the average HU density only has to be less than 1,000.

Finally, Wiesenthal and colleagues determined that age, stone area, and SSD for renal calculi and body mass index (BMI) and stone size for ureteral calculi constituted the independent predictors of SWL success according to multivariate analysis [36].

For renal calculi they derived a mathematical equation predicting successful SWL as follows:

$$
\begin{aligned}
a = \exp[3.7432 \\
&+(1.0409)(\text{if age is between } 44-53, \text{value} = 1, \text{otherwise value} = 0) \\
&+(-0.1698)(\text{if age is between } 54-62, \text{value} = 1, \text{otherwise value} = 0) \\
&+(-0.6083)(\text{if age} > 62, \text{value} = 1, \text{otherwise value} = 0) \\
&+(-0.00703)(\text{add stone area in mm}^2) \\
&+(-0.0175)(\text{add skin-to-stone distance in mm})]
\end{aligned}
$$

Then predicted probability $= a/(1+a)$

For ureteral calculi their proposed mathematical equation predicting successful SWL is:

$$
\begin{aligned}
a = \exp\ [5.5597 \\
&+(-0.0925)(\text{BMI}) \\
&+(-1.0191)(\text{if stone area} > 45\text{mm}^2, \\
&\text{then value} = 1, \text{otherwise value} = 0)]
\end{aligned}
$$

Then predicted probability $= a/(1+a)$

These nomograms are constructed using data derived from the authors' own institutions using a particular lithotripter and therefore may not be completely generalizable. However, it is evident that a number of parameters influence the success of SWL (Table 13.1), and these nomograms represent an attempt to provide a means with which to select subgroups of patients who are not likely to be successfully treated with SWL and for whom endoscopy may represent a better first-line option.

Table 13.1 Literature review of predictors of successful SWL outcome

Author	*N*	Location	Lithotriptor	Stone volume (cc)	Mean stone attenuation (HU)	Skin-to-stone distance (cm)	Other
Joseph[a] [22]	30	Renal	Lithostar Multiline	–	Yes (<1,000, $p<0.01$)	–	Median number shocks ($p<0.001$)
Pareek [28]	64	Lower calix	Doli S	–	No	Yes (10.0, $p<0.01$)	–
Gupta [24]	112	Renal and proximal ureter	Lithostar SW System C	No	Yes (≤750[b])	–	–
Yoshida [102]	62	Renal and proximal ureter	Lithostar	No	No	No	HE ($p=0.0073$)
Perks [103]	76	Renal and ureter	Doli S	No	Yes ($p=0.01$)	–	–
El-Nahas [31]	120	Renal	Doli S	–	Yes (≤1,000, $p=0.018$)	–	BMI ($p=0.039$)
Weld [30]	200	Renal	Doli S	Yes ($p=0.04$)	Yes ($p=0.02$)	No	Location ($p<0.01$)
Perks [104]	111	Renal	Lithotron Ultra	No	Yes ($p<0.01$)	Yes ($p=0.01$)	–
Kacker[b] [35]	325	Renal and ureter	Lithotron		Yes (<500, OR = 5.88)	–	–
Jacobs [32]	85	Renal and ureter	Dornier HM3	–	–	No	–
Bandi[b] [105]	94	Renal and ureter	DoliS	Yes (<5, $p<0.001$)	Yes	No	–
Ng [33]	94	Proximal ureter	Sonolith 4000+	Yes (0.2, $p=0.01$)	Yes (593 $p=0.038$)	Yes (9.2, $p=0.026$)	–
Patel [29]	83	Renal	DoLi 50	No	No	Yes ($p=0.001$)	–
Wiesenthal [106]	422	Renal and ureteral	Lithotron Ultra	No	Yes (<900, $p<0.01$)	Yes (>1.10, $p<0.01$)	–
Park [107]	115	Renal	Compact Delta	Yes <8.5	Yes <863	Yes <1.2	–
Park [108]	573	Renal	Sonolith	No	No	Yes ($p=0.009$)	–
Graversen [109]	52	NR	Dornier U/15/50	No	–	–	BMI ($p=0.026$) FMP<35 % ($p=0.010$)

SSD skin-to-stone distance, *BMI* body mass index, *HE* hump existence, *FMP* fat mass percentage, *NR* not reported
[a]Calculus >750 HU had an OR 10.5 for needing three or more SWL procedures to achieve successful outcome
[b]Univariate analysis only

Preoperative Measures to Reduce Risk

Antibiotics

The routine use of prophylactic antibiotics to reduce the incidence of post-SWL urinary tract infections (UTIs) has been widely debated in the literature. The American Urologic Association (AUA) 2008 Best Practice Statement on Antibiotic Prophylaxis [37] cites level 1A evidence in support of the use of routine antibiotic prophylaxis for SWL based on a meta-analysis showing lower post-SWL urinary tract infections in the arm receiving antibiotics compared with a placebo or no-treatment control arm (2.1 % vs. 5.7 %, respectively) [38]. On the other hand, the EUA in their 2010 Guidelines on Urologic Infections did not recommend universal antibiotic prophylaxis for SWL, citing level 1A/1B evidence showing contradictory findings or no advantage to antibiotic treatment except in the setting of indwelling stents, catheters, and/or nephrostomy tubes or in patients with known or suspected infection stones [39].

A recent systematic review and meta-analysis by Lu et al. based on nine RCTs demonstrated no statistically significant difference in post-SWL UTIs in patient with negative preoperative urine cultures between the treatment group and control group with respect to fever (RR=0.36, 95 % CI 0.07–2.36, $p=0.31$), rate of positive urine cultures (RR=0.77, 95 % CI 0.54–1.11, $p=0.17$) and incidence of clinical UTIs (RR=0.54, 95 % CI 0.29–1.01, $p=0.05$) [40]. Only two of the studies reviewed in the analysis addressed UTI in the setting of SWL with indwelling ureteral catheters and they showed no significant difference in post-SWL UTIs (none of 15 in the prophylaxis group versus 1 in 12 control cases, $p>0.05$). The authors concluded that the routine use of prophylactic antibiotics prior to SWL has little benefit except in patients with known risk factors for infection and that additional concern for antibiotic resistance and cost argue against the routine use of antibiotic prophylaxis in this setting.

As a result of conflicting recommendations regarding antibiotic prophylaxis in patients with sterile urine prior to SWL, the decision to treat and the specific regimen utilized are at this time left to the discretion of the practitioner. However, the use of antibiotics prior to SWL in high-risk patients is not in question and this patient population is not addressed in these meta-analyses. Ultimately, large, randomized, placebo-controlled trials are needed to further delineate the role of antibiotic prophylaxis in low-risk patients.

Antioxidants and Calcium Channel Blockers

Animal data have demonstrated that SWL treatment is associated with histologic evidence of renal vascular and tubular damage [41] as well as physiologic evidence of reduction in glomerular filtration rate and renal plasma flow [42]. Although it was initially thought that these insults originated from the direct effect of shockwave energy [43], oxygen free radicals have been implicated as another potential mediator of these deleterious effects. One theory postulates that shock waves cause renal capillary disruption and subsequent tissue edema, leading to ischemia and hypoxia [44]. In this ischemia-reperfusion injury model the metabolic alterations caused by reperfusion after ischemia lead to abnormally high levels of free radicals, which cause kidney damage through lipid peroxidation and disruption of cellular membranes.

Allopurinol, an inhibitor of xanthine oxidase and a potent free radical scavenger, was shown to reduce levels of conjugated dienes, an indicator of lipid peroxidation, when given prior to SWL in a porcine model [45]. Citrate and vitamin E, two other free radical scavengers, also resulted in significantly less pronounced increases in 8-isoprostane, a marker of free radical formation, in Madin-Darby canine kidney (MDCK) cells compared to cells not pretreated with either medication [46].

Verapamil and nifedipine have been proposed as agents that can alleviate the deleterious effects of SWL on renal vasculature. In an animal model, Yaman and coworkers found minimal MRI findings and less severe histopathologic changes in the kidneys of rabbits pretreated with verapamil prior to SWL compared to control rabbits undergoing SWL without pretreatment [47].

Clinical trials evaluating the protective effect of antioxidants or calcium channel blockers, however, are few. Strohmaier and colleagues randomized 24 patients undergoing SWL to verapamil or no treatment and evaluated post-SWL urinary markers of tubular function [48]. They detected smaller increases in alpha 1-microglobulin and *N*-acetyl-beta-glucosaminidase and a smaller decrease in Tamm Horsfall protein in the verapamil-treated patients than in the untreated controls, suggesting a protective effect of verapamil against SWL-induced renal tubular dysfunction. Li and coworkers randomized 40 patients scheduled to undergo SWL to one of four groups: no medication, nifedipine-only, allopurinol-only or nifedipine plus allopurinol, in which the medications were started the night before SWL and continued for 3 days post-procedure. Urine samples collected at baseline and 1 and 3 days after SWL were assayed for markers of renal tubular function: albumin, β2-microglobulin, and Tamm-Horsfall protein. Levels of albumin and β2-microglobulin increased ($p<0.001$) and Tamm-Horsfall protein decreased ($p<0.01$) after SWL in the control group, while the two nifepine groups showed no statistically significant change in any of the three urine markers before and after SWL. Although β2-microglobulin and albumin were higher after SWL compared to baseline in the allopurinol-only group, albumin and Tamm-Horsfall protein were significantly different post-SWL compared to the unmedicated group. This study suggests that nifedipine, and to a lesser extent allopurinol, may protect against SWL-induced renal injury [49].

Despite the potential protective effects of antioxidants and calcium channel blockers, however, the benefit of periprocedural use of these agents in association with SWL has never been truly validated in clinical trials and has not been adopted into widespread practice.

Optimizing Treatment

Patient Positioning

The optimal patient position for SWL treatment of ureteral calculi has been debated. Positioning of patients with stones in the middle and distal ureter are of particular concern because of the potential attenuation of shock wave energy as it travels through the bony pelvis [50–52]. Zomorrodi reviewed 68 patients undergoing SWL for proximal ureteral calculi (mean stone size 12 mm) in either the supine ($n=35$) or prone ($n=38$) position and found comparable stone-free rates (82 % and 83 %, respectively) and total number of SWL sessions (1.9 for each) in the two groups [53]. It is likely that the lack of difference between the two groups is because the advantage afforded to prone positioning might be less applicable to proximal ureteral stones that lie outside the bony pelvis.

Hara and colleagues compared the efficacy of different patient positions for SWL treatment of patients with ureteral stones [54]. Patients with proximal ureteral stones were treated with SWL in the supine ($n=246$) or supine-rotated ($n=156$) position, where the rotated position was defined as 30° from flat, maintained by a bump. Although stone-free rates for patients with proximal ureteral stones treated in the rotated and nonrotated position were comparable (95 % and 97 %, respectively), fewer secondary procedures were required for the supine-rotated compared to the supine group to become stone free (mean 1.49 vs. 1.74, respectively, $p=0.023$). Patients with middle and primary distal ureteral stones were also treated in the prone or prone rotated positions (62 prone and 60 prone-rotated in the middle ureter and 110 prone and 98 prone-rotated in the distal ureter). Stone-free rates in both locations were higher for patients in the prone-rotated than in the prone position (95 % vs. 84 %, respectively, $p=0.046$, for middle ureter and 98 % vs. 89 %, respectively, $p=0.011$, for distal ureter).

Anesthesia

With the introduction of smaller focal zone lithotripters which are associated with less pain than the original Dornier HM3 lithotripter, general anesthesia was largely replaced by regional anesthesia, including epidural [55, 56], spinal [57], and flank infiltration with or without intercostal nerve block [58], or by monitored anesthesia care (MAC) [59–61].

Patient-controlled sedation (PCS) is a form of monitored anesthesia that allows the patient to administer his/her own amount of anesthesia/analgesia so that the ideal level of pain/anxiety control can be reached without the risk of oversedation. PCS using alfentanil for SWL has been met with good clinical results [49, 62] and high patient satisfaction [63, 64]. Combining propofol with PCS was proposed as a way to potentially increase sedation, improve analgesia, and prophylax against nausea. Joo and coworkers used remifentanil, which has a shorter half-life than alfentanil, for PCS and combined it with propofol. In a group of 120 patients undergoing SWL who were randomized to remifentanil or remifentanil-propofol PCS, the addition of propofol was associated with decreased remifentanil use (24 doses vs. 15 doses with propofol, $p<0.001$) and less reported postoperative nausea (27 % vs. 8 % with propofol, $p=0.016$). The average time to hospital discharge was comparable in both groups at 67 min (remifentanil) and 64 min (remifentanil-propofol) [65].

Despite the trend away from general anesthesia, there is evidence to suggest that some newer generation lithotripters yield better outcomes with general anesthesia as it allows for better control of patient movement and more accurate targeting of the stone. Zommick and associates reviewed 145 patients with upper urinary tract calculi who underwent SWL with the Dornier HM3 lithotripter, among whom 49 received general anesthesia and 96 were treated with intravenous sedation and pretreatment analgesia [66]. Although there was no difference in success rates (stone free or ≤3 mm residual fragments at 3 months by plain radiograph or intravenous urogram) between the two groups (93 % vs. 83 %, respectively), intravenous sedation was associated with increased fluoroscopy time compared to general anesthesia (1 min vs. 0.5 min, respectively), presumably because of greater patient movement and need for repositioning with sedation.

With smaller focal zone lithotripters, patient movement results in more time spent with the stone out of the small focal zone, and potentially poorer stone fragmentation. Sorensen and associates reported lower 3-month stone-free rates (by KUB) in patients undergoing SWL for solitary <20 mm renal or proximal ureteral calculi using a Doli 50 lithotripter with general anesthesia compared to intravenous sedation (87 % vs. 55 % respectively, $p<0.001$) [67]. Lee and colleagues performed a case control study of 660 patients treated with the Medstone STS lithotripter (Aliso Viejo, CA) under MAC ($n=330$) or general anesthesia ($n=330$) in which patients were matched for stone size, stone location, and BMI [68]. Stone-free rates were higher in patients undergoing general anesthesia compared to those treated with MAC (67 % vs. 55 %, respectively, $p<0.04$). The superiority of general anesthesia over MAC was even more pronounced for the subgroup of patients with large stones (11–20 mm, 76 % vs. 48 %, respectively, $p=0.01$) and those with upper pole stones (75 % vs. 27 %, respectively, $p=0.05$).

Coupling

It is essential that the treatment head be optimally coupled to the patient to provide for efficient transmission of shock waves from the shock wave generator to the stone without loss of energy. The presence of air pockets in the coupling gel has been shown in experimental conditions to reduce shock wave amplitude by a mean of 20 % and to decrease stone breakage [69]. Furthermore, breaking and reestablishing contact, as commonly occurs with patient repositioning or movement during treatment, was associated with a 57 % reduction in acoustic energy transmission. Application of the acoustic gel onto the treatment head in a mound, delivered from a wide-mouthed jug rather than a squeeze bottle, and allowing the gel to spread by patient contact rather than by hand lessens the chance of creating of air pockets [70].

Shock Wave Delivery

Pattern of Shock Wave Administration

The pattern of shock wave delivery has been shown in vitro and in animal models to impact the efficiency of fragmentation as well as the degree of injury to the kidney. Using a fixed rate and number of shock waves, Zhou and associates demonstrated superior fragmentation of gypsum stones using a pattern of incrementally increasing shock wave voltage compared with a pattern of either decreasing or constant voltage despite delivering equivalent total energy [71]. Maloney and coworkers subsequently confirmed improved stone fragmentation with a pattern of increasing voltage in a porcine model [72]. The benefit of initial low-voltage shock wave delivery was thought to be due to a potentiation of the effect of the subsequent high-energy shock waves.

Low energy shock wave priming was also found in animal models to reduce renal damage. In a porcine model, delivery of as few as 100 shocks at 12 kV prior to shock wave escalation was shown to reduce functional renal volume (FRV) from 6 to 0.3 % [73]. Further study suggested that low-energy shock waves followed by a brief rest period (3–4 min) may be even more important in reducing renal injury [74].

Clinical studies validating the concept of low-voltage shock wave priming prior to voltage escalation have yielded conflicting results. Demirci and colleagues randomized 50 patients with <2 cm renal or ureteral calculi to a pattern of either fixed shock wave voltage (3,000 shocks at 13 kV) or incrementally increasing voltage (3,000 shocks from 11 to 13 kV) [75]. Superior success (96 % vs. 72 %, respectively, $p<0.05$) and stone-free rates (80 % vs. 60 %, respectively, $p<0.03$) were observed in the group receiving increasing shock wave voltage compared to the control group. Lambert and coworkers also randomized 45 patients with <2 cm renal calculi to receive 2,500 total shocks at either constant (13 kV) or increasing voltage (14–18 kV) and demonstrated higher success rates in the latter group (48 % vs. 81 %, respectively, $p<0.03$) [76]. Furthermore they found evidence of less renal damage, as indicated by markers of renal tubular function β2-microglobin and microalbumin, in the increasing voltage group.

In contrast, Honey and associates found a higher success rate at 3 months in patients undergoing SWL with immediate escalation of voltage (from 14 to 23 kV) than in those undergoing a single stepwise increase in voltage (1,500 shocks at 15 kV, then a quick increase to 23 kV) (73 % vs. 55 %, respectively, $p=02$), suggesting that delayed voltage escalation does not improve stone fragmentation [77]. Consequently, although there is some evidence that a strategy of voltage escalation improves SWL success rates, the exact pattern of voltage escalation has not been established.

Shock Wave Rate

The rate of shock wave delivery has also been shown to influence SWL stone-free rates. Based on in vitro [78] and animal data [79] showing superior stone-free rates with a shock wave rate of 30 shocks/min over 120 shocks/min, Honey and colleagues reported the first randomized clinical trial that compared a shock wave rate of 60 shocks/min ($n=77$) with 120 shocks/min ($n=86$) [80]. Success rates at 3 months were superior for the group treated at the slower rare compared to the group treated at the faster rate (74.5 % vs. 60.6 %, $p=0.039$). Likewise, the auxiliary procedure rate was lower in the 60 shocks/min group compared to the 120 shocks/min group (30 % vs 45 %, $p=0.031$). Interestingly, when outcomes were stratified by stone size, slow shock wave rate showed a significant advantage only in patients with large stones (>100 mm^2, 71 % vs. 32 %, respectively, $p=0.002$). Since this initial trial, three other RCTs [81–83] have likewise compared slow with fast shock wave rate, with only one [81] of the three showing no advantage to faster shock wave rate. Semins and colleagues performed a meta-analysis evaluating shock wave rate on SWL outcomes using these four RTCs and determined that patients treated at 60 shocks/min had a 10.2 % higher likelihood of a successful outcome than patients treated at a rate of 120 shocks/min (95 % CI 3.7–16.8, $p=0.002$) [84]. Consequently, although treating at slower shock wave rate necessitates longer treatment times, there is strong (level 1A) evidence to support the practice.

Adjuvant Measures to Enhance Fragment Clearance

Mechanical Maneuvers

The limited success of SWL in the treatment of lower pole renal calculi has been attributed to impaired clearance of fragments from the dependent lower pole calices. As such, a number of investigators have described the use post-SWL mechanical maneuvers to promote clearance of fragments from the lower pole calices. Irrigation through a retrograde-directed catheter [85] or a lower pole nephrostomy tube [86] during SWL has been found to promote movement of fragments out of the lower pole calices. Kosar and colleagues reported superior stone-free rates for 51 patients with lower pole stones in whom vibration massage was performed daily for 14 days post-SWL ($n=51$) compared with 52 untreated control patients (80 % vs. 60 %, respectively, $p=0.003$) [87]. Brownlee and colleagues first described the use of percussion, inversion, and hydration therapy in a small group of patients to facilitate fragment clearance from the lower pole calices after SWL [88]. This regimen was tested in a randomized trial of 69 patients with ≤4 mm residual lower pole fragments 3 months after SWL, comparing observation with a regimen of diuresis (20 mg furosemide), 60° inversion, and mechanical chest percussion [89]. Complete fragment clearance was demonstrated in 40 % of the treatment group but in only 3 % of the control group. Chiong and colleagues performed a similar randomized trial in 108 patients with <2 cm lower pole stones but initiated the treatment regimen immediately after SWL instead of 3 months later [90]. At 3-month follow-up, 63 % of the treatment group versus 35 % of the control group demonstrated complete stone clearance ($p=0.006$). These studies provide level 1 evidence in support of adjuvant mechanical measures to enhance the clearance of fragments from the lower pole calices after SWL.

Pharmacologic Measures

Based on the success of pharmacologic agents in promoting the spontaneous passage of ureteral calculi [91], a number of medications have been tested for their efficacy in improving stone-free rates after SWL (Table 13.2). Schuler and colleagues performed a meta-analysis of four RCTs comprising 418 patients treated with SWL who received either medical therapy with tamsulosin (two trials), nifedipine (one trial), or Phyllanthus niruri (one trial) versus placebo or no treatment [92]. Combining the active treatment arms of the RCTs ($n=212$), medical therapy was associated with a 17 % higher stone-free rate than placebo or no treatment ($n=206$) (95 % CI 9–24 %).

Both tamsulosin and nifedipine, which have demonstrated efficacy as medical expulsive agents for ureteral stones, have been evaluated for their efficacy in promoting the clearance of fragments after SWL of renal and/or ureteral calculi. Gravina and coworkers randomized 130 patients with nonlower pole renal calculi undergoing SWL to received either tamsulosin (0.4 mg) plus methylprednisolone or methylprednisolone alone [93]. Stone-free rates at 3 months were superior and analgesic use was significantly lower for the treatment group compared with the control group (78.5 % and 375 mg vs. 60 % and 975 mg, respectively, $p=0.037$ and $p<0.001$, respectively). When stone-free rates were stratified by stone size, the difference was insignificant for stones 4–10 mm in size (75 % vs. 68 %), but strongly favored the treatment group for stones 11–20 mm (88 % vs. 55 %, $p=0.028$). On the other hand, no difference in stone-free rates or time to stone expulsion was seen in 61 patients with ≥6 mm distal ureteral stones randomized to tamsulosin ($n=31$) or no treatment ($n=30$), although analgesic use was significantly lower in the treatment group (57 mg vs. 119 mg diclofenac, respectively, $p=0.02$) [94]. Nifidepine, however, was shown to have benefit with regard to improved stone-free rates (75 % vs. 50 %, $p=0.02$) and lower analgesic use (37.5 mg vs. 86.25 mg diclofenac, $p=0.02$) in a

Table 13.2 Summary of randomized controlled trials evaluating pharmacologic adjuncts to shockwave lithotripsy

Author	No. study/Con	Therapy study/control	Stone location	Lithotripter	Imaging modality	Follow-up	Study stone free (%)	Control stone free (%)	Passage time study/con (days)	Analgesic usage study/con
Kobayashi [110]	38/34	T 0.2 mg/NT	Ureteral	Dornier	KUB + US	28 days	32/38 (84.2)	30/34 (88.2)	15.7/35.5[a]	NR
Bhagat [111]	30/30	T 0.4 mg/P	Renal or ureteral	Dornier Compact S	Fluoro + KUB	1 mo	28/30[a] (96.6)	23/30 (79.3)	NR	1 dose/2 doses
Gravina [93]	65/65	T 0.4 mg/NT	Renal	Sonolith 4000+	US + KUB ± IVP	12 wks	51/65[a] (78.5)	39/65 (60.0)	NR	375 mg/675mg[a]
Gravas [94]	30/31	T 0.4 mg/NT	Ureteral	Dornier S II	KUB + US	1 mo	19/30 (63.3)	16/31 (51.6)	12.9/13.2	118.9 mg/56.9mg[a]
Küpeli [112]	24/24	T 0.4 mg/NT	Ureteral	Siemens Lithostar+	KUB, IVU, CT, ±US	15 days	17/24 (70.8)[a]	8/24 (33.3)	NR	NR
Naja [113]	51/65	T 0.4 mg/NT	Renal	Lithostar Multiline	KUB ± US	3 mo	48/51 (94.1)	55/65 (84.6)	35.5/47.2[a]	VAS 26.7/47.3[a]
Wang [114]	40/40	T 0.4 mg/NT	Ureteral	NR	KUB ± US	2 wks	31/40 (77.5)[a]	18/40 (45.0)	NR	5 %/20 % used analgesics[a]
Hussein [115]	67/69	T 0.4 mg/NT	Renal	Lithostar Multiline	KUB + US	3 mo	49/67 (73)[a]	38/69 (55.0)	NR	14 doses/32 doses[a]
Falahatkar [116]	70/71	T 0.4 mg/P	Renal or Ureteral	Storz	KUB + US	12 wks	50/70 (71.4)	43/71 (60.6)	10–20/20–30[a]	NR
Agarwal [117]	20/20	T 0.4 mg/NT	Ureteral	Lithostar Multiline	KUB + US	3 mo	11/20 (55)[a]	5/20 (25)	30.7/39.0	VAS 25.3–38.3
Moursy[c] [118]	44/44	T 0.4 mg/NT	Ureteral	Siemens Lithostar+	KUB + US	28 days	32/44 (72.7)[a]	25/44 (56.8)	12.7/15.1	4.39/6.11
Georgiev [119]	99/87	T 0.4 mg/NT	Renal or ureteral	NR	KUB + US, ±IVU, CT	12 wks	90/99 (91.3)[a]	65/87 (74.6)	39/71[a]	NR
Porpiglia [95]	40/40	N 30 mg/NT	Ureteral	Sonolith 4000+	KUB + US	45 days	30/40 (75)[a]	20/40 (50.0)	NR	37.6 mg/86.25mg[a]
Micali [120]	28/21	T 0.4 mg or N 30 mg/NT	Ureteral	Dornier S	KUB, US, ±IVU	60 days	T 23/28[a] N 30/35[a]	27/50	NR	NR
Vicentini [121]	38, 35/38	T 0.4 mg or N 20 mg/P	Renal	Dornier Compact Delta	US	30 days	T 23/38 N 17/35[d]	14/38	15.3/16.7/15.9	2, 3/1.5 doses
Soygür[b] [96]	46/44	PC 60 mEq/NP	Renal	Dornier MPL 9000	KUB + US	12 mo	46/46 (100)[a]	26/44 (60.0)	NR	NR
Arrabal-Martín[b] [97]	50/50	HCTZ 50 mg/P	NR	NR	US	36 mo	36/50 (72)[a]	18/50 (36.0)	NR	NR
Total							T 78 % N 70 % PC 100 % HCTZ 72 %	59 %		

Study study group, *Control and con* control group, *MET* mean expulsion time, *NT* no treatment, *P* placebo, *NR* not reported, *T* tamsulosin, *N* nifedipine, *PC* potassium citrate, *HCTZ* hydrochlorothiazide, *KUB* kidneys/ureter/bladder plain radiography, *US* ultrasonography, *IVU* intravenous urography, *CT* computed tomography, *mo* months, *wks* weeks, *VAS* visual analog scale

[a]Statistical significance ($p \leq 0.05$)

[b]Studies that assessed pharmacologic agents that alter urinary levels of stone-forming elements

[c]Study population included only post-SWL patients with steinstrasse

[d]Stratified according to stone size (5–9 and 10–20 mm), a significant difference in success rate was observed for 10–20-mm stones: tamsulosin 61.9 %, nifedipine 60 %, and placebo 26.1 %, ($p = 0.02$)

group of 60 patients with ureteral calculi randomized to nifedipine plus deflazacort compared to an untreated control group [95].

Several agents that influence urine composition have been shown to enhance stone-free rates after SWL. Soygür and associates evaluated the effect of potassium citrate therapy (20 mEq twice daily) on stone recurrence and stone clearance in 110 patients with lower pole stones started on medication or receiving no additional treatment 4 weeks post-SWL and assessed 1 year later [96]. Among 56 patients rendered stone free, none of the treatment group and 28 % of the control group developed new stones ($p<0.05$). Among 34 patients left with residual fragments, 44.5 % of the treated patients versus 12.5 % of control patients showed resolution of their stones ($p<0.05$). Likewise, hydrochlorothiazide 50 mg daily was shown to be superior to placebo in enhancing the clearance of residual fragments over 36 months in a randomized trial of 100 patients with residual fragments 3 months after SWL [97]. "Global expulsion of fragments" occurred in 72 % of the thiazide patients compared with 36 % of the control patients ($p=0.001$), although the analysis was complicated by retreatment with SWL in 18 % of the former patients and 42 % of the latter. The mechanism by which thiazides and potassium citrate enhance fragment passage is not clear and may be independent of their mechanism for stone prevention.

Medical Therapy to Reduce the Impact of Residual Fragments

Because SWL relies on spontaneous passage of fragments after treatment, this modality may be associated with higher rates of residual fragments than therapies involving manual retrieval or aspiration of fragments, potentially leaving a nidus for further stone growth. Because these fragments are frequently small and asymptomatic, they are often left untreated, although natural history studies show a 21–49 % chance of becoming symptomatic within 2–4 years of treatment [98–100]. The initiation of medical therapy may change the natural history of these residual fragments and reduce the likelihood of stone progression. Fine and colleagues reviewed 80 patients at a mean of 43 months post SWL and separated them into those rendered stone free and those left with residual fragments, then further identified those treated with medical therapy and those who were not [101]. For both patients rendered stone free ($n=31$) and those left with residual fragments ($n=49$), stone recurrence rates were lower among those on medical therapy compared with those not treated medically: 0.09 stones/patient/year versus 0.67 stones/patient/year in the stone-free group, respectively, and 0.47 stones/patient/year versus 3.09 stones/patient/year in the residual fragment group, respectively. These findings suggest that medical therapy can reduce stone growth, even in high-risk patients with residual fragments.

Conclusions

Despite relatively little progress in lithotripter technology, improvements in SWL outcomes may be realized through refinement in patient selection, optimization of treatment parameters, use of adjuvant mechanical and pharmacological measures and initiation of post-SWL directed medical therapy. In doing so, selected patients with a high likelihood of success may be treated in a way that maximizes stone fragmentation and clearance and reduces the impact of residual fragments on the chance of stone recurrence.

References

1. Pearle MS, Calhoun EA, Curhan GC. Urologic Diseases of America Project. Urologic diseases in America project: urolithiasis. J Urol. 2005;173(3): 848–57.
2. Lotan Y, Cadeddu JA, Pearle MS. International comparison of cost effectiveness of medical management strategies for nephrolithiasis. Urol Res. 2005;33(3): 223–30.
3. Matlaga BR. America Board of Urology. Contemporary surgical management of upper urinary tract calculi. J Urol. 2009;181(5):2152–6.
4. Ogan K, Pearle MS. Shock wave lithotripsy for urinary stones and non-calculus applications. In: Moore

RG, Bischoff JT, Loening S, Docimo SG, editors. Minimally invasive urologic surgery. London: Taylor and Francis; 2005. p. 614–55.

5. Preminger GM, Assimos DG, Lingeman JE, Nakada SY, Pearle MS, Wolf JS Jr. Chapter 1: AUA guideline on management of staghorn calculi: diagnosis and treatment recommendations. J Urol. 2005; 173(6):1991–2000.
6. Preminger GM, Tiselius HG, Assimos DG, Alken P, Buck C, Gallucci M, et al. 2007 guideline for the management of ureteral calculi. J Urol. 2007;178(6):2418–34.
7. Lingeman JE, Siegel YI, Steele B, Nyhuis AW, Woods JR. Management of lower pole nephrolithiasis: a critical analysis. J Urol. 1994;151(3):663–7.
8. Pearle MS, Lingeman JE, Leveillee R, Kuo R, Preminger GM, Nadler RB, et al. Prospective, randomized trial comparing shock wave lithotripsy and ureteroscopy for lower pole caliceal calculi 1 cm or less. J Urol. 2005;173(6):2005–9.
9. Türk C, Knoll T, Petrik A, Sarica K, Straub M, Seitz C. Guidelines on urolithiasis. European Association of Urology. 2011;1–104. Available from: http://www.uroweb.org/gls/pdf/18_Urolithiasis.pdf
10. Tuckey J, Devasia A, Murthy L, Ramsden P, Thomas D. Is there a simpler method for predicting lower pole stone clearance after shockwave lithotripsy than measuring infundibulopelvic angle? J Endourol. 2000;14(6):475–8.
11. Elbahnasy AM, Clayman RV, Shalhav AL, Hoenig DM, Chandhoke P, Lingeman JE, et al. Lower-pole caliceal stone clearance after shockwave lithotripsy, percutaneous nephrolithotomy, and flexible ureteroscopy: impact of radiographic spatial anatomy. J Endourol. 1998;12(2):113–9.
12. Gupta NP, Singh DV, Hemal AK, Mandal S. Infundibulopelvic anatomy and clearance of inferior caliceal calculi with shock wave lithotripsy. J Urol. 2000;163(1):24–7.
13. Keeley Jr FX, Moussa SA, Smith G, Tolley DA. Clearance of lower-pole stones following shock wave lithotripsy: effect of the infundibulopelvic angle. Eur Urol. 1999;36(5):371–5.
14. Madbouly K, Sheir KZ, Elsobky E. Impact of lower pole renal anatomy on stone clearance after shock wave lithotripsy: fact or fiction? J Urol. 2001;165(5):1415–8.
15. Sahinkanat T, Ekerbicer H, Onal B, Tansu N, Resim S, Citgez S, et al. Evaluation of the effects of relationships between main spatial lower pole calyceal anatomic factors on the success of shock-wave lithotripsy in patients with lower pole kidney stones. Urology. 2008;71(5):801–5.
16. Sumino Y, Mimata H, Tasaki Y, Ohno H, Hoshino T, Nomura T, et al. Predictors of lower pole renal stone clearance after extracorporeal shock wave lithotripsy. J Urol. 2002;168(4 Pt 1):1344–7.
17. Dretler SP. Stone fragility–a new therapeutic distinction. J Urol. 1988;139(5):1124–7.
18. Saw KC, Lingeman JE. Lesson 20 - management of calyceal calculi. AUA Update Series. 1999;20: 154–9.
19. Nakada SY, Hoff DG, Attai S, Heisey D, Blankenbaker D, Pozniak M. Determination of stone composition by noncontrast spiral computed tomography in the clinical setting. Urology. 2000;55(6):816–9.
20. Mostafavi MR, Ernst RD, Saltzman B. Accurate determination of chemical composition of urinary calculi by spiral computerized tomography. J Urol. 1998;159(3):673–5.
21. Saw KC, McAteer JA, Monga AG, Chua GT, Lingeman JE, Williams Jr JC. Helical CT of urinary calculi: effect of stone composition, stone size, and scan collimation. AJR Am J Roentgenol. 2000; 175(2):329–32.
22. Joseph P, Mandal AK, Singh SK, Mandal P, Sankhwar SN, Sharma SK. Computerized tomography attenuation value of renal calculus: can it predict successful fragmentation of the calculus by extracorporeal shock wave lithotripsy? A preliminary study. J Urol. 2002;167(5):1968–71.
23. Shah K, Kurien A, Mishra S, Ganpule A, Muthu V, Sabnis RB, et al. Predicting effectiveness of extracorporeal shockwave lithotripsy by stone attenuation value. J Endourol. 2010;24(7):1169–73.
24. Gupta NP, Ansari MS, Kesarvani P, Kapoor A, Mukhopadhyay S. Role of computed tomography with no contrast medium enhancement in predicting the outcome of extracorporeal shock wave lithotripsy for urinary calculi. BJU Int. 2005;95(9): 1285–8.
25. Manglaviti G, Tresoldi S, Guerrer CS, Di Leo G, Montanari E, Sardanelli F, et al. In vivo evaluation of the chemical composition of urinary stones using dual-energy CT. AJR Am J Roentgenol. 2011;197(1):W76–83.
26. Stolzmann P, Kozomara M, Chuck N, Muntener M, Leschka S, Scheffel H, et al. In vivo identification of uric acid stones with dual-energy CT: diagnostic performance evaluation in patients. Abdom Imaging. 2010;35(5):629–35.
27. Fung GS, Kawamoto S, Matlaga BR, Taguchi K, Zhou X, Fishman EK, et al. Differentiation of kidney stones using dual-energy CT with and without a tin filter. AJR Am J Roentgenol. 2012;198(6):1380–6.
28. Pareek G, Hedican SP, Lee Jr FT, Nakada SY. Shock wave lithotripsy success determined by skin-to-stone distance on computed tomography. Urology. 2005; 66(5):941–4.
29. Patel T, Kozakowski K, Hruby G, Gupta M. Skin to stone distance is an independent predictor of stone-free status following shockwave lithotripsy. J Endourol. 2009;23(9):1383–5.
30. Weld KJ, Montiglio C, Morris MS, Bush AC, Cespedes RD. Shock wave lithotripsy success for renal stones based on patient and stone computed tomography characteristics. Urology. 2007;70(6): 1043–6. discussion 1046–7.

31. El-Nahas AR, El-Assmy AM, Mansour O, Sheir KZ. A prospective multivariate analysis of factors predicting stone disintegration by extracorporeal shock wave lithotripsy: the value of high-resolution noncontrast computed tomography. Eur Urol. 2007;51(6): 1688–93. discussion 1693–4.
32. Jacobs BL, Smaldone MC, Smaldone AM, Ricchiuti DJ, Averch TD. Effect of skin-to-stone distance on shockwave lithotripsy success. J Endourol. 2008; 22(8):1623–7.
33. Ng CF, Siu DY, Wong A, Goggins W, Chan ES, Wong KT. Development of a scoring system from noncontrast computerized tomography measurements to improve the selection of upper ureteral stone for extracorporeal shock wave lithotripsy. J Urol. 2009;181(3):1151–7.
34. Kanao K, Nakashima J, Nakagawa K, Asakura H, Miyajima A, Oya M, et al. Preoperative nomograms for predicting stone-free rate after extracorporeal shock wave lithotripsy. J Urol. 2006;176(4 Pt 1):1453–6. discussion 1456–7.
35. Kacker R, Zhao L, Macejko A, Thaxton CS, Stern J, Liu JJ, et al. Radiographic parameters on noncontrast computerized tomography predictive of shock wave lithotripsy success. J Urol. 2008;179(5): 1866–71.
36. Wiesenthal JD, Ghiculete D, Ray AA, Honey RJ, Pace KT. A clinical nomogram to predict the successful shock wave lithotripsy of renal and ureteral calculi. J Urol. 2011;186(2):556–62.
37. Wolf Jr JS, Bennett CJ, Dmochowski RR, Hollenbeck BK, Pearle MS, Schaeffer AJ. Best practice policy statement on urologic surgery antimicrobial prophylaxis. J Urol. 2008;179(4):1379–90.
38. Pearle MS, Roehrborn CG. Antimicrobial prophylaxis prior to shock wave lithotripsy in patients with sterile urine before treatment: a meta-analysis and cost-effectiveness analysis. Urology. 1997;49(5): 679–86.
39. Graber M, Bjerklund-Johansen TE, Botto H, Cek M, Naber KG, Tenke P, et al. Guidelines on urological infection. European Association of Eurology. 2010;1–112. Available from: http://www.uroweb.org/gls/pdf/Urological Infections 2010.pdf
40. de Cógáin M, Krambeck AE, Rule AD, Li X, Bergstralh EJ, Gettman MT, et al. Shock wave lithotripsy and diabetes mellitus: a population-based cohort study. Urology. 2012;79(2):298–302.
41. Delius M, Enders G, Xuan ZR, Liebich HG, Brendel W. Biological effects of shock waves: kidney damage by shock waves in dogs–dose dependence. Ultrasound Med Biol. 1988;14(2):117–22.
42. Willis LR, Evan AP, Connors BA, Fineberg NS, Lingeman JE. Effects of SWL on glomerular filtration rate and renal plasma flow in uninephrectomized minipigs. J Endourol. 1997;11(1):27–32.
43. Morris JS, Husmann DA, Wilson WT, Preminger GM. Temporal effects of shock wave lithotripsy. J Urol. 1991;145(4):881–3.
44. Cohen TD, Durrani AF, Brown SA, Ferraro R, Preminger GM. Lipid peroxidation induced by shockwave lithotripsy. J Endourol. 1998;12(3):229–32.
45. Munver R, Delvecchio FC, Kuo RL, Brown SA, Zhong P, Preminger GM. In vivo assessment of free radical activity during shock wave lithotripsy using a microdialysis system: the renoprotective action of allopurinol. J Urol. 2002;167(1):327–34.
46. Delvecchio FC, Brizuela RM, Khan SR, Byer K, Li Z, Zhong P, et al. Citrate and vitamin E blunt the shock wave-induced free radical surge in an in vitro cell culture model. Urol Res. 2005;33(6):448–52.
47. Yaman O, Sarica K, Ozer G, Soygur T, Kutsal O, Yaman LS, et al. Protective effect of verapamil on renal tissue during shockwave application in rabbit model. J Endourol. 1996;10(4):329–33.
48. Strohmaier WL, Bichler KH, Koch J, Balk N, Wilbert DM. Protective effect of verapamil on shock wave induced renal tubular dysfunction. J Urol. 1993;150(1):27–9.
49. Chin CM, Tay KP, Ng FC, Lim PH, Chng HC. Use of patient-controlled analgesia in extracorporeal shockwave lithotripsy. Br J Urol. 1997;79(6):848–51.
50. Delakas D, Karyotis I, Daskalopoulos G, Lianos E, Mavromanolakis E. Independent predictors of failure of shockwave lithotripsy for ureteral stones employing a second-generation lithotripter. J Endourol. 2003;17(4):201–5.
51. Lingeman JE, Kim SC, Kuo RL, McAteer JA, Evan AP. Shockwave lithotripsy: anecdotes and insights. J Endourol. 2003;17(9):687–93.
52. Troy A, Jones G, Moussa SA, Smith G, Tolley DA. Treatment of lower ureteral stones using the Dornier Compact Delta lithotripter. J Endourol. 2003;17(6): 369–71.
53. Zomorrodi A, Elahian A, Ghorbani N, Tavoosi A. Extracorporeal shock wave lithotripsy in prone and supine positions for patients with upper ureteral calculi. Urol J. 2006;3(3):130–3.
54. Hara N, Koike H, Bilim V, Takahashi K, Nishiyama T. Efficacy of extracorporeal shockwave lithotripsy with patients rotated supine or rotated prone for treating ureteral stones: a case-control study. J Endourol. 2006;20(3):170–4.
55. Duvall JO, Griffith DP. Epidural anesthesia for extracorporeal shock wave lithotripsy. Anesth Analg. 1985;64(5):544–6.
56. Kopacz DJ, Carpenter RL, Mulroy MF. The reliability of epidural anesthesia for repeat ESWL: a study of changes in epidural compliance. Reg Anesth. 1990;15(4):199–203.
57. London RA, Kudlak T, Riehle RA. Immersion anesthesia for extracorporeal shock wave lithotripsy. Review of two hundred twenty treatments. Urology. 1986;28(2):86–94.
58. Malhotra V, Long CW, Meister MJ. Intercostal blocks with local infiltration anesthesia for extracorporeal shock wave lithotripsy. Anesth Analg. 1987; 66(1):85–8.

59. Monk TG, Rater JM, White PF. Comparison of alfentanil and ketamine infusions in combination with midazolam for outpatient lithotripsy. Anesthesiology. 1991;74(6):1023–8.
60. White PF, Negus JB. Sedative infusions during local and regional anesthesia: a comparison of midazolam and propofol. J Clin Anesth. 1991;3(1):32–9.
61. Monk TG, Boure B, White PF, Meretyk S, Clayman RV. Comparison of intravenous sedative-analgesic techniques for outpatient immersion lithotripsy. Anesth Analg. 1991;72(5):616–21.
62. Kortis HI, Amory DW, Wagner BK, Levin R, Wilson E, Levin A, et al. Use of patient-controlled analgesia with alfentanil for extracorporeal shock wave lithotripsy. J Clin Anesth. 1995;7(3):205–10.
63. Osborne GA, Rudkin GE, Jarvis DA, Young IG, Barlow J, Leppard PI. Intra-operative patient-controlled sedation and patient attitude to control. A crossover comparison of patient preference for patient-controlled propofol and propofol by continuous infusion. Anaesthesia. 1994;49(4):287–92.
64. Uyar M, Uyar M, Uğur G, Bilge S, Ozyar B, Ozyurt C. Patient-controlled sedation and analgesia during SWL. J Endourol. 1996;10(5):407–10.
65. Joo HS, Perks WJ, Kataoka MT, Errett L, Pace K, Honey RJ. A comparison of patient-controlled sedation using either remifentanil or remifentanil-propofol for shock wave lithotripsy. Anesth Analg. 2001;93(5):1227–32.
66. Zommick J, Leveillee R, Zabbo A, Colasanto L, Barrette D. Comparison of general anesthesia and intravenous sedation-analgesia for SWL. J Endourol. 1996;10(6):489–91.
67. Sorensen C, Chandhoke P, Moore M, Wolf C, Sarram A. Comparison of intravenous sedation versus general anesthesia on the efficacy of the Doli 50 lithotriptor. J Urol. 2002;168(1):35–7.
68. Lee C, Weiland D, Ryndin I, Ugarte R, Monga M. Impact of type of anesthesia on efficacy of medstone STS lithotripter. J Endourol. 2007;21(9):957–60.
69. Pishchalnikov YA, Neucks JS, VonDerHaar RJ, Pishchalnikova IV, Williams Jr JC, McAteer JA. Air pockets trapped during routine coupling in dry head lithotripsy can significantly decrease the delivery of shock wave energy. J Urol. 2006;176(6 Pt 1):2706–10.
70. Neucks JS, Pishchalnikov YA, Zancanaro AJ, VonDerHaar JN, Williams Jr JC, McAteer JA. Improved acoustic coupling for shock wave lithotripsy. Urol Res. 2008;36(1):61–6.
71. Zhou Y, Cocks FH, Preminger GM, Zhong P. The effect of treatment strategy on stone comminution efficiency in shock wave lithotripsy. J Urol. 2004; 172(1):349–54.
72. Maloney ME, Marguet CG, Zhou Y, Kang DE, Sung JC, Springhart WP, et al. Progressive increase of lithotripter output produces better in-vivo stone comminution. J Endourol. 2006;20(9):603–6.
73. Willis LR, Evan AP, Connors BA, Handa RK, Blomgren PM, Lingeman JE. Prevention of lithotripsy-induced renal injury by pretreating kidneys with low-energy shock waves. J Am Soc Nephrol. 2006;17(3):663–73.
74. Connors BA, Evan AP, Blomgren PM, Handa RK, Willis LR, Gao S. Effect of initial shock wave voltage on shock wave lithotripsy-induced lesion size during step-wise voltage ramping. BJU Int. 2009; 103(1):104–7.
75. Demirci D, Altiok E, Gulmez I, Ekmekçioğlu O, Poyrazoğlu HM. Stepwise shock wave lithotripsy: results of initial study for the treatment of urinary stones in childhood. Int Urol Nephrol. 2006;38(2): 189–92.
76. Lambert EH, Walsh R, Moreno MW, Gupta M. Effect of escalating versus fixed voltage treatment on stone comminution and renal injury during extracorporeal shock wave lithotripsy: a prospective randomized trial. J Urol. 2010;183(2):580–4.
77. Honey RJ, Ray AA, Ghiculete D. University of Toronto Lithotripsy Associates, Pace KT. Shock wave lithotripsy: a randomized, double-blind trial to compare immediate versus delayed voltage escalation. Urology. 2010;75(1):38–43.
78. Evan AP, McAteer JA, Connors BA, Blomgren PM, Lingeman JE. Renal injury during shock wave lithotripsy is significantly reduced by slowing the rate of shock wave delivery. BJU Int. 2007;100(3):624–7. discussion 627–8.
79. Paterson RF, Kuo RL, Lingeman JE. The effect of rate of shock wave delivery on the efficiency of lithotripsy. Curr Opin Urol. 2002;12(4):291–5.
80. Honey RJ, Schuler TD, Ghiculete D, Pace KT, Canadian Endourology Group. A randomized, double-blind trial to compare shock wave frequencies of 60 and 120 shocks per minute for upper ureteral stones. J Urol. 2009;182(4):1418–23.
81. Davenport K, Minervini A, Keoghane S, Parkin J, Keeley FX, Timoney AG. Does rate matter? The results of a randomized controlled trial of 60 versus 120 shocks per minute for shock wave lithotripsy of renal calculi. J Urol. 2006;176(5):2055–8. discussion 2058.
82. Madbouly K, El-Tiraifi AM, Seida M, El-Faqih SR, Atassi R, Talic RF. Slow versus fast shock wave lithotripsy rate for urolithiasis: a prospective randomized study. J Urol. 2005;173(1):127–30.
83. Yilmaz E, Batislam E, Basar M, Tuglu D, Mert C, Basar H. Optimal frequency in extracorporeal shock wave lithotripsy: prospective randomized study. Urology. 2005;66(6):1160–4.
84. Semins MJ, Trock BJ, Matlaga BR. The effect of shock wave rate on the outcome of shock wave lithotripsy: a meta-analysis. J Urol. 2008;179(1):194–7. discussion 197.
85. Nicely ER, Maggio MI, Kuhn EJ. The use of a cystoscopically placed cobra catheter for directed irrigation of lower pole caliceal stones during extracorporeal shock wave lithotripsy. J Urol. 1992;148(3 Pt 2):1036–9.

86. Graham JB, Nelson JB. Percutaneous caliceal irrigation during extracorporeal shock wave lithotripsy for lower pole renal calculi. J Urol. 1994;152(6 Pt 2):2227.
87. Kosar A, Oztürk A, Serel TA, Akkus S, Unal OS. Effect of vibration massage therapy after extracorporeal shockwave lithotripsy in patients with lower caliceal stones. J Endourol. 1999;13(10):705–7.
88. Brownlee N, Foster M, Griffith DP, Carlton Jr CE. Controlled inversion therapy: an adjunct to the elimination of gravity-dependent fragments following extracorporeal shock wave lithotripsy. J Urol. 1990;143(6):1096–8.
89. Pace KT, Tariq N, Dyer SJ, Weir MJ, D'A Honey RJ. Mechanical percussion, inversion and diuresis for residual lower pole fragments after shock wave lithotripsy: a prospective, single blind, randomized controlled trial. J Urol. 2001;166(6):2065–71.
90. Chiong E, Hwee ST, Kay LM, Liang S, Kamaraj R, Esuvaranathan K. Randomized controlled study of mechanical percussion, diuresis, and inversion therapy to assist passage of lower pole renal calculi after shock wave lithotripsy. Urology. 2005;65(6):1070–4.
91. Hollingsworth JM, Rogers MA, Kaufman SR, Bradford TJ, Saint S, Wei JT, et al. Medical therapy to facilitate urinary stone passage: a meta-analysis. Lancet. 2006;368(9542):1171–9.
92. Schuler TD, Shahani R, Honey RJ, Pace KT. Medical expulsive therapy as an adjunct to improve shockwave lithotripsy outcomes: a systematic review and meta-analysis. J Endourol. 2009;23(3):387–93.
93. Gravina GL, Costa AM, Ronchi P, Galatioto GP, Angelucci A, Castellani D, et al. Tamsulosin treatment increases clinical success rate of single extracorporeal shock wave lithotripsy of renal stones. Urology. 2005;66(1):24–8.
94. Gravas S, Tzortzis V, Karatzas A, Oeconomou A, Melekos MD. The use of tamsulozin as adjunctive treatment after ESWL in patients with distal ureteral stone: do we really need it? Results from a randomised study. Urol Res. 2007;35(5):231–5.
95. Porpiglia F, Destefanis P, Fiori C, Scarpa RM, Fontana D. Role of adjunctive medical therapy with nifedipine and deflazacort after extracorporeal shock wave lithotripsy of ureteral stones. Urology. 2002;59(6):835–8.
96. Soygür T, Akbay A, Küpeli S. Effect of potassium citrate therapy on stone recurrence and residual fragments after shockwave lithotripsy in lower caliceal calcium oxalate urolithiasis: a randomized controlled trial. J Endourol. 2002;16(3):149–52.
97. Arrabal-Martín M, Fernández-Rodríguez A, Arrabal-Polo MA, Garcií-Ruiz MJ, Zuluaga-Gómez A. Extracorporeal renal lithotripsy: evolution of residual lithiasis treated with thiazides. Urology. 2006;68(5):956–9.
98. Streem SB, Yost A, Mascha E. Clinical implications of clinically insignificant store fragments after extracorporeal shock wave lithotripsy. J Urol. 1996; 155(4):1186–90.
99. El-Nahas AR, El-Assmy AM, Madbouly K, Sheir KZ. Predictors of clinical significance of residual fragments after extracorporeal shockwave lithotripsy for renal stones. J Endourol. 2006;20(11): 870–4.
100. Osman MM, Alfano Y, Kamp S, Haecker A, Alken P, Michel MS, et al. 5-year-follow-up of patients with clinically insignificant residual fragments after extracorporeal shockwave lithotripsy. Eur Urol. 2005;47(6):860–4.
101. Fine JK, Pak CY, Preminger GM. Effect of medical management and residual fragments on recurrent stone formation following shock wave lithotripsy. J Urol. 1995;153(1):27–32. discussion 32–3.
102. Yoshida S, Hayashi T, Ikeda J, Yoshinaga A, Ohno R, Ishii N, et al. Role of volume and attenuation value histogram of urinary stone on noncontrast helical computed tomography as predictor of fragility by extracorporeal shock wave lithotripsy. Urology. 2006;68(1):33–7.
103. Perks AE, Gotto G, Teichman JM. Shock wave lithotripsy correlates with stone density on preoperative computerized tomography. J Urol. 2007;178(3 Pt 1): 912–5.
104. Perks AE, Schuler TD, Lee J, Ghiculete D, Chung DG, D'A Honey RJ, et al. Stone attenuation and skin-to-stone distance on computed tomography predicts for stone fragmentation by shock wave lithotripsy. Urology. 2008;72(4):765–9.
105. Bandi G, Meiners RJ, Pickhardt PJ, Nakada SY. Stone measurement by volumetric three-dimensional computed tomography for predicting the outcome after extracorporeal shock wave lithotripsy. BJU Int. 2009;103(4):524–8.
106. Wiesenthal JD, Ghiculete D, D'A Honey RJ, Pace KT. Evaluating the importance of mean stone density and skin-to-stone distance in predicting successful shock wave lithotripsy of renal and ureteric calculi. Urol Res. 2010;38(4):307–13.
107. Park YI, Yu JH, Sung LH, Noh CH, Chung JY. Evaluation of possible predictive variables for the outcome of shock wave lithotripsy of renal stones. Korean J Urol. 2010;51(10):713–8.
108. Park BH, Choi H, Kim JB, Chang YS. Analyzing the effect of distance from skin to stone by computed tomography scan on the extracorporeal shock wave lithotripsy stone-free rate of renal stones. Korean J Urol. 2012;53(1):40–3.
109. Graversen JA, Korets R, Hruby GW, Valderrama OM, Mues AC, Katsumi HK, et al. Evaluation of bioimpedance as novel predictor of extracorporeal shockwave lithotripsy success. J Endourol. 2011; 25(9):1503–6.
110. Kobayashi M, Naya Y, Kino M, Awa Y, Nagata M, Suzuki H, et al. Low dose tamsulosin for stone expulsion after extracorporeal shock wave lithotripsy: efficacy in Japanese male patients with ureteral stone. Int J Urol. 2008;15(6):495–8.
111. Bhagat SK, Chacko NK, Kekre NS, Gopalakrishnan G, Antonisamy B, Devasia A. Is there a role for

tamsulosin in shock wave lithotripsy for renal and ureteral calculi? J Urol. 2007;177(6):2185–8.
112. Küpeli B, Irkilata L, Gürocak S, Tunc L, Kirac M, Karaoglan U, et al. Does tamsulosin enhance lower ureteral stone clearance with or without shock wave lithotripsy? Urology. 2004;64(6):1111–5.
113. Naja V, Agarwal MM, Mandal AK, Singh SK, Mavuduru R, Kumar S, et al. Tamsulosin facilitates earlier clearance of stone fragments and reduces pain after shockwave lithotripsy for renal calculi: results from an open-label randomized study. Urology. 2008;72(5):1006–11.
114. Wang HJ, Liu K, Ji ZG, Li HZ. Application of Alpha1-adrenergic antagonist with extracorporeal shock wave lithotripsy for lower ureteral stone. Zhongguo Yi Xue Ke Xue Yuan Xue Bao. 2008; 30(4):506–8.
115. Hussein MM. Does tamsulosin increase stone clearance after shockwave lithotripsy of renal stones? A prospective, randomized controlled study. Scand J Urol Nephrol. 2010;44(1):27–31.
116. Falahatkar S, Khosropanah I, Vajary AD, Bateni ZH, Khosropanah D, Allahkhah A. Is there a role for tamsulosin after shock wave lithotripsy in the treatment of renal and ureteral calculi? J Endourol. 2011;25(3): 495–8.
117. Agarwal MM, Naja V, Singh SK, Mavuduru R, Mete UK, Kumar S, et al. Is there an adjunctive role of tamsulosin to extracorporeal shockwave lithotripsy for upper ureteric stones: results of an open label randomized nonplacebo controlled study. Urology. 2009;74(5):989–92.
118. Moursy E, Gamal WM, Abuzeid A. Tamsulosin as an expulsive therapy for steinstrasse after extracorporeal shock wave lithotripsy: a randomized controlled study. Scand J Urol Nephrol. 2010;44(5):315–9.
119. Georgiev MI, Ormanov DI, Vassilev VD, Dimitrov PD, Mladenov VD, Popov EP, et al. Efficacy of tamsulosin oral controlled absorption system after extracorporeal shock wave lithotripsy to treat urolithiasis. Urology. 2011;78(5):1023–6.
120. Micali S, Grande M, Sighinolfi MC, De Stefani S, Bianchi G. Efficacy of expulsive therapy using nifedipine or tamsulosin, both associated with ketoprofene, after shock wave lithotripsy of ureteral stones. Urol Res. 2007;35(3):133–7.
121. Vicentini FC, Mazzucchi E, Brito AH, Chedid Neto EA, Danilovic A, Srougi M. Adjuvant tamsulosin or nifedipine after extracorporeal shock wave lithotripsy for renal stones: a double blind, randomized, placebo-controlled trial. Urology. 2011;78(5): 1016–21.

14 Complications of Shock Wave Lithotripsy

Mitra R. de Cógáin and Amy E. Krambeck

Renal Effects

Hematoma/Hemorrhage

Gross hematuria occurs frequently in patients receiving greater than 200 shocks, and may be an indicator of acute renal damage [5]. In most patients the hematuria resolves without further sequelae within 12 h [6]. However, acute or sustained renal injury may also occur. The area of injury to the kidney parenchyma produced by SWL appears to be dependent on number of shock waves administered and power of the lithotripter [8]. The most frequently identified complication of SWL is acute subcapsular hematoma formation. The occurrence of this complication varies with the type of lithotripter, with a reported incidence of 0.6–12 % [7]. In one porcine study by Willis and colleagues, SWL-related renal injury extended from the renal capsule to the medulla [9]. Small venules appear to be especially at risk to injury with SWL; however, other renal vascular constituents, namely vasa recta, cortical capillaries, intralobular, and arcuate vessels are also susceptible to injury [9].

Studies focusing on the development of symptomatic perirenal hematoma following SWL note an incidence of this complication in 0.2–1.5 % of patients (Fig. 14.1) [5, 7, 10, 11]. Although most studies have focused on results from treatment with the HM3, newer model lithotripters, which have smaller focal area and thus higher peak pressures, still appear to have significant rates of posttreatment hematoma formation [12]. Occasionally, large hematomas can lead to the need for blood transfusions or even angioembolization [10, 13]. Such hemorrhage may produce a state of acute renal failure, and if the condition is not identified in a timely fashion, even death [14]. Fortunately, most hematomas are clinically insignificant. Post-SWL routine screening with computed tomography (CT) or magnetic resonance imaging (MRI) has demonstrated perirenal hematoma rates ranging up to 20–25 % [6, 11]. In addition, 63–85 % of kidneys 24 h following SWL were found to have edema or contained hemorrhage [6, 10]. Both the edema and subclinical hemorrhage were found most often to dissipate without permanent effects. Perirenal fluid absorbs quickly, resolving within days, while subcapsular fluid or hemorrhage can take up to 6 months to disappear [10].

Subcapsular hematoma formation following SWL appears to be associated with certain risk factors including: hypertension, pretreatment urinary tract infection (UTI), diabetes, coronary artery disease, obesity, and age [10, 11, 15]. Not only is hypertension associated with the incidence of hematoma following SWL, the severity of hypertension also appears to be significant, as Knapp and colleagues demonstrated [10]. Patients

M.R. de Cógáin, M.D. (✉) • A.E. Krambeck, M.D.
Department of Urology, Mayo Clinic Rochester, Rochester, MN, USA
e-mail: decogain.mitra@mayo.edu

S.Y. Nakada and M.S. Pearle (eds.), *Surgical Management of Urolithiasis: Percutaneous, Shockwave and Ureteroscopy*, DOI 10.1007/978-1-4614-6937-7_14,

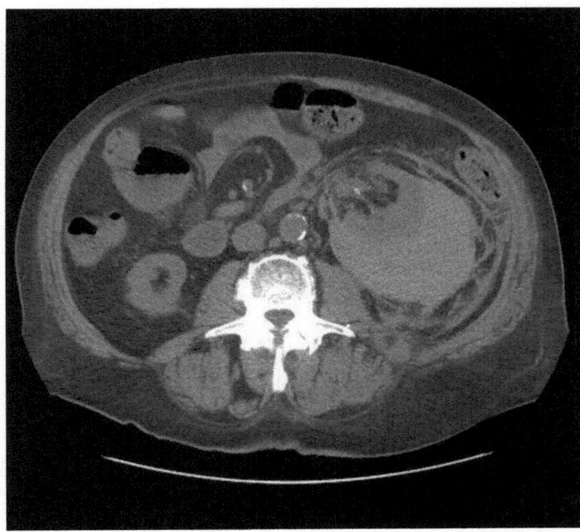

Fig. 14.1 Perirenal hematoma following SWL. Noncontrast CT of the abdomen coronal cuts demonstrating a severe perinephric hematoma following SWL

with poorly controlled hypertension experienced post-SWL hematoma formation at a rate of 3.8 % as compared to patients with well-controlled hypertension, with a rate of 2.5 % [10]. Rates of post-SWL hematoma are also directly proportional to age [16]. In a multivariate analysis performed by Dhar and associates in 2004, excluding patients with bleeding disorders, the risk of subcapsular hematoma formation doubled with each decade of life [16].

Patients with bleeding diathesis are at particular risk for hemorrhage and large volume retroperitoneal bleed. If the coagulopathy can be appropriately corrected prior to treatment, SWL may be safely employed as treatment for urolithiasis [17]. However, if the patient's medical condition precludes reversal, as in cases of a mechanical heart valve or drug eluting cardiac stents, ureteroscopy should instead be employed. Watterson and colleagues demonstrated ureteroscopy to be a safe and effective treatment in patients with bleeding diathesis or need for anticoagulation without the need for anticoagulation reversal [18].

Functional Renal Injury

Changes in renal function related to SWL therapy may be categorized into short- and long-term (sustained) effects. The mechanism(s) of SWL-related renal dysfunction is not completely defined but may stem from multiple pathways. Cavitation forces, among other causes, play a significant role in early tissue changes, while sustained deleterious effects on renal function are likely related to parenchymal scar formation following the initial insult to the kidney [19]. This idea is substantiated by a murine in vivo study by Dalecki and colleagues, which demonstrated an increase in renal hemorrhage with injection of Albunex®, a microbubble contrast agent that provides a nucleus for cavitation, into the circulation during SWL [20]. Shear forces also appear to contribute to parenchymal injury, particularly at fast shock wave rates. SWL performed in pigs using a modified HM3 lithotripter fitted with a cavitation suppressing reflector demonstrated a reduction in vascular renal injury [21]. However, bleeding was still noted from the renal papillae following SWL, pointing to causes other than cavitation alone as a source of injury.

Renal biopsies obtained from patients 1 week post-SWL demonstrate acute histologic changes, namely, marked tubular, vascular, and interstitial damage [22]. Rigatti and colleagues showed that glomeruli localized to the plane of shock waves were injured, while the rest of the nephron demonstrated degenerative changes. The microvascular structure was also altered, demonstrated by dilation of veins with endothelial damage and thrombus formation. Intraparenchymal hemorrhage at the corticomedullary junction was noted by Seitz in a 1991 study of four patients treated with piezoelectric SWL [23]. The severity of hemorrhage was directly related to the number of shock waves administered. In a cadaveric study, therapeutic SWL was found to consistently injure nephrons, as well as small- to medium-sized blood vessels [24]. Again, these effects appear to correlate with the number of shocks delivered.

Not only have initial parenchymal changes following SWL been noted on the microscopic level, but the noted insults to renal structure may also translate into demonstrable transient deterioration of renal function. Renal plasma flow is decreased by 30 % immediately following SWL, as determined by nuclear renal scan [6].

Furthermore, Grantham and colleagues noted delayed intravenous contrast excretion following SWL of unobstructed kidneys [25]. The degree of renal dysfunction in these studies correlates with the number of shocks delivered.

Although acute changes in kidney architecture and renal function are demonstrable immediately following SWL, these alterations would not be of significant clinical importance without sustained effects on renal function. Data in the arena of sustained dysfunction is limited; however, some indirect evidence does confirm the existence of long-term consequences of SWL therapy. The acute vascular lesions, as noted above, can progress to scarring of the renal parenchyma, with loss of nephron function.

One month following SWL therapy with the HM3 lithotripter, canines were found to have fibrosis of the kidney [26]. Furthermore, scar severity correlated with the number of shock waves delivered. These findings were substantiated by a study in which scar volume at 1 month was nearly tenfold higher in rabbits treated with 2,000 shock waves compared to 100 shock waves [27]. A porcine model demonstrated the inner medullary portion of the kidney to be the most sensitive to scar formation and damage from SWL therapy, with complete atrophy of treated papilla at 3 months following SWL [7]. Scar formation has also been radiographically apparent in humans following SWL therapy. Photon Emission CT was employed to evaluate parenchymal changes in patients 30 days following SWL treatment for nephrolithiasis [28]. All kidneys studied had poor vascular perfusion with scarring and loss of Technicium-99 uptake following SWL.

Although renal scarring following SWL has been documented, it is unclear if this noted parenchymal change is clinically relevant, with a related decline in renal function. Karlsen and Berg found a significant decline in glomerular filtration rate in patients with solitary kidneys 3 months following SWL therapy [29]. This effect may be sustained in the long term, as demonstrated in another solitary kidney study by Brito and colleagues, where patients were found to have an elevated serum creatinine 5 years following SWL treatment [30]. In addition, various studies have documented decreases in renal plasma flow, worsened creatinine clearance, and increased transit time of ^{131}I-Hippuran following SWL therapy [31, 32]. However, in a study performed by Chaussy and Fuchs, patients actually had an improvement in renal function from 3 months to 1 year following SWL [2]. Two additional later studies, with follow-up of 5 years or greater also noted no apparent deterioration in renal function after SWL [33, 34].

Hypertension

The link between SWL and renal scar formation has been documented in the literature (as outlined above); therefore, there is significant concern for the possible development of new-onset hypertension following SWL treatment. This topic has been widely evaluated and debated in the literature, and there are multiple conflicting reports (Table 14.1) [2, 19, 31, 33–47].

In a 1986 study, Peterson and Finlayson first described an increase in blood pressure following SWL and since that time multiple investigators have evaluated the association between SWL and hypertension [33]. In another study by Janetschek and colleagues, patients aged 60 years or greater were found to be at increased risk for elevated renal resistive indices following SWL, as measured by ultrasound [34]. Forty-five percent of patients (almost exclusively all older than 60 years) had elevated resistive indices in the 26 month follow-up period, with new onset hypertension noted in 17.5 %, prompting concern over the use of SWL in the elderly population [34].

An increased risk of hypertension was also noted in post-SWL patients as compared to those undergoing conservative management for urolithiasis, in 19 years of follow-up, with increased risk in those who had undergone bilateral treatment [36]. Since that study, however, two reports have been published showing no correlation between SWL and hypertension. A study by Sato and colleagues, comparing SWL patients undergoing SWL for renal calculi to those undergoing SWL for ureteral calculi, demonstrated no

Table 14.1 Hypertension and shock wave lithotripsy

Study	Length of study (months)	Mean # of shock waves	Incidence of hypertension	Change in diastolic blood pressure
Krambeck et al. [73]	104	–	No change	–
Sato et al. [39]	204	928	No change	–
Krambeck et al. [36]	228	1,125	Increased	–
Elves et al. [43]	26.4	5,281	No change[a]	No change[a]
Strohmaier et al. [38]	24	–	Increased	Increased
Jewett et al. [44]	24	4,411	No change	No change
Janetschek et al. [34]	26	2,735	Increased[b]	Increased[b]
Yokoyama et al. [46]	19	–	–	Increased
Lingeman et al. [41]		1,289	No change	Increased
Montgomery et al. [37]	29	1,429	Increased	No change
Puppo et al. [47]	12	1,380	No change	No change
Liedl et al. [40]	40	1,043	No change	–
Williams et al. [31]	21	1,400	Increased	Increased

[a]Compared to control group not undergoing SWL
[b]Change noted in patients aged 60–80 years only

increased risk of hypertension [39]. A large, population-based study also noted no increased risk of hypertension in patients undergoing SWL as compared to other treatment modalities for urolithiasis at 8.7 years of follow-up [45].

Diabetes Mellitus

Multiple studies have demonstrated that the pancreas may be vulnerable to injury at the time of SWL; however, it is unclear if the risk of developing diabetes is increased with SWL therapy. Kirkali and colleagues found increased serum amylase, serum lipase, and urinary amylase, with elevated values sustained for up to 1 week post-SWL in the absence of overt pancreatitis, and other case studies have reported symptomatic pancreatitis following SWL [45–51]. Furthermore, pancreatic hematomas and microvascular changes have been noted after SWL in patients who are asymptomatic [52].

A recent population based study demonstrated that previous SWL did not increase the risk of diabetes in a univariate or multivariate analysis accounting for age, gender, and obesity, over a period of nearly 9 years of follow-up [53]. Further, an earlier study by Sato and associates demonstrated no appreciable difference in the risk for the development of diabetes of patients undergoing SWL for ureteral calculi as compared to those being treated for SWL for renal calculi at 17 years of follow-up [39]. However, in a 2006 retrospective review, patients treated with SWL were more likely to develop diabetes mellitus at 19 years of follow-up, as compared to conservatively managed stone patients [36]. Furthermore, the development of diabetes was associated with number of shocks administered and total intensity of the treatment.

Age-Related Renal Considerations

Although complications may arise in any age group, certain patient populations including elderly patients and children may be at increased risk for adverse effects from SWL therapy. In these vulnerable groups, as well as in patients with preexisting renal insufficiency and hypertension, care should be taken to limit the number and energy of shock waves delivered. In a 2004 study by Dhar and colleagues, older patients were more likely to suffer a subcapsular hematoma following SWL [16]. In another study, patients aged 60 years or greater were found to be at increased risk for elevated renal resistive indices following SWL and for new onset hypertension [34].

Furthermore, elderly patients are more likely to have significant comorbid conditions and polypharmacy, putting them at greater risk for other SWL complications [54, 55]. However, if appropriate patient selection is undertaken and changes in shock wave delivery are made to minimize the impact of SWL, this treatment can be safely performed in the elderly without increased complication rates.

Although not approved by the FDA for use in children, SWL is a common first-line treatment for pediatric urolithiasis. Thus, there is concern over the possible sustained effects of SWL on renal growth and renal function in the pediatric population. There does appear to be an impact of SWL on juvenile renal growth, as demonstrated by Lifshitz and colleagues. In a 1998 study, they found that children treated with SWL experienced a decrease in renal size not only of the treated kidney, but also of the contralateral kidney, at 9 years of follow-up [56]. Neal and associates compared SWL in adult and infant rhesus monkeys, and found a significant decrease in effective renal plasma flow in the infant group at 6 months following SWL [57]. In addition, intraparenchymal hemorrhage volume was found to be significantly higher in juvenile pigs as compared to adult pigs undergoing SWL therapy (7 % vs. 2 %) [58]. Mean arterial blood pressure was also found to increase significantly at 4 and 8 weeks after SWL therapy in immature rabbits, as compared to controls [59]. Although SWL does appear to have an impact on renal growth and function, it is still considered acceptable first-line therapy for children with urolithiasis.

Fragment Side Effects

Steinstrasse

Steinstrasse, the term used to define the accumulation of stone fragments in the ureter, is a known complication of SWL, with overall reported rates ranging from 2 to 10 % (Fig. 14.2) [7, 60]. Steinstrasse can be categorized into simple, defined as less than 5 cm in length without infection, or complex, if a longer length of ureter is involved or infection is present. Simple steinstrasse can be managed with symptomatic treatment and observation or ureteroscopic intervention. However, if complex steinstrasse is present, it should be managed with emergent collecting system decompression. The clinical presentation of steinstrasse is variable, with some patients experiencing symptoms within hours, and others within months following SWL. The most common symptoms of steinstrasse include renal colic, urinary tract infection, and renal insufficiency. Other patients may be asymptomatic. 70 % of all steinstrasse occurs in the distal ureter [7, 15, 61].

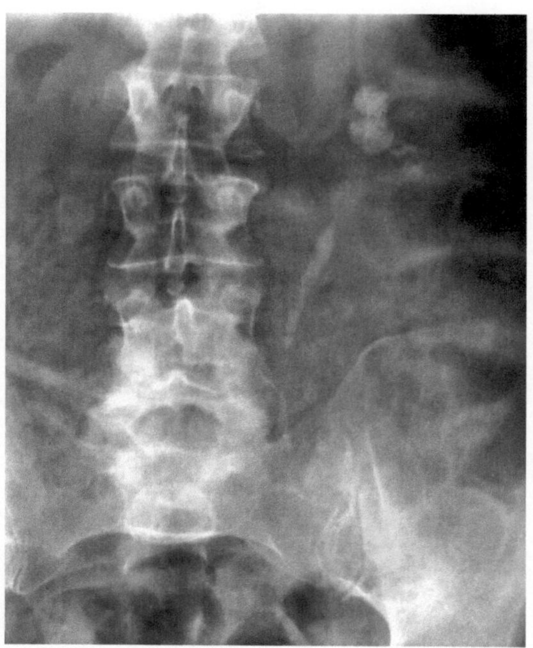

Fig. 14.2 X-ray of the abdomen demonstrating steinstrasse along the length of the left proximal and mid-ureter after shock wave lithotripsy

An early study by Weinerth and associates demonstrated that the risk of steinstrasse following SWL increased with large calculus size, staghorn calculi, bilateral SWL treatment, and preexisting ureteral obstruction [62]. Also, the occurrence of steinstrasse is directly related to stone size, as the risk increases with increasing stone burden [7]. Madbouly and colleagues evaluated 4,600 patients undergoing SWL and identified stone size >2 cm, a dilated renal unit, shock wave voltage greater than 22 kV, and renal stone treatment as risk factors for the development of steinstrasse in a multivariate analysis [61].

Placement of a ureteral stent prior to SWL therapy may decrease the occurrence or limit symptoms from, but will not eliminate the risk of steinstrasse [63, 64]. A prospective, randomized study performed by Al-Awadi and associates compared the results of SWL with or without stent placement for renal calculi ranging from 1.5 to 3.5 cm [64]. As discussed previously, patients with a higher stone burden had increased risk of steinstrasse; however, the incidence of steinstrasse was significantly decreased with stent placement [64]. Another study, which focused on SWL for stones greater than 2.0 cm, found the incidence of steinstrasse was significantly decreased in patients with ureteral stenting prior to SWL (15 % versus 38 %) [65]. In addition, patients who had preoperative stenting required fewer hospital admissions following SWL. Although there is some data to support ureteral stenting prior to SWL, other studies demonstrate no benefit, with no significant difference in steinstrasse, and potential worsened postoperative course, due to stent-related discomfort and decreased stone clearance [63, 66, 67]. Pre-SWL stent placement remains a controversial practice, and the greatest benefit is likely to be observed in patients with large renal calculi or those with a solitary kidney [7, 15]. Of note, the 2007 American Urological Association/European Urological Association ureteral calculus consensus guidelines noted no benefit to ureteral stent placement prior to SWL of ureteral stones [60].

Asymptomatic patients with simple steinstrasse can be treated conservatively, as spontaneous stone passage occurs in 60–80 % of patients [7]. However, patients with complex steinstrasse, recalcitrant discomfort, large stone fragments, bilateral obstruction or obstruction of a solitary kidney, as well as those who have failed initial conservative management, should be managed with urinary tract decompression by ureteral stenting, percutaneous nephrostomy tube placement, or ureteroscopic intervention [15, 62]. Percutaneous nephrostomy tube placement alone has been reported to allow for spontaneous passage of all stone fragments in up to 75 % of patients with steinstrasse [15].

If steinstrasse persists following 3–4 weeks of urinary tract decompression, further intervention is warranted. Options include repeat SWL, retrograde or antegrade ureteroscopy, with success rates near 100 % [7, 15, 62]. However, ureteroscopy for steinstrasse can be technically challenging, with a risk for ureteral perforation. Further, stone-free rates for primary ureteroscopy near only 60 %, with significantly higher success following urinary tract decompression [62].

Multiple Treatments

In general, increased stone size and total stone burden are associated with lower stone-free rates, and an increased requirement for repeat SWL or additional stone procedures [7]. The mean stone-free rate for SWL for stones 1 cm or less is 79.9 % (range 63–90 %), 64.1 % (range 50–82.7 %) for stones 1–2 cm, and 53.7 % (range 33.3–81.4 %) for stones larger than 2 cm [7]. The requirement for additional stone treatment increases from 10 % for SWL of stones 1–2 cm in size to 33 % for SWL of stones 2–3 cm [68]. Furthermore, the success rate of SWL decreases with each subsequent treatment, such that the cumulative stone-free rate with two treatments is 76 % and with three only marginally increases to 77 % overall [69]. Due to the disparity in retreatment rates, the 1988 National Institutes of Health Consensus Conference recommended that all patients with stones larger than 2 cm be treated initially with percutaneous nephrolithotomy (PCNL), which is further supported by the decreased efficacy noted in repeat SWL patients [70].

Ureteral Stricture Disease

The development of ureteral stricture following SWL has been cited as a concern; however, this appears to be of low likelihood, despite the risks of renal parenchymal injury, steinstrasse, and multiple treatments as noted above. Rates of ureteral stricture following SWL documented in a meta-analysis ranged from 0 % for distal calculi, to 1 % for mid-ureteral stones and 2 % for proximal calculi [60].

Stone Recurrence

Multiple studies have documented increased rates of stone recurrence in patients treated with SWL over other treatment modalities. In a study comparing 298 SWL patients to 62 PCNL patients who were all initially stone free, Carr and colleagues found that SWL patients were at an increased risk for new stone formation within 1 year of treatment as compared to those treated with PCNL [71]. A later study confirmed this finding, with increased rates of stone recurrence in patients treated with SWL compared to patients undergoing PCNL, at 19 years of follow-up [72].

In a study of residual stone fragments less than 0.5 cm following SWL, Bucholz and associates found that although after a mean follow-up of 2.5 years 12.7 % of residual stone fragments had not passed spontaneously, only 2 % demonstrated appreciable growth, and no stone recurrences occurred following the initial procedure [73]. Based on this study, the group recommended no further intervention to completely clear residual small fragments following SWL. However, Streem and colleagues argue that a significant number of SWL patients with small residual stone fragments are at risk for stone recurrence and recommend that these fragments not be categorized as clinically insignificant [74].

Brushite Stones

SWL therapy has also been associated with the development of brushite stones, which are notoriously resistant to fragmentation. As compared to other stone formers, patients with brushite stones have a significant amount of renal tissue damage noted on histopathologic examination. It has been theorized that brushite stone formation is more likely following SWL due to SWL-induced tissue damage and resultant defects in urine acidification [75]. Furthermore, patients undergoing treatment for brushite stones have a significantly decreased stone-free rate following SWL [76]. Parks and associates also noted that calcium phosphate (brushite and apatite) stone formers required a higher number of SWL procedures as compared to calcium oxalate stone formers [77]. Furthermore, the brushite stone formers had received a significantly greater number of SWL treatments than patients with apatite stones. However, to date no direct causal association between SWL and development of brushite stone disease has been identified.

Extrarenal Damage

Pain

The earliest lithotripter models could incite significant pain at the site of treatment. Patients undergoing SWL with an unmodified HM3 lithotripter at 18–24 kV commonly complain of localized flank pain at the site of shock wave entry and may have petechia or bruising [35]. Parr and colleagues noted increased creatine phosphokinase within 24 h following SWL, suggesting muscular trauma secondary to treatment [78]. Since the development of initial lithotripters, subsequent generation models have been modified to decrease patient discomfort. Specifically, the aperture at the shock source was widened to spread pulse energy over a broader area of the body; this, in turn, narrowed the focal zone and generated increased peak pressures at the target site.

Urinary Tract Infection (UTI) and Sepsis

The risk of sepsis following an uneventful SWL is low (less than 1 %), but increases significantly (2.7–56 %) when SWL is performed for staghorn calculi [5]. In a study by Duvdevani and colleagues, they identified several risk factors for the development of fever following SWL, which included a positive urine culture, an indwelling nephrostomy tube or stent at the time of SWL, renal or proximal ureteral location, preoperative symptomatic urinary tract infection or sepsis [79]. In addition, the risk of overt sepsis after SWL is increased with a positive preoperative urine culture or urinary system obstruction, and thus SWL should only be performed in the absence of these clinical characteristics [7].

For high risk patients (i.e. history of UTI, urinary diversion, immunocompromised, instrumentation

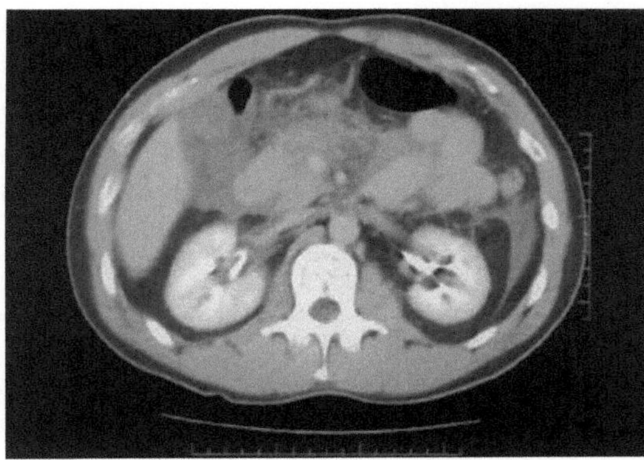

Fig. 14.3 Contrast-enhanced CT scan of the abdomen demonstrating acute pancreatitis following SWL

at time of SWL) prophylactic antibiotic therapy peri-procedurally should be considered, but is not indicated in all patients [79, 80]. Furthermore, a UTI in the presence of urolithiasis can be difficult to completely eradicate unless all stone fragments are completely removed, due to stone material harboring bacteria. Therefore, if a patient has an infected stone, PCNL or ureteroscopic intervention after directed antibiotic therapy should be considered for definitive stone management over SWL, as these procedures have higher stone clearance rates [12].

Visceral Organ Injury

Abdominal organ injury, although rare, has been reported following SWL with first-, second-, and third-generation lithotripters. As mentioned previously, acute pancreatitis, associated with a significant increase in serum amylase and lipase levels have been reported following SWL, and even in the absence of symptomatic pancreatitis, increased amylase levels have been noted (Fig. 14.3) [35, 48, 51]. In addition, a study by Kirkali and associates described elevations in serum and urinary pancreatic enzymes up to 1 week after SWL of proximal ureteral and renal stones [51]. Of note, pancreatic enzymes were not elevated when distal ureteral stones were treated. Wendt-Nordahl and colleagues, however, performed a prospective evaluation of 12 patients undergoing SWL which failed to show a change in pancreatic enzymes following SWL therapy [81]. Other investigators have noted microvascular damage to the pancreas and small pancreatic hematomas in post-SWL patients [52].

Hepatic injury following SWL is a known entity, as evidenced by elevated bilirubin, lactate dehydrogenase, and serum aspartate transaminase within 24 h of SWL therapy [35]. Liver enzymes start to trend downward at 3–7 days following SWL and generally normalize at 3 months. Furthermore, subcapsular hepatic hematomas and hepatic hematomas associated with hepatic vein thrombosis requiring emergent exploration have been described following SWL therapy [82]. The spleen can also be injured at time of SWL, and splenic hematoma prompting splenectomy post-SWL has also been reported [83].

Bowel complications are well documented following SWL. An early report by Al Karawi and associates reported an 80 % incidence of gastric and duodenal erosion after SWL [84]. Hematochezia, secondary to colonic mucosal damage from SWL, has also been reported. This complication is typically self-limiting and usually resolves without further sequelae [85]. However, more serious gastrointestinal complications, including large and small bowel perforation, have also been reported [86].

Cardiac and Vascular Injury

The cardiovascular system appears to be at risk of complications due to SWL treatment, with reports of myocardial infarctions as well as cerebral vascular accidents [7]. Early Dornier HM models were found to induce cardiac arrhythmias, an observation that eventually led to electrocardiographic synchronization with R-wave triggering [5]. Minor, non-life-threatening cardiac arrhythmias have also been noted with spark gap and piezoelectric generators when they are not synchronized to the electrocardiogram [7]. Synchronization is not required with newer-generation lithotripters, and patients with preexisting cardiac arrhythmias and pacemakers can undergo SWL safely. However, dual-chamber pacemakers should be reprogrammed to single-chamber mode and rate-responsive pacemakers should be reprogrammed to non-rate-responsive mode prior to SWL [87].

Patients with a calcified abdominal aortic aneurysm (AAA) may be at risk for aneurysm rupture with SWL, which is a known, reported complication [88]. However, multiple studies have demonstrated the safety of SWL in the presence of AAA. Vasavada and colleagues performed an vitro study on tissue harvested from calcified human aortic aneurysms at the time of elective repair, and then compared the tissue response following SWL to untreated tissue [89]. With the administration of a maximum of 1,000 shock waves, no appreciable difference in tissue disruption was noted. SWL therapy has been accomplished safely in patients with AAAs and renal aneurysms [90]. SWL is thought to be permissible in patients if their aneurysm is asymptomatic, with a maximal diameter of 2 cm for a renal aneurysm and 5 cm for an AAA. The stone to aneurysm distance should be a minimum of 5 cm and the aneurysm should not lie parallel to the shock wave access, to ensure minimal pressure on the aneurysm, with a maximum of an 18 kV (or the equivalent) energy setting [90]. Although SWL has been demonstrated as a safe and efficacious treatment for urolithiasis in aneurysm patients, the authors still advocate for treatment with ureteroscopy or PCNL instead of SWL in this population, as the consequences of thromboembolic events or aneurysm rupture can be life-threatening [12].

Pulmonary Injury

As the lung parenchyma has the highest attenuation coefficient of any human tissue, it is particularly vulnerable to shock wave injury [2]. In addition, pediatric patients may be at increased risk of pulmonary injury during SWL, due to closer proximity of the lung base to the kidney, as compared to adults [91]. SWL-induced hemoptysis has been reported in both adults and children, and is generally inconsequential; however, severe hypoxemia and death after SWL have been reported [91, 92]. Protective maneuvers, such as shielding the lungs with shock absorbing pads or alternative ventilation techniques, have been proposed to limit the risk of lung injury with SWL therapy; however, there is a paucity of supporting clinical data for these suggested changes in technique [92].

Fetal and Reproductive Organ Injury

Pregnancy remains a contraindication to SWL therapy, although inadvertent SWL treatment of pregnant patients has been reported, without subsequent detrimental effects to the fetus [93]. Ureteroscopy with holmium laser lithotripsy and basket stone extraction remains the primary treatment of choice in pregnant women, with proven safety and efficacy [7]. If a pregnant patient desires SWL for treatment of her urinary calculus, she should be temporized with an indwelling ureteral stent until after delivery, at which time SWL can be completed.

A prospective study performed by Gulum and colleagues evaluated semen parameters of young men before and after SWL for distal ureteral stones, and compared the results to men undergoing SWL for proximal ureteral stones. They found a statistically significant difference in sperm parameters, total semen oxidant, and antioxidant status and the DNA damage score in patients undergoing distal ureteral SWL, while these changes were not appreciated in the proximal ureteral control population. Semen changes normalized at 3 months following treatment [94]. Thus, selection of an alternative treatment modality may be appropriate in men with fertility concerns.

A similar concern exists in women of childbearing age. Erturk and associates evaluated 39 young women treated with SWL for distal ureteral calculi. No reports of infertility were made in the ten women who attempted pregnancy following SWL [95]. However, some clinicians elect to avoid SWL in women of childbearing age due to the potential for injury to reproductive organs.

Mechanisms to Reduce Adverse Effects

Renal hemorrhage occurs in three general locations: perirenal, subcapsular, and intraparenchymal, always at or near the treatment focal point (F2). Histopathologic evaluation at the hemorrhage location demonstrates rupture of small veins, arteries and glomerular, and peritubular capillaries [9]. In addition, nearby nephrons demonstrate evidence of direct damage from shock waves and ischemic changes. Renal hematomas increase in number as the number of shock waves administered rises [9]. Furthermore, as the energy level of SWL increases, there is a related decrease in renal blood flow, with an increase in the volume of renal damage [28]. SWL also appears to impact not only the treated kidney, but the contralateral kidney as well, by inducing significant vasoconstriction [7, 96]. In animal models, a large number of shocks, a high power setting, a condensed therapy period, treatment of a juvenile kidney and treatment of a kidney with impaired function all correlate with an increased degree of renal trauma [7]. Evan and colleagues also report that acute pyelonephritis may potentiate the renal injury sustained during SWL [97]. Thus, some patient, kidney and treatment properties can significantly alter the risk for SWL-related side effects.

Protective Pretreatment/Treatment Protocols

While there are patient and SWL therapy characteristics that cannot be changed, there are others that may be modified, in an attempt to decrease the risk of SWL-related complications. Certain aspects of shock wave delivery may be changed to minimize the amount of renal trauma sustained during SWL treatment (Table 14.2). So-called priming protocols, where one area of the kidney is treated with low energy shock waves prior to being treated with a therapeutic shock wave regimen, have been shown to decrease renal tissue damage in a porcine model [96]. Willis and associates treated female farm pigs with the HM3 lithotripter, at a clinical dose of 2,000 shock waves at 24 kV (120 shock waves per minute), which created a lesion measuring approximately 6 % of the functional renal volume (FRV). This area of tissue damage was decreased to 0.3 % of the FRV by priming the kidney with as few as 100 shock waves at 12 kV before completion of the therapeutic regimen [96]. The priming protocol may induce vasoconstriction, which in turn may decrease blood vessel susceptibility to shock wave stress. However, a later study by Connors demonstrated that it is not the low volume priming dose but rather the interruption of shock wave delivery that is protective [98]. In that study, the noted renal lesion was the same size when the priming dose was delivered at 12, 18, or 24 kV [98]. However, only when a 3–4 min delay was instituted following the priming dosing before resuming treatment SWL was renal protection observed.

Table 14.2 Alterations in SWL treatment protocols that have been found to be protective to the renal unit

Ensure no distal ureteral obstruction
Treat UTI prior to SWL
Delivery of priming protocol, with 100 shocks at low voltage (i.e. 12 kV)
Institute 3–4 min pause following priming protocol
Decrease rate of shock wave delivery (30–60 shocks/min)
Perform frequent imaging to assess for stone fragmentation
Discontinue treatment once stone comminution is achieved

In another porcine study, decreasing the rate of shock waves also appeared to decrease renal damage [99]. Reducing the rate of shock wave delivery to 30 shocks per minute reduced the renal lesion to less than 0.1 % of the FRV [99]. The effects on renal tissue damage seen with slowed shock wave frequency are similar to those noted with institution of a priming protocol. An added benefit of the decreased rate of shock wave delivery is improved stone fragmentation. A meta-analysis of 589 patients demonstrated that slow-rate SWL (60 shock waves per minute) garnered improved success over fast-rate SWL (120 shock waves per minute) [100]. Canine studies have also demonstrated a benefit to reducing the number of total shock waves delivered [26]. When the number of shocks delivered was increased from 1,000 to 2,000, the size of the renal scar increased from 1.4 to 12.8 %. Therefore, frequent fluoroscopic observation of a stone during SWL is recommended, to allow for timely discontinuation of therapy when acceptable fragmentation of the stone has been achieved.

Conclusions

SWL has become a widely used, first-line therapy for ureteral and renal calculi since its introduction in the early 1980s. It is an increasingly attractive treatment option to both patients and physicians, due to its minimally invasive nature, and outpatient capabilities. However, SWL does have notable short- and long-term complications, including injury to the kidney parenchyma and other vulnerable adjacent structures. Appropriate patient selection, optimization of treatment variables, and close Urologic follow-up should allow for safe, efficacious use of SWL for treatment of urolithiasis. Modifications of SWL treatment parameters including the use of low voltage priming protocols, treatment pause, slow shock wave rate delivery, and limited number of shock waves administered may help prevent adverse events following SWL.

References

1. Chaussy C, Schniedt E, Jocham D, Brendel W, Forssmann B, Walther V. First clinical experience with extracorporeally induced destruction of kidney stones by shockwaves. J Urol. 1982;127(3):417–20.
2. Chaussy C, Fuchs G. Extracorporeal lithotripsy in the treatment of renal lithiasis. 5 years' experience. J Urol. 1986;92(6):339–43.
3. Pearle MS, Calhoun EA, Curhan GC, Urologic Diseases of America Project. Urologic diseases in America project: urolithiasis. J Urol. 2005;173(3): 848–57.
4. McAteer JA, Evan AP. The acute and long-term adverse effects of shockwave lithotripsy. Semin Nephrol. 2008;28(2):200–13.
5. Chaussy C, Schüller J, Schmiedt E, Brandl H, Jocham D, Liedl B. Extracorporeal shock-wave lithotripsy (ESWL) for treatment of urolithiasis. Urology. 1984;23:59–66.
6. Kaude JV, Williams CM, Millner MR, Scott KN, Finlayson B. Renal morphology and function immediately after extracorporeal shock-wave lithotripsy. AJR Am J Roentgenol. 1985;145:305–13.
7. Lingeman JE, Matlaga BR, Evan AP. Surgical management of upper urinary tract calculi. In: Kavoussi LR, Novick AC, Partin AW, et al., editors. Campbell-Walsh urology. 9th ed. Philadelphia, PA: Saunders-Elsevier; 2007. p. 1431–507.
8. Connors BA, Evan AP, Blomgren PM, Willis LR, Handa RK, Lifshitz DA, et al. Reducing shock number dramatically decreases lesion size in a juvenile kidney model. J Endourol. 2006;20(9):607–11.
9. Willis LR, Evan AP, Connors BA, Blomgren P, Fineberg NS, Lingeman JE. Relationship between kidney size, renal injury, and renal impairment induced by shock wave lithotripsy. J Am Soc Nephrol. 1999;10(8):1753–62.
10. Knapp PM, Kulb TB, Lingeman JE, Newman DM, Mertz JH, Mosbaugh PG, et al. Extracorporeal shock wave lithotripsy-induced perirenal hematomas. J Urol. 1988;139(4):700–3.
11. Newman LH, Saltzman B. Identifying risk factors in development of clinically significant post-shock-wave lithotripsy subcapsular hematomas. Urology. 1991;38(1):35–8.
12. Krambeck A, Lingeman JE. Clinical implications and bioeffects of shock wave lithotripsy. AUA Update Series. 2009;28(25):230–2.
13. Baumgartner BR, Dickey KW, Ambrose SS, Walton KN, Nelson RC, Bernardino ME. Kidney changes after extracorporeal shock wave lithotripsy: appearance on MR imaging. Radiology. 1987;163(2):531–4.
14. Uemura K, Takahashi S, Shintani-Ishida K, Nakajima M, Saka K, Yoshida K. A death due to perirenal hematoma complicating extracorporeal shockwave lithotripsy. J Forensic Sci. 2008;53(2):469–71.
15. Coptcoat MJ, Webb DR, Kellett MJ, Fletcher MS, McNicholas TA, Dickinson IK, et al. The complications of extracorporeal shockwave lithotripsy: management and prevention. Br J Urol. 1986;58(6): 578–80.
16. Dhar NB, Thornton J, Karafa MT, Streem SB. A multivariate analysis of risk factors associated with subcapsular hematoma formation following electromagnetic shock wave lithotripsy. J Urol. 2004; 172(6 Pt 1):2271–4.
17. Streem SB, Yost A. Extracorporeal shock wave lithotripsy in patients with bleeding diatheses. J Urol. 1991;144(6):1347–8.
18. Watterson JD, Girvan AR, Cook AJ, Beiko DT, Nott L, Auge BK, et al. Safety and efficacy of holmium:YAG laser lithotripsy in patients with bleeding diatheses. J Urol. 2002;168(2):442–5.

19. Lingeman J, Delius M, Evan A, Gupta M, Sarica K, Strohmaier W. Bioeffects and physical mechanisms of SW effects in SWL. In: Segura J, Conort P, Khoury S, et al., eds. Stone disease: first international consultation on stone disease. Paris: Heath Publications; 2003, p. 251-86.
20. Dalecki D, Raeman CH, Child SZ, Penney DP, Mayer R, Carstensen EL. The influence of contrast agents on hemorrhage produced by lithotripter fields. Ultrasound Med Biol. 1997;23(9):1435–9.
21. Evan AP, Willis LR, McAteer JA, Bailey MR, Connors BA, Shao Y, et al. Kidney damage and renal functional changes are minimized by waveform control that suppresses cavitation in SWL. J Urol. 2002;168(4 Pt 1):1556–62.
22. Rigatti P, Colombo R, Centemero A, Francesca F, Di Girolamo V, Montorsi F, et al. Histological and ultrastructural evaluation of extracorporeal shock wave lithotripsy-induced acute renal lesions: preliminary report. Eur Urol. 1989;16(3):207–11.
23. Seitz G, Pletzer K, Neisius D, Dippel W, Gebhardt T. Pathologic-anatomic alterations in human kidneys after extracorporeal piezoelectric shock wave lithotripsy. J Endourol. 1991;5(1):17–20.
24. Brewer SL, Atala AA, Ackerman DM, Steinbock GS. Shock wave lithotripsy damage in human cadaver kidneys. J Endourol. 1988;4:333–9.
25. Grantham JR, Millner MR, Kaude JV, Finlayson B, Hunter 2nd PT, Newman RC. Renal stone disease treated with extracorporeal shock wave lithotripsy: short-term observations in 100 patients. Radiology. 1986;158(1):203–6.
26. Newman R, Hackett R, Senior D, Brock K, Feldman J, Sosnowski J, et al. Pathological effects of ESWL on canine renal tissue. Urology. 1987;29(2): 194–200.
27. Morris JS, Husmann DA, Wilson WT, Preminger GM. Temporal effects of shock wave lithotripsy. J Urol. 1991;145(4):881–3.
28. Lechevallier E, Siles S, Ortega JC, Coulange C. Comparison by SPECT of renal scars after extracorporeal shock wave lithotripsy and percutaneous nephrolithotomy. J Endourol. 1993;7(6):465–7.
29. Karlsen SJ, Berg KJ. Acute changes in renal function following extracorporeal shock wave lithotripsy in patients with a solitary functioning kidney. J Urol. 1991;145(2):253–6.
30. Brito CG, Lingeman JE, Newman DM, Newman DE, Kight JL, Heck LL. Long-term follow-up of renal function in ESWL treated patients with a solitary kidney. J Urol. 1990;143(Suppl):299.
31. Williams CM, Kaude JV, Newman RC, Peterson JC, Thomas WC. Extracorporeal shock-wave lithotripsy: long-term complications. AJR Am J Roentgenol. 1988;150(2):311–5.
32. Orestano F, Caronia N, Gallo G. Functional aspects of the kidney after shock wave lithotripsy. In: Lingeman JE, Newman DM, editors. Shock Wave Lithotripsy. New York: Plenum Press; 1989. p. 15–7.
33. Peterson JC, Finlayson B. Effects of ESWL on blood pressure. In: Gravenstein JS, Peter K, editors. Extracorporeal shock wave lithotripsy for renal stone disease: technical and clinical aspects. Boston, MA: Butterworths; 1986. p. 145–50.
34. Janetschek G, Frauscher F, Knapp R, Höfle G, Peschel R, Bartsch G. New onset hypertension after extracorporeal shock wave lithotripsy: age related incidence and prediction by intrarenal resistive index. J Urol. 1997;158:346–51.
35. Lingeman JE, Newman D, Mertz JH, Mosbaugh PG, Steele RE, Kahnoski RJ, et al. Extracorporeal shock wave lithotripsy: the Methodist Hospital of Indiana experience. J Urol. 1986;135(6):1134–7.
36. Krambeck AE, Gettman MT, Rohlinger AL, Lohse CM, Patterson DE, Segura JW. Diabetes mellitus and hypertension associated with shock wave lithotripsy of renal and proximal ureteral stones at 19 years of follow-up. J Urol. 2006;175:1742–7.
37. Montgomery BS, Cole RS, Plafrey EL, Shuttleworth KE. Does extracorporeal shockwave lithotripsy cause hypertension? Br J Urol. 1989;64(6):567–71.
38. Strohmaier WL, Schmidt J, Lahme S, Bichler KH. Arterial blood pressure following different types of urinary stone therapy Presented at the 8th European Symposium on Urolithiasis, Parma, Italy, 1999. Eur Urol. 2000;38:753–7.
39. Sato Y, Tanda H, Kato S, Ohnishi S, Nakajima H, Nanbu A, et al. Shock wave lithotripsy for renal stones is not associated with hypertension and diabetes mellitus. J Urol. 2008;71(4):586–91.
40. Liedl B, Jocham D, Lunz C, Schuster C, Schmiedt E. Five year follow-up of urinary stone treatment with extracorporeal shock wave lithotripsy. J Endourol. 1988;2:157–62.
41. Lingeman JE, Woods JR, Toth PD. Blood pressure changes following extracorporeal shock wave lithotripsy and other forms of treatment for nephrolithiasis. JAMA. 1990;263(13):1789–94.
42. Puppo P, Germinale F, Ricciotti G, Caviglia C, Saffoti S, Pontremoli P. Hypertension after extracorporeal shock wave lithotripsy: a false alarm. J Endourol. 1988;3:401–4.
43. Elves AW, Tilling K, Menezes P, Wills M, Rao PN, Feneley RC. Early observations of the effect of extracorporeal shockwave lithotripsy on blood pressure: a prospective randomized control clinical trial. BJU Int. 2000;85(6):611–5.
44. Jewett MA, Bombardier C, Logan AG, Psihramis KE, Wesley-James T, Mahoney JE, et al. A randomized controlled trial to assess the incidence of new onset hypertension in patients after shock wave lithotripsy for asymptomatic renal calculi. J Urol. 1998;160(4): 1241–3.
45. Krambeck AE, Rule AD, Li X, Bergstralh EJ, Gettman MT, Lieske JC. Shock wave lithotripsy is not predictive of hypertension among community stone formers at long-term followup. J Urol. 2011;185:164–9.

46. Yokoyama M, Shoji F, Yanagizawa R, Kanemura M, Kitahara K, Takahasi S, et al. Blood pressure changes following extracorporeal shock wave lithotripsy for urolithiasis. J Urol. 1992;147(3):553–7.
47. Puppo P, Germinale F, Ricciotti G, Caviglia C, Saffioti S, Pontremoli P, et al. Hypertension after Extracorporeal Shock Wave Lithotripsy: A False Alarm. J. Endourol. 1989;3(4):401–404.
48. Hassana I, Zietlow SP. Acute pancreatitis after extracorporeal shock wave lithotripsy for a renal calculus. Urology. 2002;60(6):1111.
49. Abe H, Nisimura T, Osawa S, Miura T, Oka F. Acute pancreatitis caused by extracorporeal shock wave lithotripsy for bilateral renal pelvic calculi. Int J Urol. 2000;7(2):65–8.
50. Karakayali F, Sevmis S, Ayvaz I, Tekin I, Boyvat F, Moray G. Acute necrotizing pancreatitis as a rare complication of extracorporeal shock wave lithotripsy. Int J Urol. 2006;13:613–5.
51. Kirkali Z, Kirkali G, Tanci S, Tahiri Y. The effect of extracorporeal shock wave lithotripsy on pancreatic enzymes. Int Urol Nephrol. 1994;26:405–8.
52. Hung SY, Chen HM, Jan YY. Common bile duct and pancreatic injury after extracorporeal shock wave lithotripsy for renal stone. Hepatogastroenterology. 2000;47(34):1162–3.
53. de Cógáin MR, Krambeck AE, Rule AD, Li X, Bergstralh EJ, Gettman MT, et al. Shock wave lithotripsy and diabetes mellitus: a population-based cohort study. Urology. 2012;79(2):298–302.
54. Simunovic D, Sudarevic B, Galic J. Extracorporeal shockwave lithotripsy in elderly: impact of age and comorbidity on stone-free rate and complications. J Endourol. 2010;24(11):1831–7.
55. Sighinolfi MC, Micali S, Grande M, Mofferdin A, De Stefani S, Bianchi G. Extracorporeal shock wave lithotripsy in an elderly population: how to prevent complications and make the treatment safe and effective. J Endourol. 2008;22(10):2223–6.
56. Lifshitz DA, Lingeman JE, Zafar FS, Hollensbe DW, Nyhuis AW, Evan AP. Alterations in predicted growth rates of pediatric kidneys treated with extracorporeal shockwave lithotripsy. J Endourol. 1998;12(5):469–75.
57. Neal DE, Harmon E, Hlavinka T, Morvant A, Richardson E, Thomas R. Effects of multiple sequential extracorporeal shock wave treatments on renal function: a primate model. J Endourol. 1991;5:217–21.
58. Evan AP, Willis LR, Lingeman JE, McAteer JA. Renal trauma and the risk of long-term complications in shock wave lithotripsy. Nephron. 1998;78(1):1–8.
59. Feagins BA, Alexander M, Dollar M, Husmann DA, Preminger GM. Prevention of lithotripsy-induced hypertension in a juvenile animal model. J Urol. 1991;145:258.
60. Preminger GM, Tiselius HG, Assimos DG, Alken P, Buck AC, Gallucci M, et al. 2007 guideline for the management of ureteral calculi. Eur Urol. 2007;52(6):1610–31.
61. Madbouly K, Sheir KZ, Elsobky E, Eraky I, Kenawy M. Risk factors for the formation of a steinstrasse after extracorporeal shock wave lithotripsy: a statistical model. J Urol. 2002;167(3):1239–42.
62. Weinerth JL, Flatt JA, Carson 3rd CC. Lessons learned in patients with large steinstrasse. J Urol. 1989;142(6):1425–7.
63. Lucio 2nd J, Korkes F, Lopes-Neto AC, Silva EG, Mattos MH, Pompeo AC. Steinstrasse predictive factors and outcomes after extracorporeal shockwave lithotripsy. Int Braz J Urol. 2011;37(4):477–82.
64. Al-Awadi K, Abdul Halim H, Kehinde EO, Al-Tawheed A. Steinstrasse: a comparison of incidence with and without J stenting and the effect of J stenting on subsequent management. BJU Int. 1999;84(6):618–21.
65. Sulaiman MN, Buchholz NP, Clark PH. The role of ureteral stent placement in the prevention of Steinstrasse. J Endourol. 1999;13(3):151–5.
66. Pryor JL, Jenkins AD. Use of double-pigtail stents in extracorporeal shock wave lithotripsy. J Urol. 1990;143(3):475–8.
67. Argyropoulos AN, Tolley DA. Ureteric stents compromise stone clearance after shockwave lithotripsy for ureteric stones: results of a matched-pair analysis. BJU Int. 2009;103(1):76–80.
68. Lingeman JE, Coury TA, Newman DM, Kahnoski RJ, Mertz JH, Mosbaugh PG, et al. Comparison of results and morbidity of percutaneous nephrostolithotomy and extracorporeal shock wave lithotripsy. J Urol. 1987;138(3):485–90.
69. Pace KT, Weir MJ, Tariq N, Honey RJ. Low success rate of repeat shock wave lithotripsy for ureteral stones after failed initial treatment. J Urol. 2000;164(6):1905–7.
70. Consensus conference. Prevention and treatment of kidney stones. JAMA. 1988;260(7):977–81.
71. Carr LK, D'A Honey J, Jewett MA, Ibanez D, Ryan M, Bombardier C. New stone formation: a comparison of extracorporeal shock wave lithotripsy and percutaneous nephrolithotomy. J Urol. 1996;155(5):1565–7.
72. Krambeck AE, LeRoy AJ, Patterson DE, Gettman MT. Long-term outcomes of percutaneous nephrolithotomy compared to shock wave lithotripsy and conservative management. J Urol. 2008;179(6):2233–7.
73. Buchholz NP, Meier-Padel S, Rutishauser G. Minor residual fragments after extracorporeal shockwave lithotripsy: spontaneous clearance or risk factor for recurrent stone formation? J Endourol. 1997;11(4):227–32.
74. Streem SB, Yost A, Mascha E. Clinical implications of clinically insignificant stone fragments after extracorporeal shock wave lithotripsy. J Urol. 1996;155(4):1186–90.
75. Krambeck AE, Handa SE, Evan AP, Lingeman JE. Brushite stone disease as a consequence of lithotripsy? Urol Res. 2010;38(4):293–9.

76. Klee LW, Brito CG, Lingeman JE. The clinical implications of brushite calculi. J Urol. 1991;145(4): 715–8.
77. Parks JH, Worcester EM, Coe FL, Evan AP, Lingeman JE. Clinical implications of abundant calcium phosphate in routinely analyzed kidney stones. Kidney Int. 2004;66:777–85.
78. Parr KL, Lingeman JE, Jordan M, Coury TA. Creatinine kinase concentrations and electrocardiographic changes in extracorporeal shock-wave lithotripsy. Urology. 1988;32(1):21–3.
79. Duvdevani M, Lorber G, Gofrit ON, Latke A, Katz R, Landau EH, et al. Fever after shockwave lithotripsy–risk factors and indications for prophylactic antimicrobial treatment. J Endourol. 2010;24(2): 277–81.
80. Bierkens AF, Hendrikx AJ, Ezz el Din KE, de la Rosette JJ, Horrevorts A, Doesburg W, et al. The value of antibiotic prophylaxis during extracorporeal shock wave lithotripsy in the prevention of urinary tract infections in patients with urine proven sterile prior to treatment. Eur Urol. 1997;31(1): 30–5.
81. Wendt-Nordahl G, Kramobach P, Hannak D, Häcker A, Michel MS, Alken P, et al. Prospective evaluation of acute endocrine pancreatic injury as collateral damage of shock-wave lithotripsy for upper urinary tract stones. BJU Int. 2008;100(6): 1339–43.
82. Gordetsky J, Hislop S, Orloff M, Butler M, Erturk E. Subcapsular hepatic hematoma with right hepatic vein thrombosis: a complication of shock wave lithotripsy. Can Urol Assoc J. 2008;2(1):61–3.
83. White WM, Morris SA, Klein FA, Waters WB. Splenic rupture following shock wave lithotripsy. Can J Urol. 2008;15:4196–9.
84. Al Karawi MA, Mohamed AR, el-Etaibi KE, Abomelha MS, Seed RF. Extracorporeal shock-wave lithotripsy (ESWL)-induced erosions in upper gastrointestinal tract. Prospective study in 40 patients. Urology. 1987;30(3):224–7.
85. Cass AS. Colonic injury with ESWL for an upper ureteral calculus. In: Lingeman JE, Newman DM, editors. Proceedings of the 4th symposium on shock wave lithotripsy: state of the art. New York: Plenum Press; 1988.
86. El-Faqih SR. Small bowel perforation after extracorporeal shockwave lithotripsy for ureteric stone: a case report and review of the literature. Saudi J Gastroenterol. 2002;8:59–61.
87. Albers DD, Lybrand 3rd FE, Axton JC, Wendelken JR. Shockwave lithotripsy and pacemakers: experience with 20 cases. J Endourol. 1995;9(4):301–3.
88. Lazarides MK, Drista H, Arvanitas DP, Dayantas JN. Aortic aneurysm rupture after extracorporeal shock wave lithotripsy. Surgery. 1996;122(1):112–3.
89. Vasavada SP, Streem SB, Kottke-Marchant K, Novick AC. Pathological effects of extracorporeally generated shock waves on calcified aortic aneurysm tissue. J Urol. 1994;152(1):45–8.
90. Carey SW, Streem SB. Extracorporeal shock wave lithotripsy for patients with calcified ipsilateral renal arterial or abdominal aortic aneurysms. J Urol. 1992;148(1):18–20.
91. Miller RD, Cucchiara RF, Miller ED, Reves JG, Roizen MF, Savarese JJ. Anesthesia. 5th ed. Philadelphia, PA: Churchill Livingstone; 2000. p. 1950–1.
92. Tiede JM, Lumpkin EN, Wass CT, Long TR. Hemoptysis following extracorporeal shock wave lithotripsy: a case of lithotripsy-induced pulmonary contusion in a pediatric patient. J Clin Anesth. 2003;15:530–3.
93. Frankenschmidt A, Sommerkamp H. Shock wave lithotripsy during pregnancy: a successful clinical experiment. J Urol. 1998;159(2):501–2.
94. Gulum M, Yeni E, Kocyigit A, Taskin A, Savas M, Ciftci H, et al. Sperm DNA damage and seminal oxidative status after shock-wave lithotripsy for distal ureteral stones. Fertil Steril. 2011;96(5):1087–90.
95. Erturk E, Ptak AM, Monaghan J. Fertility measures in women after extracorporeal shockwave lithotripsy of distal ureteral stones. J Endourol. 1997;11(5):315–7.
96. Willis LR, Evan AP, Connors BA, Handa RK, Blomgren PM, Lingeman JE. Prevention of lithotripsy-induced renal injury by pretreating kidneys with low-energy shock waves. J Am Soc Nephrol. 2006;17(3):663–73.
97. Evan AP, Connors BA, Pennington DJ, Blomgren PM, Lingeman JE, Fineberg NS, et al. Renal disease potentiates the injury caused by SWL. J Endourol. 1999;13(9):619–28.
98. Connors BA, Evan AP, Blomgren PM, Handa RK, Willis LR, Gao S. Effect of initial shock wave voltage on SWL-induced lesion size during step-wise voltage ramping. BJU Int. 2009;103(1):104–7.
99. Evan AP, McAteer JA, Connors BA, Pm B, Lingeman JE. Renal injury during shock wave lithotripsy is significantly reduced by slowing the rate of shock wave delivery. BJU Int. 2007;100(3):624–7. discussion 627–8.
100. Crow P, Keeley FX. Does the rate of shock wave delivery affect outcomes in patients receiving shock wave lithotripsy for urinary calculi? Nat Clin Pract Urol. 2008;5(9):478–9.

Index

S.Y. Nakada and M.S. Pearle (eds.), *Surgical Management of Urolithiasis: Percutaneous, Shockwave and Ureteroscopy*, DOI 10.1007/978-1-4614-6937-7, © Springer Science+Business Media New York 2013

N

O

P

V

W

MIX
Papier aus verantwortungsvollen Quellen
Paper from responsible sources
FSC® C105338

If you have any concerns about our products,
you can contact us on
ProductSafety@springernature.com

In case Publisher is established outside the EU,
the EU authorized representative is:
Springer Nature Customer Service Center GmbH
Europaplatz 3, 69115 Heidelberg, Germany

Printed by Libri Plureos GmbH
in Hamburg, Germany